W9-DHY-806

JOHN F. KENNEDY INSTITUTE
MEDICAL LIBRARY

SCIENCE AND EPILEPSY

NEUROSCIENCE GAINS IN
EPILEPSY RESEARCH

AND SO, SINCE ONE GENERATION TEACHES ANOTHER,
IT HAS BECOME RATHER CLEAR TO THE RULERS OF
STATES THAT,
FOR THE PRESERVATION AND ADVANCEMENT OF THE
PHYSICAL HEALTH OF A PEOPLE,
MEDICINE
OUGHT TO BECOME A MATTER OF
COMMON RIGHT
SETTING HEALTH AND PHYSICAL PERFECTION
OF A WHOLE PEOPLE AS ITS GOAL
INVOKING FOR THAT PURPOSE PUBLIC AUTHORITIES
AND EXECUTIVE POWERS,
SO THAT WHAT THE SCATTERED EFFORTS OF
INDIVIDUALS
HAVE ATTEMPTED IN VAIN MAY BE BROUGHT ABOUT.

JAN EVANGELISTA PURKINJE (1787–1869)
From *Commentatio de Examine
Physiologico Organi Viscus
et Systematis Cutanei . . .
December 22, 1823.*
(Translated by N. J. Twombly, S.J.)

Science and Epilepsy
Neuroscience Gains in Epilepsy Research

James L. O'Leary, Ph.D., M.D.
*Professor Emeritus of Neurology
and Experimental Neurological
Surgery*

Sidney Goldring, M.D.
*Professor and Head of
Neurological Surgery*

*Department of Neurology and Neurological Surgery
Washington University School of Medicine
St. Louis, Missouri*

One of a series of historical monographs sponsored by the Committee on Brain Sciences, Division of Medical Sciences, Assembly of Life Sciences, National Research Council

Raven Press ■ New York

© 1976 by Raven Press Books, Ltd. All rights reserved. This book is protected by copyright. No part of it may be reproduced, stored in a retrieval system, or transmitted, in any form or by any means, electronic, mechanical, photocopying, recording, or otherwise, without the prior written permission of the publisher. However, this work may be reproduced in whole or in part for the official use of the U.S. Government on the condition that copyright notice is included with such official reproduction.

Made in the United States of America

International Standard Book Number 0-89004-072-9
Library of Congress Catalog Card Number 75-21860

The project that is the subject of this report was approved by the Governing Board of the National Research Council, acting in behalf of the National Academy of Sciences. Such approval reflects the Board's judgment that the project is of national importance and appropriate with respect to both the purposes and resources of the National Research Council.

The members of the committee who were selected to undertake this project and prepare this report were chosen for recognized scholarly competence and with due consideration for the balance of disciplines appropriate to the project. Responsibility for the detailed aspects of this report rests with that committee.

Each report issuing from a study committee of the National Research Council is reviewed by an independent group of qualified individuals according to procedures established and monitored by the Report Review Committee of the National Academy of Sciences. Distribution of the report is approved, by the President of the Academy, upon satisfactory completion of the review process.

Acknowledgments

The work on which this publication is based was performed pursuant to Contract No. HSM–42–71–94 with the National Institute of Mental Health, Health Services and Mental Health Administration, Department of Health, Education, and Welfare and Contract No. PH–43–64–44 Task Order 67, National Institute of Neurological and Communicative Disorders and Stroke, National Institutes of Health, Department of Health, Education, and Welfare.

Dedication

This volume, which was largely the work of James O'Leary, stands as a tribute to his deep commitment to the study of the nervous system, his broad knowledge of the field, and his own extensive contributions to scientific knowledge in this field.

Foreword

Within what environment and under what circumstances is scientific advance most likely to occur? A projection for the future is most securely based upon a study of the past. With this in mind, the Committee on Brain Sciences of the National Academy of Sciences commissioned a series of reviews of the events leading up to certain major advances in scientific knowledge that have been of practical significance to society. Among those reviews selected for study was improvement in the diagnosis and treatment of convulsive disorders, exemplified by the use of electroencephalography and drugs and neurosurgery in control of the epilepsies.

For this task, the Committee has been fortunate to enlist a scientist and clinician who has actively participated in this area of science, and who has been a friend of many of those about whom he has written. His authoritative review serves to document, as few others could, the breadth of the base from which our current knowledge has been built. It also highlights the diversity of background, interest, and approach of the outstanding men and women who have participated in advancing this frontier of knowledge. Some made their contribution through a lifetime of caring for the sick; others systematically attacked the fundamental questions of biology; still others seem only to have been satisfying their curiosity, or attempting to solve an intriguing puzzle. We are indebted to them all. We are also indebted to Dr. James O'Leary not only for this volume, but for his many contributions to our understanding of the brain and its functions.

Richard L. Masland, M.D.

Preface and Acknowledgments

In developing the content of this volume on the historical perspectives of epilepsy and related neuroscience areas, matters related to professionalism in science have been kept to a minimum. Scientists have been presented as human beings and science as a human activity. Scientists are always enthusiastic about their work. However, at the beginnings of science the inadequacies of available technology resulted in advances occurring with exasperating slowness. Today, by comparison, a productive technological advance can be exploited to the full more rapidly than one can imagine.

Chapter I provides initial explanatory material of a very general nature. It defines epilepsy, provides some statistics, and describes an attack. The importance of science in advancing knowledge of epilepsy is stressed. Since the volume concerns the advances of neurological science that have improved both the diagnosis and treatment of epilepsy over the past two centuries, a purview of the methods of science and the importance of international cooperation in studies of epilepsy are emphasized. Chapter II introduces a series of case reports in order to provide both a current view of the diagnosis and treatment of epilepsy and an opportunity to introduce items of nomenclature.

Chapter III covers selected aspects of the history of epilepsy extending from ancient to modern times. The material selected provides the necessary background against which to judge the neuroscience developments of the nineteenth and twentieth centuries. I am especially indebted to the scholarly treatise of Oswei Temkin, *The Falling Sickness,* which is based largely on primary sources. That work covers the social, religious, and magical, as well as the medical and scientific history of epilepsy and was an indispensable guide to the development of this, in many ways the most difficult, aspect of the material presented.

The historical objective of the present study has been to relate developments in the several neuroscientific disciplines and their technologies to the advance in basic science and medical understanding of epileptic disorders as measured by a large increase in diagnostic acumen, the discovery of many reliable therapeutic agents, and vastly improved insights into the aberrations of neural mechanisms that permit the occurrence of epileptic attacks. The broader outlook relates to the advances in neuroscientific understanding that have contributed to making the lives of many epileptics bearable, a status not achieved in ancient times, the Middle Ages, the Renaissance, or the Enlightenment.

Of the succeeding chapters, several of historical import commence with assorted observations drawn from nature that serve to introduce the beginnings of the particular neuroscientific area to be traced. Others open with observations relating to how the scientific area is currently understood. Many chapters end with a Comment, which either recapitulates the highlights of a scientific development, relates to lessons learned from misinterpretations that were made, or discusses a scientific personality whose discoveries played an important role in that science's development. Chapters X to XIV cover the more recent history of neuroscientific advance. Chapter XV deals with matters that concern the development of antiepileptic drugs; Chapter XVI, with the surgical treatment of epilepsy. The latter was written by Dr. Sidney Goldring. The final chapter presents an outlook on future research planning in epilepsy.

A glossary is provided at the end of the book for those unfamiliar with terminology in the medical and especially the neuroscientific areas. Other definitions are given in the text or in the Notes at the end of each chapter.

This work was made possible by the support of the National Institute of Neurological and Communicative Disorders and Stroke and of the National Institute of Mental Health. I am especially indebted to Louise Marshall, Ph.D. (National Research Council); J. Kiffin Penry, M.D. (Chief, Applied Neurological Research Branch, and Head, Section of Epilepsy, Collaborative and Field Research, National Institute of Neurological and Communicative Disorders and Stroke); and Lyle W. Bivens, Ph.D., and Fred Almadjian, Ph.D. (National Institute of Mental Health) for their continuing advice and counsel. I am also thankful to all members of the Committee and the Subcommittee who helped in the writing and provided innumerable suggestions concerning content and sources. Several Committee members who provided specialized advice are mentioned below.

As noted previously, I am greatly indebted to Temkin's classical history of epilepsy. Dr. Philip R. Dodge, Professor and Head of Pediatrics, Washington University School of Medicine, contributed the historical account of salaam attacks. Professor Jan Bureš (Czechoslovak Academy of Sciences, Prague) supplied the picture of J. Marek. Professor Vladislav Kruta (University J. E. Purkyně, Brno, Czechoslovakia) gave me much of the material used relating to Purkinje. Professor Richard Jung (Freiburg) provided the historical material on the early Berlin electrophysiologists and an original tracing from Hans Berger's work.

For the chapter on animal electricity and electrophysiology, I received valuable suggestions from the following: Hallowell Davis (Professor Emeritus of Audiology and Physiology, the Central Institute for the Deaf and Washington University, St. Louis); Albert and Ellen Grass (Grass Instrument Company, Quincy, Mass.) and Alberta Dawson (formerly with Grass Instrument Company); Leslie Geddes (Baylor University School of Medicine, Houston); and Arthur Gilson (Professor Emeritus of Physiology, Washington University School of Medicine). Stuart Snider (Department of Neurology, College of Physicians and Surgeons, Columbia University, New York) aided on the chapter concerning neurotransmitters.

In the field of electroencephalography, I was helped immensely by Mary A. B. Brazier (Professor of Physiology and Anatomy, University of California, Los Angeles); Hallowell Davis; Ralph W. Gerard (neurophysiologist, formerly of

Irvine and now deceased); Robert A. Cohen (National Institute of Mental Health); Donald B. Lindsley (Professor of Psychology, University of California, Los Angeles); John R. Knott (Department of Psychology, University of Iowa, Iowa City); Charles E. Henry (Cleveland Clinic); Robert Cohn (Professor of Neurology, Howard University Medical School, Washington, D.C.); Joseph Hughes (Medical College of Pennsylvania, Philadelphia); and Melvin Thorner (Veterans Administration, Traverse City, Mich.).

Sidney Goldring (Professor of Neurological Surgery) who wrote the chapter on surgical treatment of epilepsy; Irwin Levy (Professor of Neurology); and Arthur Prensky (Associate Professor of Pediatrics and of Neurology, Washington University, St. Louis) all contributed to the Case Reports in Chapter II. J. Kiffin Penry gave much direct aid and other cooperation on clinical aspects of the work. Mary A. B. Brazier contributed a number of pictures from her historical collection of neuroscience investigators, much sound criticism, and constant encouragement.

I am much indebted to Viola Graeler and Sally Kraus for expert secretarial assistance, to Thomas Spagnolia for art work, and to Cramer Lewis and his staff for photography related to the illustrations. My wife, Nancy B. O'Leary, gave me much editorial assistance. Estelle Brodman and her associates at Washington University School of Medicine Library also gave much invaluable assistance. The National Library of Medicine, Washington, D.C., the St. Louis University Medical School Library, and the Library of the University of Missouri School of Medicine, Columbia, aided the work through the loan of books. The St. Louis Medical Society loaned books from its historical collection. The *Neurosciences Research Symposium Summaries* of F. O. Schmitt *et al.* provided a reliable source of up-to-date material on neuroscience advances.

Finally, Mr. Ernest Kirschten of St. Louis read and reread the manuscript and directed me in simplifying it for nonmedical readers. I shall be forever grateful to him.

James O'Leary, M.D.

Contents

Committee on Brain Sciences, 1972–1974*

ELIOT STELLAR, *University of Pennsylvania, Philadelphia, Pennsylvania [Chairman]*

FLOYD E. BLOOM, *National Institute of Mental Health, St. Elizabeths Hospital, Washington, D.C.*

VICTOR H. DENENBERG, *University of Connecticut, Storrs, Connecticut*

PETER B. DEWS, *Harvard Medical School, Boston, Massachusetts*

DANIEL X. FREEDMAN, *Pritzker School of Medicine, University of Chicago, Chicago, Illinois*

HOWARD F. HUNT, *Columbia University, New York, New York*

JEROME KAGAN, *Harvard University, Cambridge, Massachusetts*

SEYMOUR S. KETY, *Harvard Medical School and Massachusetts General Hospital, Boston, Massachusetts*

RICHARD T. LOUTTIT, *University of Massachusetts, Amherst, Massachusetts*

RICHARD L. MASLAND, *College of Physicians and Surgeons, Columbia University, New York, New York*

NEAL E. MILLER, *The Rockefeller University, New York, New York*

WILFRID RALL, *National Institutes of Health, Bethesda, Maryland*

MARK R. ROSENZWEIG, *University of California, Berkeley, California*

FREDERIC G. WORDEN, *Neurosciences Research Program, Massachusetts Institute of Technology, Brookline, Massachusetts*

Advisory Panel on Diagnosis and Treatment of Convulsive Disorders

RICHARD L. MASLAND, *Moses Professor of Neurology and Chairman, Department of Neurology, College of Physicians and Surgeons, Neurological Institute, Columbia University, New York, New York [Chairman of Panel]*

FLOYD E. BLOOM, *Chief, Laboratory of Neuropharmacology, National Institute of Mental Health, St. Elizabeths Hospital, Washington, D.C.*

MARY A. B. BRAZIER, *Professor of Anatomy and Physiology, Department of Anatomy, School of Medicine, University of California, Los Angeles, California*

RALPH W. GERARD [deceased], *Professor and Dean Emeritus, University of California, Irvine, Corona del Mar, California*

GILBERT H. GLASER, *Professor of Neurology, Department of Neurology, Yale University School of Medicine, New Haven, Connecticut*

---

* These members guided the planning and development of *Science and Epilepsy—Neuroscience Gains in Epilepsy Research*. The current Committee on Brain Sciences reflects a rotation of membership.

HERBERT H. JASPER, *Professor of Neurophysiology, Department of Physiology, University of Montreal, Montreal, P. Q., Canada*

JAMES L. O'LEARY [deceased], *Lecturer, Department of Neurology and Neurological Surgery, Washington University School of Medicine, St. Louis, Missouri*

GEORGE ROSEN, *Professor of History of Medicine and Epidemiology and Public Health, Department of History of Medicine, Yale University School of Medicine, New Haven, Connecticut*

DIXON M. WOODBURY, *Professor and Acting Head, Department of Pharmacology, College of Medicine, University of Utah, Salt Lake City, Utah*

Staff

LYLE W. BIVENS, *Behavioral Sciences Research Branch, National Institute of Mental Health, Rockville, Maryland*

LOUISE H. MARSHALL, *Professional Associate, National Research Council, National Academy of Sciences, Washington, D.C.*

J. KIFFIN PENRY, *Chief, Applied Neurologic Research Branch, and Head, Section on Epilepsy, Collaborative and Field Research, National Institute of Neurological and Communicative Disorders and Stroke, Bethesda, Maryland*

Contributors and Reviewers

JAN BUREŠ, *Czechoslovak Academy of Sciences, Prague, Czechoslovakia*

ROBERT A. COHEN, *National Institute of Mental Health, Bethesda, Maryland*

ROBERT COHN, *Howard University, Washington, D.C.*

HALLOWELL DAVIS, *Central Institute for the Deaf, St. Louis, Missouri*

ALBERTA DAWSON, *84 Lincoln Avenue, Wollaston, Massachusetts*

PHILIP R. DODGE, *Washington University School of Medicine, St. Louis, Missouri*

LESLIE A. GEDDES, *Baylor University College of Medicine, Houston, Texas*

ARTHUR S. GILSON, *Washington University School of Medicine, St. Louis, Missouri*

ALBERT M. GRASS, *Grass Instrument Company, Quincy, Massachusetts*

ELLEN R. GRASS, *Grass Instrument Company, Quincy, Massachusetts*

CHARLES E. HENRY, *Cleveland Clinic, Cleveland, Ohio*

JOSEPH F. HUGHES, *Medical College of Pennsylvania, Philadelphia, Pennsylvania*

RICHARD JUNG, *University of Freiburg, West Germany*

ERNEST H. KIRSCHTEN [deceased], *St. Louis, Missouri*

JOHN R. KNOTT, *University of Iowa, Iowa City, Iowa*

VLADISLAV KRUTA, *University J. E. Purkyně, Brno, Czechoslovakia*

Y. M. F. LAPORTE, *Collège de France, Paris*

IRWIN LEVY, *Washington University School of Medicine, St. Louis, Missouri*

DONALD B. LINDSLEY, *University of California, Los Angeles, California*

H. HOUSTON MERRITT, *College of Physicians and Surgeons, Columbia University, New York, New York*

ALBERT POPE, *McLean Hospital, Belmont, Massachusetts*

ARTHUR PRENSKY, *Washington University School of Medicine, St. Louis, Missouri*

ZDENĚK SERVÍT, *Institute of Physiology, Czechoslovak Academy of Sciences, Prague, Czechoslovakia*

STUART R. SNIDER, *College of Physicians and Surgeons, Columbia University, New York, New York*

OSWEI TEMKIN, *Johns Hopkins University, Baltimore, Maryland*

MELVIN W. THORNER, *Veterans Administration, Traverse City, Michigan*

NEIL J. TWOMBLY, S. J., *Georgetown University, Washington, D.C.*

Chapter I

INTRODUCTION

Epilepsy is a chronic brain disorder causing seizures that recur irregularly and unexpectedly. Its name is derived from the ancient Greek word *epilepsia,* which means "seizure," and the disorder itself probably was recognized prior to the development of the earliest of civilizations. Today it afflicts about 1% of the American population, or 2,200,000 people. About 7% (more than 15,000,000 persons) suffer at least one convulsion in a lifetime. An estimated 30,000,000 cases of epilepsy for the present entire world population seems probable; however, we know little of its incidence in India and China.

The usual epileptic seizure is of short duration, characterized by a fall, a jerky and rather violent contraction of the body musculature, and a loss of awareness of surroundings. Unless immediately ended by a physiological intervention still beyond our understanding, a seizure runs its course and thereafter subsides rather abruptly. The brain energy necessary to maintain a seizure has then, presumably, been exhausted. Because this energy is not rapidly replenished, a stupor or brief sleep may follow. Epilepsy refers to a recurrence of such seizures. Of course, this explanation is an oversimplification. Chapter II will provide several case histories illustrating manifestations of the disorder.

To date, medical science has not explained satisfactorily why seizures occur in one person and not in another. There is a strong suspicion, however, that the cause of most epilepsy lies in a covert defect of the brain that becomes overt in the epileptic and not in others with the defect. Some tangible clues, as yet untestable, suggest that epileptic attacks may occur as a result of heredity, but knowledge of the genetics of seizures does not yet provide a certain answer to this complex problem. Parents with no epileptic inheritance might possibly produce an epileptic child as the result of a genetic error occurring during embryological development. Deoxyribonucleic acid (DNA), the heredity carrier, programs molecular organization to the minutest detail, including how the embryo and the brain within it will develop; yet minute errors may occur in the implementation of the genetic code. As a result, of two individuals with structurally normal brains, one may have spontaneously occurring seizures and the other not.

Epilepsy is not an "end-of-the-road disease." Although it often develops in early life, it does not alter the life expectancy of the majority of epileptics. Were it a common cause of death, like cancer, heart disease, and stroke, it undoubtedly would receive greater support to facilitate research for better understanding of its causes and for a more effective repertoire of drugs for its treatment. Such work surely would enhance an epileptic's productivity and enjoyment of life.

If severe seizures recur unabated, uncontrolled epilepsy can be a disorder of attrition and ruin prospects for a satisfactory life. Some such cases may be brought under control, usually through an effective combination of several drugs, although they may require continuing medical treatment throughout life. Fortunately, many seizures can now be partially or completely controlled. This is, of course, in sharp contrast to the past, when for thousands of years the only recourse was to semimedical, magical, or religious therapies. Although our knowledge is less than complete, we have come a long way toward understanding the epileptic's illness and promoting his welfare. Whatever subtle defects of brain organization are at its roots, epilepsy need not affect the overall working capacity of the brain. Uncontrolled, seizures can occur unexpectedly in a variety of circumstances. Even during periods of frequent seizures, many epileptics continue to function quite effectively. This has been demonstrated through the centuries by writers, artists, musicians, political and military leaders, and scientists who overcame the handicap of their sporadic seizures. Julius Caesar is a classic example.

Seizures often commence in early childhood, and youth is the period of their highest incidence. Even though they disappear spontaneously or become controlled in adult life, these attacks may have a lasting effect upon normal social development. The reactions of unknowledgeable or ill-informed associates can cause epileptic children to avoid normal activities. Also, safety factors may limit their participation in sports and, at adolescence, may prohibit them from such endeavors as driving an automobile. Thus, childhood epilepsy requires the continuation of research to broaden the range of effective drugs available to the physician. It is in childhood that ineffective seizure control hurts most. The adult epileptic also has problems, but the growing child must remain the major focus of our attention.

Were it available, a detailed biological specification of the cause of epilepsy would greatly ease the search for more effective medications. Fortunately, there is good reason to believe that an interdisciplinary neuroscientific approach, employing greatly improved methods of fine structure analysis, electrophysiology, and neuropharmacology, undertaken separately or in combination, will ultimately clarify the cause or causes of epilepsy. Such an effort should lead to more specific knowledge of normal brain structure and function, however complex these may be. This also is true of the psychopharmacological approach. Indeed, the greater our knowledge of the normal brain, the greater is the prospect for understanding its maladies.

This book is intended to present an account of the neuroscientific disciplines that have added so greatly to contemporary knowledge of the basic mechanisms of epilepsy. These considerable achievements can be appreciated only by looking back at the long and patient search, one that must continue at an accelerating pace and, nopefully, with accelerating results. The present is a middle ground from which past trends can be perceived and future ones projected.

Scientific knowledge is acquired by efforts to solve particular problems. But ordinarily it neither emerges from observations alone nor from the mere accretion of facts.[1] Facts must be validated and compared to other presumed facts with which they are either consistent or conflicting. Finally, as best as possible, facts should be tagged for later use. Technologies subordinate to science play an important role in fact accumulation, and over the past century the biological sciences have become dependent on the physical sciences for much of their instrumentation.

Historically, the biosciences emerged from an obscurity in which facts were so scarce that it was hardly possible to cross-check them, or even to establish the simplest interrelationships among them. Given this inadequacy, absurd errors were made, some of which persisted tenaciously. Thus, the road of scientific advance often was rough, and progress was unsustained; yet science did advance remarkably and has now reached its golden age of promise. Today, further progress depends on the motivation and the training of those who take up the work. Scientific training perforce is so prolonged, exacting, and expensive that promising individuals are deterred from entering the field. Too often they fear that lack of sufficient support may doom them to an unproductive career.

Training to cope with the complexities of modern science must satisfy at least two objectives: a scientist must know how to develop original ideas, and he must become a superior craftsman.[2] He requires understanding of the uses and limitations of technology in amassing facts that lead to the solution of problems. Furthermore, to utilize facts properly he must be able to combine his personal experience with that of others. He must read widely. He needs many personal contacts with fellow scientists in his own and related disciplines, and he must be able to communicate with them accurately and effectively.

Scientific research may be discipline- or mission-oriented. Neuroanatomy, neurophysiology, neurochemistry, neuropharmacology, and neuropathology are examples of disciplines among the neurosciences. Work related to the conquest of a disease, an example of mission orientation, sometimes seems to counter today's trend toward discipline orientation. Discipline-oriented research requires special concentration on the technologies of a particular specialty, on a limited number of current and fertile ideas, and on a close familiarity with specialized literature. The mission-oriented investigator proceeds from a broader base. He may not have the depth of understanding in one field that characterizes the discipline-oriented scientist, but apply several technologies, instead of a single one, to a problem. The problem of epilepsy requires both kinds of scientists. It needs not only specialized research, but also the broader, more fundamental research on which it is based.

Both depend on public support and better communication between scientist and citizen. It is regrettable that this mutual understanding depends so largely on the good offices of a relatively small number of people who, although they work in other fields, possess an appreciation of the scientific method which they gained in the course of their education. (An obvious example is those physicians who have had research training before going into the practice of medicine.) In this regard, it is not merely self-serving to say that there must be a realization in the community at large that the progress of science depends on public support of professional scientists. As long as science was the pursuit of a few, training and working in the field was made possible by a few enlightened patrons—by appointment as court physicians or astronomers, for example, or by the interest of groups such as the Royal Society, established in the seventeenth century. More than a few were intellectually curious "amateurs" of independent means. Such capricious support, of course, is hopelessly inadequate today. It has been replaced partly by the support of foundations, universities, and, in a more limited way, by industry. Yet even this support is not sufficient to maintain the impetus of contemporary scientific endeavor. Generous governmental support for both research and training is necessary if the pace of progress is to be maintained.

A European science foundation, comparable to our own National Science Foundation, is said by a correspondent in a British science weekly to be in formation (*Nature*, 1973). Starting with a relatively small budget, it promises greater cooperation within the world scientific community and offers further evidence that nationally supported scientific enterprises should not be nationally circumscribed. Such a cooperative venture in association with our own National Science Foundation could bring about wider integration of research. It could lead to an international community transcending the frustrations of "national security." Even the most specifically mission-oriented researcher abhors being "boxed in." He knows that however brilliant the contribution of an individual may be, the progress and the benefits of research depend on the efforts of many people, in many places, and at many times.

NOTES

[1] *(From Ravetz, Chapter 6, p. 181):* "Once we have achieved the slightest historical perspective on science, and cease to view it as the steady and certain accumulation of increasing heaps of true facts about the natural world, a number of paradoxes present themselves to us. First, there is the contrast between the highly personal endeavour required for a penetrating inquiry into the natural world, always fallible and governed by mainly tacit craft methods; and the public, objective, impersonal knowledge which eventually issues from that work. Similar to this contrast is that between the ephemeral structures in which scientific inquiry is undertaken, problems succeeding each other with great rapidity and theories and concepts being ploughed under at a perceptible rate, against the steadily increasing depth and power of the knowledge which somehow remains and grows amidst the swirling currents of the day-to-day work. And, finally, we have already observed the impossibility of 'proving' a single result in science, or even of establishing its 'probability' of being true; and yet the stock of permanent knowledge, absorbing all reinterpretations and surviving all attempts at refutation survives and grows."

[2] *(From Ravetz, Chapter 3, p. 77):* "In this work with pieces of physical equipment, the scientist is a very special sort of craftsman, for the objects he is dealing with are highly artificial. The relation of the readings taken off the apparatus to the objects of his inquiry is not at all immediate; the establishment of their relevance requires another set of operations. The experimental apparatus itself is frequently a complex affair, designed for the production of very special effects. A purely 'practical' mastery of the technique of standard manipulations will be sufficient only for the most routine work. Without a deeper knowledge of the operation of the apparatus, the scientist may well fall into the first pitfall of experimental research, that of too easily accepting readings which are stable for reports which are sound."

REFERENCES AND BIBLIOGRAPHY

"European Science Foundation inevitable" Sir Brian says. *Nature* 243:254, 1973.
Ravetz, J. R. *Scientific Knowledge and Its Social Problems.* Oxford: Clarendon Press, 1971. 449 pp.

Chapter II

Case Reports

The succeeding, simplified case reports should serve to acquaint the reader with some of the problems of epilepsy. To aid understanding, a simple seizure classification is provided, followed by a brief version of how an epilepsy suspect is handled during a diagnostic office visit and a summary of other procedures for which hospitalization might be recommended.

SIMPLE CLASSIFICATION OF SEIZURES

I. *Generalized Seizures Without Focal Onset, but with Bilateral Symmetry and Loss of Consciousness.*
1. Grand mal (tonic-clonic movement sequence; variants of pure tonic or pure clonic character).
2. Petit mal (*absences,* sometimes called staring spells). When occurring with myoclonic jerks (rapid involuntary jerks of a body part) and/or akinetic spells (sudden loss of power), they are referred to as the Lennox *petit mal triad.*

II. *Local Motor, Extending into Generalized Seizures.*

III. *Partial Seizures Without Impairment of Consciousness.*
1. With motor march over one side of the body arising either in thumb-index finger, hallux, or side of face (called Jacksonian motor).
2. With sensory march over the body from a local origin (called Jacksonian sensory).

IV. *Partial Seizures with Temporal Lobe Symptomatology (Generally with Impairment but not Loss of Consciousness), Characterized by:*
Automatisms (often called psychomotor seizures).
Hallucinations, sometimes called psychical seizures, or *déjà vu* interludes.
Autonomic (visceral) accompaniments.

An initial office visit includes the taking of a case history followed by a general physical and a neurological examination. In addition, referral may be made for: (1) electroencephalogram (EEG) of 24-minutes duration that includes 3 minutes of deep, rapid breathing (hyperventilation), and may include a sleep interval as well; and (2) X-rays of the skull. Psychological tests are required in some instances. A lumbar puncture, which may be deferred unless hospitalization is required, can be recommended for diagnostic purposes when it is believed helpful in ruling out a brain tumor or other neurological impairment as a cause of seizures. The procedures conducted during hospital inpatient study may also

5

include a brain scan, pneumoencephalography, and arteriography. In some instances a neuro-ophthalmological evaluation is also desirable. Brain scans and computerized transaxial tomography (CTT), the latter providing a two-dimensional view of the brain obtained by scanning the head with X-rays and computing the resulting data, can be done on an in- or outpatient basis. The CTT is entirely painless and does not even require an injection. In epilepsy without other complicating factors, hospital work-ups for the diagnostic purpose indicated are believed necessary in less than one-quarter of all cases examined.

The following facts illustrate the extent to which science recently has relatively improved diagnosis and treatment of the epileptic. Even the technique of the neurological examination was not developed until the latter half of the nineteenth century. X-ray diagnosis became feasible after the discovery of X-rays by Wilhelm C. Roentgen (1845–1923) in 1895. Pneumoencephalography, basically an X-ray procedure, was introduced by Walter Dandy (1886–1946) in 1918. Egas Moniz (1874–1955) first used arteriography in 1927. In 1947 at the University of Minnesota, George Moore developed brain scans. He first injected radioactive phosphorus (^{32}P) during surgery and localized tumors with a Geiger counter. Subsequently, he used iodine (^{131}I) for preoperative detection (Moore, 1947 and 1948). The EEG, which will be treated in detail in later chapters, arose out of the successes of Hans Berger of Germany in 1929. None of these technological advances were available to nineteenth-century physicians who cared for epileptics.

Similarly, modern medication for epilepsy commenced with the use of the first synthetic organic compound, phenobarbital, by A. Hauptmann in 1912. At present 13 antiepileptic drugs, all approved by the U.S. Food and Drug Administration (FDA) and all of synthetic derivation, are in use (see Chapter XV). These also provide strong evidence of the importance of relatively recent scientific developments to the improved care of epileptics.

The following case reports, it is hoped, will clarify features that distinguish different types of epileptic attacks; diagnostic procedures used in particular cases to rule out an organic cause for seizures; the fact that in cases where single drugs currently in use have proved ineffective, moderate to large doses of several drugs in different combinations may be required; and other difficulties encountered during treatment. It is also hoped that they will acquaint the reader with technical terminology.

CASE I

A young girl without prior history of head injury, encephalitis, or seizure had shown normal development and school performance up to age 12. Then she began to have staring spells at school, a few a day, during which time she would be out of touch with those around her. Diphenylhydantoin (DPH) and phenobarbital were prescribed but proved ineffective in ordinary dosages; in fact, the patient's entire course of treatment was marked by difficulties with medication.

Steadily worsening over a 7-year period, the girl developed psychomotor-type (temporal lobe) seizures, characterized by shuffling gait, fanning of fingers, fumbling with clothes, occasional speech arrest, and convulsive flexor muscular spasms of both arms. She was admitted to the hospital at age 19. A combination of DPH, thioridazine, diazepam, and primidone was administered, but the attacks continued. EEGs, previously unavailable, showed a generalized, slow abnormality with frequent right-side, spike-wave discharges of temporal predominance. X-ray plates of the skull were not considered abnormal. A pneumoencephalogram was read as normal, although the temporal horns of the lateral ventricles appeared mildly dilated. An arteriogram showed occlusion of a branch of the right anterior choroidal artery, which ordinarily supplies the Ammon's horn territory of the temporal lobe. It appeared that the patient's nondominant right hemisphere was primarily involved.

On the basis of these findings, it was decided to explore her right temporal lobe by electrocorticography (direct electrical brain recording) and, if necessary, to remove it.

Superficial and deep recordings revealed no sharply localized epileptogenic lesion, but the right temporal lobe showed abnormal electrical activity and was removed. Pathological evaluation of the tissue indicated neuronal loss and gliosis in the Sommer sector of Ammon's horn (see Chapter XI), compatible with old anoxic degenerative changes.

Postoperatively, the patient exhibited no symptoms other than a minimal weakness in the left arm and leg. She was discharged and prescribed a combination of DPH, diazepam, and phenobarbital.

Comment

This case belongs to the category of temporal lobe seizures of psychomotor type. Semipurposive, short-duration movements during unresponsive intervals are the chief manifestations—very different from the involuntary, severe, generalized spasms of grand mal attacks, with loss of consciousness. The frequency of this girl's attacks, and their refractoriness to usual antiepileptic medication, led to a disabling seizure state for which surgery was the only effective remedy.

Both the type of seizure and the localized pathological changes have been recognized since the early nineteenth century. Residual anoxic lesions, presumably as a result of birth injury in this case, are also described in the early literature.

CASE II

A 21-year-old man suffered from uncontrolled grand mal seizures for 11 years, along with transient lapses of awareness described as petit mal attacks. The grand mal attacks, severe and incapacitating, occurred about four times a month, but as many as 20 petit mal attacks could happen in 1 day. Reports that the petit mal attacks were sometimes brought on by looking at the sun suggested visual sensitivity as a factor.

Four years earlier, a craniotomy to remove a portion of the man's motor cortex had left his attack pattern unchanged, except that in addition he began to suffer attacks of Jacksonian focal origin starting in his left hand; he also experienced residual weakness, such as that which occurs after the hand area of the motor cortex is removed.

Upon hospitalization, skull X-rays showed no abnormalities, an EEG registered a mixed fast- and slow-frequency pattern with bursts of three-per-second, nonfocal spike-waves; and a pneumoencephalogram indicated some dilation of the ventricular system.

What was unusual about this patient, before and during treatment, was the unresponsiveness of his seizures to ordinarily effective drugs given to him in large doses and in various combinations: DPH, phenobarbital, mephobarbital, mephenytoin, trimethadione, were all tried with mediocre success, until administered in combination with an experimental drug that was used with the permission of the FDA. Although combinations with the experimental drug proved efficacious, it had to be discontinued because the manufacturer could not afford the long and expensive tests required to have the drug licensed. The patient could not serve as a test case anyway, because, in view of the severity of his seizures, it would have been undesirable to withdraw the established drugs and depend on the experimental one alone.

Comment

Despite the use of many drugs in various combinations and dosages, this patient never achieved optimum anticonvulsant control. No physician could have given him a favorable prognosis for achieving an abundant life, although the last information from him indicated that he had just completed 20 years of service in a responsible position with a business concern. However, no indication of whether or not his seizures were controlled was given.

The case demonstrates two important points. First, even when prognosis is not favorable, the rare patient may achieve a state of control that permits regular work of high quality. Second, the financial risk incurred in testing a potentially valuable drug may deter a manufacturer from continuing trials of promising products.

CASE III

A 34-year-old man had been under the care of the same physician since his first attacks began at age 12 when recovering from measles. As a boy he had been a leader in school, and throughout his adult life he had been continuously employed.

In the beginning, the attacks had occurred as often as 20 times a day. They were minor in character, typical of petit mal; showed no significant premonitory or postseizure event; and consisted of upward turning of the eyes, fluttering of the lids, and speech arrest, lasting from 5 to 10 seconds. Occasionally during a seizure he could say, "I'm all right."

As a youngster, he was normal neurologically. His skull X-ray films showed a mild craniofacial disproportion of questionable significance, and his EEGs registered runs of three-per-second spike-waves typical of petit mal epilepsy. Treatment with trimethadione or paramethadione, acetazolamide, and phenobarbital reduced his attacks to four or six a day. During late adolescence, he enjoyed at least one period free from seizures. Thereafter, attacks occurred intermittently.

Several years later, he began having generalized attacks as well. The first ended in a fall, with interruption of consciousness, accompanied by a cry, but no biting of the tongue occurred, no loss of sphincter control, and no tonic or clonic muscular contractions, or postseizure event. DPH was added to his other medicines, but the attacks continued with a tonic-clonic component, clearly grand mal in character. A recent EEG showed moderately fast waves and contained intermittent, atypical spike-waves, nonfocal in their occurrence.

Comment

This is a common history of combined petit and grand mal attacks. The subject was treated over a long period with various combinations of conventionally used drugs, but he has yet to achieve complete freedom from seizures. The onset of petit mal attacks preceded those of grand mal, which is the usual order. During the prolonged treatment, he had several episodes of skin sensitivity, none of which could be attributed to any of the antiepileptics used, for each was removed, one at a time, without affecting the rash.

CASE IV

A 25-year-old man with a long history of epilepsy was admitted to the hospital for consideration of surgery to relieve his seizures. At 18 months of age he had suffered a compound skull fracture, which was treated surgically. For several years thereafter he experienced grand mal attacks, followed by a few years of remission, until age 12. After the reappearance of grand mal, he began to have temporal lobe (psychomotor) seizures, four to eight a month, during which he might run *(epilepsia cursiva)*, become aggressive, eat nonedible things, or otherwise act aimlessly. Each seizure lasted 5 to 7 minutes, after which he might find himself in a strange place without knowing how he got there.

All efforts to control his seizures had been ineffective. At the time of hospitalization, he was taking primidone, mephenytoin, diazepam, and phenobarbital, all in rather large dosages. On that medication, he had great difficulty in holding a job.

General physical and neurological examinations were within normal limits. A recent EEG on an outpatient basis had been nonlocalizing, but a repeat in the hospital showed a mixed, fast and slow disorder attributable, in part, to his antiepileptic regimen but with no localizing features. Skull X-rays were within normal limits. A right carotid arteriogram was normal, and a WADA test[1] revealed the right hemisphere *not to be the dominant one.* A pneumoencephalogram indicated mild right ventricular dilation.

Depth-electrode implants were made in each mesial temporal region as a presurgical diagnostic procedure. The right electrode of the pair showed continuous spiking activity indicative of an epileptogenic focus in the anteromedial temporal area; the left one showed no spiking activity. Electrical stimulation on the right side did not occasion the premonitory aura of a seizure, nor was there activation of a continuous seizure discharge. Because of the right-sided brain localization of abnormal spiking activity and long-existing difficulty in medical control, a resection of the right anterior temporal lobe was undertaken.

The involved area of the anterior temporal lobe was removed, including the Ammon's horn region. About 1 week later, the patient developed a left facial and arm weakness. An arteriogram showed spasms (localized contractions of the arterial wall) of the right internal carotid and proximal right-middle cerebral arteries.[2] During the next week, the left arm and face weakness improved, leaving only a facial asymmetry. He had no seizures postoperatively and was discharged on routine antiepileptic medication.

Microscopic study of the principal specimen showed fibrous toughening of Ammon's horn with loss of neurons and gliosis. Remaining neurons were shrunken.

Comment

We believe that the damage to the right medial temporal lobe resulted in this instance from the compound skull fracture that occurred in early life. The temporal lobe seizures described were typical of that origin. Waking EEG records taken during interseizure intervals showed no convulsive activity. With classical seizures of temporal lobe type and refractoriness to medication, resort to depth electrodes for preoperative confirmation of the existence of a temporal epileptogenic focus seemed justified.

CASE V

A 35-year-old man was admitted to the neurosurgical service for investigation of focal seizures that had begun a month before. The initial one occurred at night. He awakened with the feeling that his lower jaw was being pulled to the right; his head began turning in that direction; and he heard a roaring in both ears. The same seizure pattern recurred early the next morning, accompanied by numbness and weakness of the right shoulder and arm and followed by transient speech impairment.

Skull X-rays proved negative, but an EEG showed a left, mid-temporal, slow-wave focus, presumably arising from the convex outer surface of the brain. Pneumoencephalograms were normal. DPH and phenobarbital were prescribed, and the patient was discharged.

The attacks continued at irregular intervals, and the patient was readmitted 2 years later. At that time skull X-rays showed a tiny calcification in the left parietal region. Neurological examination was negative, except for a slight, right facial asymmetry and hesitation of speech. An EEG and an arteriogram were normal, but a pneumoencephalogram revealed a slight symmetrical dilatation of the lateral ventricles and of the third ventricle as well.

While in the hospital, the patient had several focal seizures consisting of tonic and clonic movements of the right face with adversive movements of the eyes to the right. After one of them, a temporary paralysis of the right arm developed. A prescription of chloral hydrate, DPH, and phenobarbital controlled the seizures. The patient became less drowsy, his speech improved, and his right arm recovered its function. But he continued to show a right facial weakness with protrusion of the tongue to the right.

Since the seizures clearly interfered with the patient's work, it was decided to perform an exploratory operation. A left parietal craniotomy with electrocorticography showed a spiking epileptogenic focus arising from a very small area of cortex belonging to the lower part of the precentral gyrus, just above the Sylvian fissure. A very small block of tissue was removed for biopsy. Microscopic sections through it revealed a tiny, centrally situated lesion with a stream of malignant cells extending toward one edge. It was a typical glioblastoma surrounded by nontumorous tissue.

In a second operation, a significantly wider area was removed. Immediately thereafter, the patient experienced a severe aphasia with a weakness of the right side of his body. Rapid improvement of the aphasia and of the right arm and face followed, and antiepileptic medication prevented the recurrence of seizures. The man was then discharged from the hospital.

Comment

When focal (or generalized) epilepsy strikes an adult with no prior history of attacks, the possibility exists that it is caused by a cerebral tumor until proven otherwise. This is even more true when the history is one of progressive neurological deficit. In this case, the usual diagnostic tests were negative, except for one focally abnormal EEG, which pointed to the site of the lesion, and the even more definitive electrocorticography. The underlying tumor had remained tiny despite a presumed 2 years of growth; without surgical exploration, it may not have been discovered for a much longer period of time. In right-handed persons, motor aphasia is not unusual in cases of left frontotemporal lesions; and, in this instance, the remainder of the neurological findings also indicated the possibility of a tumor in that locale.

CASE VI

A girl began having epileptic attacks at age 11. Described as "dazes," at first they occurred infrequently. An EEG taken at that time showed the typical three-per-second, spike-wave discharges of petit mal. Initially, she was treated with phenobarbital, later replaced by methsuximide, because it caused headaches.

The attacks continued over the next 3 years; in the last year they increased from a few to 50 or 60 a day. Toward the end of that year, the girl began to have a series of myoclonic jerks, lasting 15 to 20 minutes each, without loss of consciousness, for which she was treated with DPH. Less than a month later, she had a grand mal attack that began as a focal seizure of the left side of her mouth. Primidone was added to the DPH medication, and in 1969, at the age of 14, she was admitted to St. Louis Children's Hospital.

Physical and neurological examinations conducted at the hospital showed no abnormalities, but a petit mal attack lasting 15 seconds was precipitated by hyperventilation, i.e., rapid deep breathing. An EEG revealed bursts of three-per-second spike-waves in the resting trace; one such burst occurred in the overventilation phase of the record.

The patient's DPH was increased, and ethosuximide was substituted for the primidone. During the following 2 years, she continuously took these medicines. In the first year no seizures were observed; during the second, she did reasonably well, averaging one to three brief myoclonic jerks on getting up in the morning and two to three staring spells ("dazes") per week.

Thereafter, she was not observed for a year or more, during which time she continued to have brief myoclonic jerks in the morning. One akinetic spell occurred when she was crossing the street.

Later, she stopped taking her medicine because she felt "drugged." She had no difficulty until a month later when she returned to Children's Hospital for a checkup. At that time she experienced six or seven "drop attacks," each of which lasted only a few seconds. Treatment with DPH and ethosuximide was reinstituted.

Comment

Several types of seizures have been recounted here. Except for the single grand mal, tonic-clonic, generalized attack of focal origin, all were consistent with Lennox's *petit mal triad,* which may include staring spells *(absences),* myoclonic jerks, and drop attacks.

The following observations are noteworthy. The patient's intellectual and social development was usual for her age. Attacks, for whatever reason, frequently increased in number on visiting the physician, a not unusual occurrence. A petit mal attack brought on by hyperventilation should never be overlooked in the neurological evaluation of such a case.

The ultimate prognosis would appear good.

CASE VII

A 14-year-old girl had suffered head injury twice within a brief period. A short time later she showed the following signs of illness: stumbling and falling on the stairs in the early morning, often before breakfast; jerking movements of her eyes; and occasional involuntary jerking of her right leg or throwing of her right arm upwards and outwards. No aura preceded such spells, though some began with a turning of the head and eyes to the left. A cousin was an epileptic.

Skull X-rays, a fasting blood sugar, and an EEG were interpreted as normal; and the girl was given phenobarbital. Some time later she had her first grand mal seizure, at 7:00 A.M., consisting of generalized tonic-clonic movements and urinary incontinence followed by confusion and drowsiness. Additional skull films still appeared normal, but a brain scan suggested a radioactive uptake in the right parieto-occipital area. DPH was prescribed instead of the phenobarbital; later phenobarbital was again prescribed with the DPH.

The patient continued having three to four short-lived attacks a month, akinetic in type. Just before one such attack, she experienced jumping objects in her right visual field, and after each jerk, she felt she was whirling around. She was having frequent headaches, experiencing feelings of *déjà vu,* and sleeping more; she saw her friends less; she was also depressed about low grades at school.

Because of the possibility of a brain tumor, she was admitted to the children's service for a series of studies, including skull X-rays, lumbar puncture, brain scan, and tests to rule out collagen disease, the results of which were within normal limits. Her DPH plasma concentration was then 21.3 $\mu g/ml$; her phenobarbital level was 23.9 $\mu g/ml$. DPH, phenobarbital, acetazolamide, dextroamphetamine sulfate, and amitriptyline hydrochloride were prescribed. She was discharged from the hospital on continuing observation.

A month later she was much better, was far less lethargic, and was again going out with friends. She had missed no school, and her grades had improved. During the following 5 months, she had only one spell, in which her right arm flung outward and her eyes rolled upwards momentarily. She complained of drawing sensations in the fingers of her right hand, but no movements took place. Her prescription was not changed. During another 3 months, she had one questionable grand mal seizure in her sleep. In addition, she had awakened several times to find her tongue severely bitten.

Nine months later, when she reported having several grand mal seizures in the morning just before awakening, the phenobarbital was increased. Subsequently, she experienced a grand mal convulsion every month, usually related to her menstrual period, and often occurring in the morning. Simultaneously, her drug doses were gradually increased. However, her DPH plasma level was only 4.5 $\mu g/ml$, probably because she had not been taking her medicine regularly. The importance of taking every dose was emphasized strongly.

Two years after hospitalization, the patient's seizure condition had worsened. She had had three grand mal seizures at night. The DPH dosage was reduced because her eyes were crossing and she was having trouble with her balance. Several weeks later, she was hospitalized a second time. Her general physical examination was satisfactory, but she was staggering markedly, which suggested DPH intoxication. Two EEGs were abnormally slow. A brain scan and lumbar puncture were normal. DPH plasma concentration was 25 μg/ml. The dosages of both drugs were reduced. As her DPH plasma level dropped, the staggering disappeared. Upon discharge at an effective but lower level of medication, she had no significant remaining neurological abnormality.

Comment

This case demonstrates well the ups and downs of treating the epileptic adolescent in out- and inpatient practice. When first seen, the girl was having both grand mal and akinetic seizures. The involuntary flinging movements of her right arm could well have been interpreted as a partial seizure manifestation of myoclonic type. As it does not infrequently, the question of brain tumor arose, but there was no evidence of progressive neurological deficit in this instance. At one point, the patient's plasma DPH fell quite low, probably indicating that she was not taking her medicine regularly. On another occasion, DPH evidently exceeded the limits of toxicity, the resultant neurological signs disappearing when the dosage was reduced.

NOTES

[1] A test to establish cerebral dominance. Threshold doses of a barbiturate are injected into each carotid artery (supplying a side of the brain) in turn. The left carotid, supplying the usually dominant left hemisphere, is injected first. Dominance is indicated by garbling of speech due to a direct effect of the barbiturate upon the motor speech center. If speech remains unaffected, the right side is similarly tested.

[2] Experience teaches that such spasms are often suggestive of neighborhood intracranial pathology.

REFERENCES

Moore, G. W. Fluorescein as agents in differentiation of normal and malignant tissues. *Science* 106:130–131, 1947.

Moore, G. W. Use of radioactive diiodofluorescein in the diagnosis and localization of brain tumors. *Science* 107:569–571, 1948.

Chapter III

Epilepsy over the Millennia

All men are delighted to look back

Dante

An object of pity and horror in antiquity, often a social outcast, the epileptic also fell prey to religious superstition, especially that stemming from a fear of witches and demons. Traditional remedies handed down from ancient Greek or earlier physicians and the valueless cures that quacks were forever proposing continued to be used in the Middle Ages and later, supplemented by equally as preposterous new "cures," talismans, incantations, and rituals. Yet there were always physicians who conscientiously sought the underlying cause of disorders and diseases. The failure of seemingly reasonable and time-tested remedies forced them to the conclusion that chronic epilepsy was a difficult, if not impossible, condition to cure. Because of a dearth of well-trained physicians, but even more because science was still in its infancy, the empirical treatment of epilepsy, as well as the miseries of its victims, persisted into the nineteenth century. Only with the advance of science did real help come to those who suffered repeated convulsions. Thus, a backward glance provides a necessary base for assessing the impact of the rise of the neurosciences on the improved treatment and social acceptance of the epileptic. Temkin (1971) has rightly said that the history of epilepsy epitomizes the long struggle between magical and scientific concepts of disease, and only over the last two centuries has the epileptic found himself wearing the winner's colors with increasing frequency.

EPILEPSY IN ANCIENT MEDICINE

Authorities on the history of epilepsy see no reason to believe that it spared prehistoric man. In France, for example, Stone Age cave paintings suggest that trephinings may have been used to help epileptics. Mesopotamians were familiar with epilepsy. An Akkadian text of 2000 B.C. describes a person in an attack which the exorcist ascribed to the god Sin (Temkin, 1971). The London neurologist, Hughlings Jackson (1835–1911), has said that satanic possession is the oldest alleged cause of epilepsy (Taylor, 1931, p. 252). Even today, public fascination over the topic of satanic possession has not waned, as evidenced by the success of the controversial motion picture, *The Exorcist.*

GREEK VIEWS OF EPILEPSY

In ancient Greece, the word *epilepsia* referred to a variety of convulsive diseases popularly thought of as inflictions of the gods; later writings came to describe the seizures of epilepsy much as we know them today. Because its causes were unknown and because it was usually attributed to the supernatural, it was commonly known as the "Sacred Disease."

In his authoritative work, *The Falling Sickness,* Oswei Temkin (1971) begins with an account of the earliest known treatise on epilepsy. Hippocratic writings dealing with the subject date from about 400 B.C. One of them, entitled *On the Sacred Disease,* includes a survey of beliefs and practices and a vigorous attack on the magicians and charlatans who called the disease "sacred" as a shelter for their own ignorance and fraud. The following oft-quoted passage from *On the Sacred Disease* is from the translation found in H. J. Muller's *The Loom of History* (1958, p. 122):

> It seems to me that the disease is no more divine than any other. It has a natural cause just as other diseases have. Men think it is divine merely because they do not understand it. But if they called everything divine which they do not understand, why there would be no end of divine things.

This is a fair sample of the thinking of Greek physicians of the fifth century B.C., who by their resistance to magic laid the foundation for the medical interpretation of all diseases as natural disturbances of the body. They had observed and correctly inferred much about epilepsy. The writer of *On the Sacred Disease* ascribed the trouble to a cold, moist humor (phlegm) and clearly recognized that epilepsy originated in the brain. To the contrary, the writer of *On Breaths,* another of the Hippocratic writings as paraphrased by E. B. Levine (1971), attributed the cause to a combination of air and blood.[1]

The Greeks knew that epilepsy occurs most frequently in early life, that its initial appearance after age 20 is unusual, and that the disorder can be innate. Certain Hippocratic writings even characterized it as hereditary and agreed that it could be precipitated by a variety of factors.

According to Temkin (1971, p. 28), ancient authors defined epilepsy as a "convulsion of the whole body together with an impairment of its leading functions," which succinctly distinguished it from other spasms or fits. They recognized three types of attack; one in which the subject was initially overcome by a deep sleep, another by a convulsion, and a third in which convulsion was followed by sleep. The description of the *aura* as the upward sweep of a breeze through the body is understandable today, if not taken too literally.

The ancients separated symptoms premonitory of an attack, such as stupor, dizziness, and slurred speech, from those that immediately preceded it. The latter included such sensory hallucinations as lights before the eyes, ringing in the ears, bad odors, or a feeling in hand or foot that crept slowly toward the head. For the latter, the ancients understood that a constriction placed about an arm or leg might slow or stop an advancing seizure.

They knew the dangers of suffocation and the chance of biting the tongue, and understood that a generalized seizure tends to build toward a maximum and may cause incontinence during abatement. They even mentioned the epileptic cry (since shown to result from expulsion of air against a partially closed larynx). All of these symptoms are similar to those known today. Furthermore, the ancients understood that an isolated attack could occur without repetition.

On one score the clinical acuity of the Hippocratic writings is difficult to evaluate. E. C. Streeter (1922, p. 8) quotes Hippocrates on epilepsy as follows: "Observe the goat for that animal is most prone to this disease." E. B. Levine (1971, p. 109) states the following: "The disease was thought by the author to be endemic in domestic animals as well as in man, but especially common among goats. . . ."

Without denying that strains of goats may have a high incidence of epilepsy, that species is also prone to another illness that equally deserves the name "falling sickness"—as epilepsy became known in the Middle Ages. To casual inspection its manifestations could well be mistaken for an attack of epilepsy. The illness is *myotonia congenita,* a hereditary condition afflicting certain goat herds in middle Tennessee, adjoining states, and a part of Texas. When a myotonic animal tries to run, it becomes rigid in part or in all of its voluntary musculature, falls over, and lies outstretched and stiff as if in an epileptic seizure. But only its musculature, not its nervous system, is involved in the generalized spasm, which a practiced eye can distinguish as myotonia, not epilepsy.[2]

Temkin (1971) indicates a decline in medical standards, by modern criteria, during the centuries following Hippocrates. A few physicians were scientists, but many acquiesced to popular superstitions. An excessive number of remedies are recorded. Temkin cites 45 for epilepsy, some of which recur over and over again in later literature. Just as now, many difficulties had to be overcome by anyone setting out to establish the efficacy of an antiepileptic agent. The praise of an influential physician for a particular remedy resulted in the undeserved popularity of many "cures." Significantly, many such remedies were difficult to obtain, particularly in quantities needed for daily consumption, as modern procedure requires.

Prescriptions were capricious, empirical, and often unappetizing, to say the least. Not infrequently, the mode of preparation was overly exacting or haphazard, and failure to produce the desired effect could be attributed to error in compounding. Often, the same remedies, peony or mistletoe roots, for example, were taken internally or worn as an amulet. Many of these "cures" had magical connotations extending into the ageless past; for example, the influence of the waxing moon on the recurrence of attacks was widely accepted and, in turn, its waning phase was thought to be the best time to gather remedies. Human blood, organs such as the liver, or ground bone from skulls were early remedies. Blood might be smeared on the mouth of an epileptic during an attack, or he might be required to drink it or suck it from the mouth of a dying gladiator. Pliny the Elder (23–79 A.D.) witnessed the latter. Religious cures were unopposed by physicians who accepted divine intervention, and some were not above accepting other nonreligious miracles. The epileptic has always had to put up with much unkindness born of ignorance. The disorder has been often looked upon with horror and disgust, and the victim has been treated as untouchable. People have feared to drink from the same cup with him. Allusions in literature to the fact that an epileptic might hide his head or run for cover when he felt an oncoming attack suggest that he feared ostracism, perhaps even violence.

EPILEPSY IN ROMAN TIMES

In the days of the Roman Republic, medicine consisted of household remedies, simple surgical manipulations, and magical formulas derived from the Etruscans; yet in at least one book of Etruscan folklore (Leland, 1963), no mention is made of the treatment of epilepsy. The chief medical practitioner of the Roman family was usually the *pater familias,* who cared for his own family, slaves, other dependents, and friends.

The conversion of the Romans to Greek medicine is attributed to Asclepiades (first century B.C.), who had both common sense and insight into human character. Even before that time, in the third century B.C., Greek physicians and midwives had begun to immigrate to Rome. They have been described as ill-trained charlatans who traded on the credulity of the people.

Typical of the Roman medical attitude toward epilepsy was Galen, who was born in Pergamum in Asia Minor about 130 A.D. and died, probably in Rome, about 200 A.D. During the Middle Ages, he became the most celebrated of the ancient physicians. That this friend of emperors and avid searcher for knowledge should have won the esteem of medieval schoolmen seems natural enough. Especially in his voluminous philosophical writings, he expressed respect for Plato, Aristotle, and advocated monotheism, even though he rejected Christianity. He was virtually a determinist, insisting that all the functions and purposes of Creation could be discovered by observing natural phenomena and their laws. A persistent dissectionist, he worked mostly on apes, and became acknowledged as "The father of physiology." William Harvey[3] (1578–1657) implied that Galen was well on the way to discovering the pulmonary circulation of blood. Yet, for all his careful work, Galen made some gross errors—attributable, perhaps, to a lack of means for closer observation, as well as to misinterpretation of some of his discoveries. Probably, the most serious of these was his hypothesis regarding the pneumata (spirits) and their role in the process of life. Thus, the work of this greatest of the ancient anatomists is a reminder of the role of speculation in research and also a warning against the premature acceptance of a hypothesis as fact. Many eager investigators have failed to heed this lesson!

Galen's opinions were derived from those popular in Greece in about 400 B.C. There, the four-humors doctrine was being promulgated in some Hippocratic writings, elaborated in *On the Nature of Man,* and associated with epilepsy in *On the Sacred Disease.* Epilepsy was explained as a stagnation of the cold humors (mostly phlegm, but also black bile[4]) within the ventricles, or cavities, of the brain (Fig. 1).

Galen held that the cerebral pneuma filled the ventricles of the brain. Why

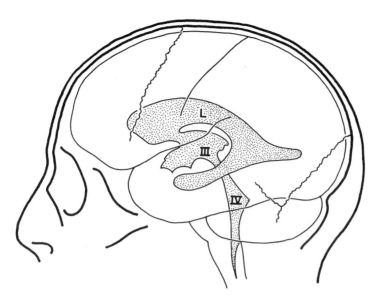

Fig. 1. Left lateral view of the brain with the ventricular system superimposed. L, lateral ventricle; III, third ventricle; IV, fourth ventricle. Lateral and third ventricles were formerly called *anterior;* IV, the *posterior.*

he thought such pneuma was involved in epilepsy remains obscure. It is probably unimportant that Galen viewed the ventricles, not the substance of the brain, as the seat of epilepsy (and of sensation and motion), for science was then in its infancy and errors were inevitable but not irreparable. However, the fact that this notion remained entrenched for more than two millennia is clear evidence of the stagnation of ideas characteristic of the long interim preceding the rise of the modern neurosciences.

Through the Middle Ages the error was perpetuated in the transcriptions of many documents without ever being put to the challenge of scientific proof. Thus, it provided the only physiological or pathological rationale for choosing one proposed epilepsy remedy over another. Essentially, the same errors persisted in the Arabic stream of knowledge; for example, *The Canon,* by Avicenna,[5] later added to the prestige of the Galenic concept in Europe. In the sixteenth century, however, some European physicians subscribed to Galenic philosophy, free of Arabic influences. This was part of the often exaggerated emphasis on the classics in the Renaissance.

Besides generalized seizures of the type known today as grand mal, Galen defined a category akin to the present Jacksonian epilepsy. He also distinguished a third type that he believed to originate in another part of the body. In this variety, which he called epilepsy by *sympathy,* he believed the brain to be only secondarily involved, seizures originating in a related organ, the stomach often being regarded as the source. Not until the writings of Thomas Willis (1621–1675) were all the phenomena of the epileptic attack, including the aura, regarded as cerebral in origin (see pp. 25–26).

Galen, noted for his sophistication in therapy, evidently used traditional Greek remedies, especially *theriaca,* which is defined in modern medical dictionaries as an effective antidote to the bites of poisonous animals. Scribonius, a Roman physician of the first century A.D., recommended the electric discharge of the torpedo fish[6] as a cure for epilepsy, headache, and gout (Hodgkin, 1964).

EPILEPSY IN MEDIEVAL TIMES—THE FALLING SICKNESS

The Greek description of epilepsy as the "Sacred Disease" arose from the belief that a god had entered the stricken one. The Latin *morbus comitialis* reflected the superstition that an attack occurring on the day of the *Comitia* (assembly) was an ominous sign. Such an attack inevitably broke up the gathering. Apuleius, the Roman author, used the term *caducus* ("falling one"), and the disease acquired the name of *passio caduca* (Temkin, 1971), which means "falling sickness" or "falling evil" in English. The latter had a broader connotation, including demoniac possession as well as epilepsy.

MEDICAL AND RELIGIOUS ASPECTS OF THE MEDIEVAL PERIOD

Since mundane help seemed of little or no avail, men in the Ages of Faith naturally turned to the intercession of the saints (Fig. 2). For relief from epilepsy, they prayed especially to St. Cornelius, St. Gilles, St. Michael, and St. Valentine

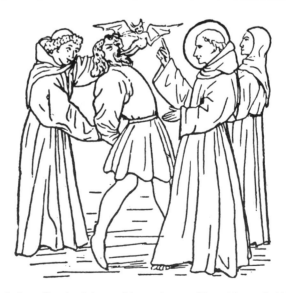

FIG. 2. A medieval saint exorcising a demon. (From Haggard, 1932.)

(Streeter, 1922). Such devotion was encouraged not only by simple parish priests but also by some of the great monastic establishments, especially those associated with shrines. They were not only the centers of culture and learning of the times but also the hospices for the traveler and the dispensaries of help to the poor and sick.

Also, because of a lack of knowledge, people often turned to charlatanism and superstition. Such "cures" as "baptism by fire" on St. John's Eve stemmed from Nordic paganism and were deeply rooted in folklore. Combined with imperfect religious notions, they sometimes erupted into mass hysteria, such as that which fanned out from Aix La Chapelle in 1374. Because of the frenzied dancing accompanying such incidences, they have been superficially associated with epilepsy, which, indeed, acquired still another name, *St. John's Disease*. But surely there are more acceptable explanations for these phenomena than have come down to us through the ages.

Some such outbreaks have been associated with a disease caused by bread made from grain containing ergot, a toxic product of fungal action. They also were characterized by convulsions, bizarre behavior, and hallucinatory experiences.[7] The latest of these experiences took place in Port St. Esprit, France, in August 1954. Even with the excellent diagnostic opportunities afforded modern physicians, the condition was not recognized immediately (Fuller, 1968). Since medieval times, however, physicians have generally provided accurate diagnoses, even when they were unable to determine a cause or prescribe a remedy.

Almost implicit in the alleviation or cure of a disease named after a saint was the handling by the afflicted person of relics associated with the saint. Under the circumstances, a monk could hardly denounce the incantations and amulets that simple folk believed to be effective in warding off attacks. Should he pit his own ignorance against theirs?[8] In general, however, the physician of medieval times seems not only to have been less questioning than the Greeks, but also more ready to accept, without doubt, the knowledge they had passed on to him.

THE RENAISSANCE AND THE ENLIGHTENMENT

The sixteenth and early seventeenth centuries presented many instances of conflicting public attitudes toward epilepsy. These played a minor role in the larger sphere of popular confusion concerning religion, witchery, black magic, and demoniac possession. In Holland, Italy, and Germany, inexplicable eruptions of hysteria occurred about 1550. In Hamburg, 43 so-called sorcerers perished at the stake together. In many cases the judges condemned convulsionaries as victims of sorcery, whereas they were actually sick people sorely in need of help. Some members of the intelligentsia, Montaigne for example, argued that to broil human beings alive was to inflate vastly the price of conjecture (Streeter, 1922). It would be incorrect to give the impression that all such victims were epileptics; but, in mass "contagions" such as were sometimes encountered, it may have been well-nigh impossible to differentiate them, one and all, from those suffering from either hysteria or what was interpreted "legalistically" as possession.

Amidst the Puritan excitement of the seventeenth century, Temkin reports that "frothing at the mouth—an accompaniment of many true seizures—was frequent among the zealots." In the Salem witchcraft trials, those afflicted by epilepsy often were regarded as contaminated by the devil or by witches. It was not a better understanding of epilepsy, however, that ended such outrages, but public revulsion from the harsh theology of the Puritan divines whose belief in their predestination allowed them to judge others. Those not so certain about their destiny were inclined to be somewhat more tolerant toward victims of a disease they did not understand.

DIAGNOSIS AND TREATMENT AS RECOMMENDED BY MEDIEVAL AND LATER PHYSICIANS

Historically, it is worth recalling the conclusions of five physicians who gave considerable attention to epilepsy and who provide examples of the practices of their times. Of these, Bernard of Gordon (Lennox, 1941), who wrote *Lilium Medicinae* in the early fourteenth century, ascribed epilepsy to a humor or coarse windiness that occluded the non-principal ventricles of the brain (III and IV in Fig. 1) and impeded the passage of breath to the members. As a cure for an attack, he recommended that the ministrant whisper a religious verse into the subject's ear. That surely did no harm, but one may wonder about other remedies, such as mistletoe, pyrethrum, and curds of a leopard's milk.

John of Gaddesden (1280–1361) (Lennox, 1939) wrote the *Rosa Medicinae.* He prescribed remedies to fit the patient's purse, sagacious in pre-Medicare days, and he also advised that the best cures be kept secret, perhaps a premonition of the proprietaries of the modern drug industry. His cures included the reading of the Gospel over the subject's head and amulets of peony, chrysanthemum, or the hair of an all-white dog, which should not be marked by the slightest black spot. In addition, he recommended swallowing of one of several unappetizing potions.

Arnold of Villanova (1234–1313) (von Storch and von Storch, 1938) derived his notions from Galen. He advised bloodletting, along with a special diet composed of items very difficult to procure. Economics to the contrary, why should rarity imply value? As important as the diet itself were abstentions: bones and brains of animals, cucumbers, lentils, cabbage, and beans were proscribed. Such was the quality of medical care given a victim of epilepsy, prince or pauper.

Antonius Guainerius (ca. 1488) (Lennox, 1940) argued that epilepsy could be due to any humor, frequently phlegm, least often yellow bile. He divided signs of epilepsy into indicative and prognostic. The former, of course, necessitated observation of an attack by the physician. Guainerius differentiated between the actions of the humors presumed to induce epilepsy. But humors could be mixed in their actions, and when they were, so were the signs. This further confused correct diagnosis. Among remedies he deemed successful in rooting out all curable epilepsy, he included *theriaca,* powder of peony root or seed, minerals, and parts of animals. The head of the cuckoo worn around the neck was supposed to prevent an epileptic from falling.[9] Animal hearts, eaten hot or powdered, were recommended in variety. In extreme cases, Guainerius favored the cautery.

A prescription by Jean Fernel (1497–1568) of Paris (Fig. 3), who, according to his biographer, C. S. Sherrington (1946), wrote the first treatise on physiology since Galen's *On the Use of the Parts,* 1,300 years previously, provides an illustration of Renaissance treatment of epilepsy. Fernel's book was issued under the title *The Natural Part of Medicine,* later changed to *Physiology.* Sherrington (1946, p. 36) quotes Fernel's famous prescription thus:

> Take mistletoe of the oak; man's skull powdered (we are told by Matthiolus the skull must be one that was never buried); peony—male peony—seeds or root (if gathered in the wane of the moon you shall find nothing better); of these 2 scruples apiece; mix.

Separating the reasonable from the impossible, Sherrington looks for meaning in Fernel's prescription and suggests: ". . . epilepsy, ailment of the brain; pituita (Lat. for 'phlegm') secretion from the brain (cold and moist); powdered skull, cold and dry . . .; gathered in the wane of the moon, drier; *human* skull versus *human* brain: contraries cure. But, of course, behind each ingredient, stretched an age-long tradition, laden with the occult" (Sherrington, 1946, p. 36). And that best summarized, from a modern point of view, the therapy of epilepsy that continued through the Renaissance.

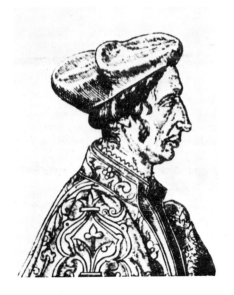

Fig. 3. Jean Fernel (1497–1558). (Underwood, 1953.)

FACTS AND FANCIES WHICH CONCERN PEONY AND MISTLETOE

Peony and mistletoe are among the most frequently mentioned and venerable ingredients of remedies for epilepsy. Each has an ancient origin. According to one source, the word "peony" was derived from the name of the divine physician of the Greek gods, *Paean,* mentioned in Homer. Bullfinch (1796–1867) (*Bullfinch's Mythology,* n.d.), however, identifies Paean as an alternative name for both Apollo and Aesculapius. For use in epilepsy, peonies were to be gathered during the wane of the moon, since epileptic attacks were presumed to occur more often as the moon waxes, according to the dogma that "contraries cure." Among the Etruscans, the root of the peony was worn in an amulet to keep away incubi. In seventeenth-century England, it was prescribed for all kinds of illnesses. The Mongols of the eighteenth century are said to have eaten its seeds and roots.

Mistletoe was held in great esteem by the Druids. If plucked on the sixth day of the new moon, it had magical virtues and was considered a cure-all (*Bullfinch's Mythology,* n.d.). Mistletoe grows worldwide in several genera and many species, but the ceremonial mistletoe of Europe is *Viscum albans.* Its range extends from northern Asia to the British Isles. Its growth on oak trees, however, is rare, which may be why the mistletoe of oak and not that of another tree was prescribed by Fernel and others. Among early Christians, mistletoe was excluded from church decorations at Christmas, perhaps because of its veneration by the Druids, whom the Christians supplanted. More recently in Sweden, a knife made with an oak mistletoe handle was carried by epileptics to ward off seizures.

EARLIEST SURGICAL TREATMENTS OF EPILEPSY

The earliest surgical procedures in treating epilepsy date from prehistory. (See Chapter XVI for modern surgical practices.) One was cauterization of the head, used in the Middle Ages and perhaps earlier. The usual site of application was the back of the head or brow, sometimes the spine, chest, or arm. It was even used on normal children as a preventative of disease. Trephination, ordinarily regarded as an extreme procedure, was only used in the most stubborn cases. A sixteenth-century trephine is shown in Fig. 4.

Skulls have been found in early neolithic burial sites in France and Peru into which holes had been bored sometime before death (Rogers, 1930). In France, bone amulets the size of a hole have been found near a trephined skull, suggesting a magical association with the practice. In Peru, the holes appear to have been bored largely for therapeutic purposes such as decompressing a fracture. More recent evidence of trephining has been discovered in many parts of the world, particularly in the South Sea Islands and North Africa. Whether the explanation be surgical treatment or the release of demons, the findings suggest the prehistoric prevalence of epilepsy.

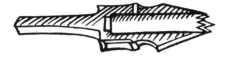

Fig. 4. A sixteenth century surgical instrument. (From Haggard, 1932.)

TRANSITION TO THE MODERN AGE

A controversial figure often heralds a new era long before his peers have divined the need for change. The epilepsy prescription of Jean Fernel was galenical. Relying on rationalization, he used the dogma of contraries to support the selection of one substance or one manner of preparation rather than another. Yet, as the fifteenth century gave way to the sixteenth, both the therapy and the alchemy of the Middle Ages were wearing thin. A new scientific chemistry was long overdue.

Paracelsus (Theophrastus Bombastus von Hohenheim) (1493–1541), predecessor of the iatrochemists (from the Greek word, *iatros,* meaning physician), was born 20 years after Copernicus, whose quincentenary was celebrated in 1973. It is Copernicus who, in addition to his contribution to the heliocentric universe, is credited with introducing the scientific revolution on which today's society is based. Paracelsus, who entered the lists on the side of radical change, became quite unpopular with the entrenched academic bureaucracy, a not unusual experience of pioneers. Unfortunately, his neoplatonic notions militated against his sounder ideas. He argued that chemistry should be based on the observation of nature, as did Aristotle before him. He publicly cast Galen's works and Avicenna's *Canon* into the flames at Basel to dramatize the need for a clear break with the beliefs of his predecessors. His philosophy, outlined simply by A. Debus (1965), never materialized in practice, hard as he tried to introduce chemical concepts and methods into both pathology and therapy.

SCHOOLS OF IATROCHEMISTRY AND IATROPHYSICS

The exponents of these new schools of medicine offered primitive chemical and physical explanations of epilepsy and its treatment. François le Boë (or Sylvius) (1614–1672) of Amsterdam and later Leyden, a leading anatomist, clinician, and bedside teacher, for whom the lateral fissure of the human brain is named, was an exemplar of the iatrochemical school. He espoused a theory involving acids, alkalis, effervescence, fermentation, and putrescence, although it did not have a sound foundation in either physiology or pathology. He spoke of an acid volatile spirit as a cause of epilepsy, and recommended antiepileptic remedies that contained a basic salt. Evidently, he had not fully escaped the influence of contraries, which so markedly characterized medieval therapy.

Thomas Willis (1621–1675), a leading London clinician, well known for his studies of the blood supply of the brain, reaffirmed in 1667 that the central nervous system is the seat and source of all convulsive processes (Streeter, 1922). His most important contribution to the knowledge of epilepsy was the affirmation that the premonition (signal) of an attack (medical, *aura,* fr. Lat., for "breath"), as well as the attack itself, emanates from the brain. He developed a chemical theory that muscular movement was caused by "spiritosaline" particles within the muscle fibers mixing with "nitrosulphurous" ones (gunpowder?) brought to the muscle by arterial blood. Local explosions of this mixture inflated and short-ened the muscle fibers. A similar theory, applied to the nervous system, was used to explain epileptic attacks.

The outstanding iatrophysicists were Italian, notably Giovanni Alfonso Borelli (1608–1679) and G. Baglivi (1668–1742). Borelli's explanation of neuromuscular action entailed a mechanical nervous juice and nerves made up of canals filled with a porous substance through which fluid commotion was passed outwards, causing droplets to enter the muscle and produce its contraction. Baglivi was a chemist, pathologist, and clinician who had done many autopsies, and from those experiences he developed a theory that the outer tough membrane covering the brain contracted in systole and relaxed in diastole, forcing a fluid arising from the brain through the body. Although these theories rested on sketchy and erroneous evidence, they were nevertheless further elaborated on before being abandoned.

BOERHAAVE (1669–1725)

An indefatigable worker and an effective and versatile teacher, clinician, and scientist (Lindeboom, 1968), Herman Boerhaave was called the Batavian Hippoc-rates. At one time he simultaneously held the academic chairs of botany, chemis-try, and medicine at Leyden. Boerhaave wrote a simple, lucid treatise on nervous diseases that was used for a century. In general, he and his followers continued to prescribe for epilepsy drugs that had been in vogue since ancient times, includ-ing black hellabore, oak mistletoe, and valerian. Boerhaave was responsible for one innovation in antiepileptic therapy, a preparation of chalcanth (blue vitriol or copper sulfate),[10] which he claimed produced incredible cures. It is extremely doubtful that its use as an antiepileptic would be considered today.

EPILEPSY IN EASTERN EUROPE

A vigorous and innovative thinker of the Enlightenment in Eastern Europe was Jan Marek (Johannes Marcu Marci) (1595–1667), a professor (later rector) at Charles University in Prague after 1630 (Fig. 5).[11] Marek defined epilepsy as including not only generalized fits but also "absences" and psychomotor seizures; he refuted mechanical and humoral theories of causation. He recognized stimuli from without the body as playing an important role in the activation of the attack.

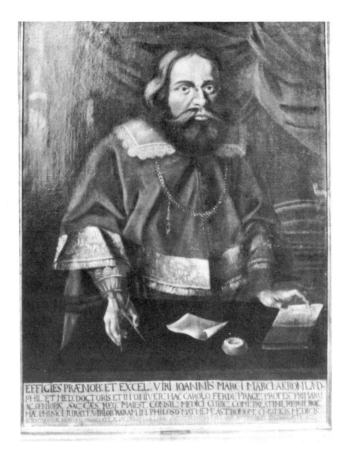

FIG. 5. Jan Marek. (Servít, 1965.)

Marek's scholarship provided a transition between mythical speculation and the origins of biomedical knowledge. He denied the existence of inherent ideas and espoused sensory perception as the basis of knowledge. The latter view allied him with John Locke (1632–1704), who is remembered for his remark that "all knowledge comes from experience."

TREATMENT OF EPILEPSY ON THE EARLY AMERICAN SCENE

American Indian folk remedies were often shrouded in secrecy. In an account dated 1725, an Indian squaw is said to have cured a French soldier of epilepsy by administering some kind of pulverized root (Vogel, 1970). The Indians used bayberry, passion flower, and stramonium seeds for treatment. Of these, stramonium is still occasionally administered for Parkinson's disease.

Sketchy reports of pre-Revolutionary treatments are to be found in lay journals, letters, and family medical books. Colonial medicine lagged behind that of

Europe, but an advertisement in a Virginia newspaper in 1737 (Blanton, 1931) touted the careful compounding of chemical and galenical medicines. In 1764 a slave with epileptic attacks and ensuing complications (Blanton, 1931) was eventually freed of them by a physician who attributed the seizures to the phases of the moon.

In 1771 George Washington, according to his household account, paid 14 pounds of Maryland currency for the treatment of a member of his household who had seizures. The treatment was less than successful since she later died of the ailment. Blanton (1931, p. 212) stated that:

> Patsy Custis, a member of Washington's household, was a victim of epilepsy. Her attacks of fits had baffled the physicians for years. Finally Washington heard of Mr. J. N. O. Johnson, who claimed to cure fits by a receipt all his own. He was summoned to Mount Vernon in August 1771, and the young lady was placed in his care. Though Washington paid the gentleman "14 pounds Maryland currency" for his services, Patsy made no improvement, and she later died in one of her fits.

In 1828 Dr. B. W. Dudley of Lexington, Ky., reported that he had trephined five epileptics to relieve pressure on the brain, resulting in the disappearance of convulsions in all of them (Packard, 1963).

Among other accounts of the treatment of epilepsy by American pioneers is one found in a medical book published in 1815 in Frankfort, Ky., by Dr. Richard Carter. Pickard and Buley, (1945, pp. 65–66) describe a prescription for childhood fits contained in that volume:

> Fits caused by worms in children should be cured by Carolina pinkroot stewed in water and sweetened with honey. Dr. Carter suggested, however, that it was "best to add to each dose about one-eighth of an ounce of manna; the importance of which addition, will appear when it is remarked, that the pink root is poisonous, and if given in too large quantities, kills the child to whom it is given." Alloes, Jesuit bark, bear's foot, table salt, wormwood, garlic, and wormseed made an effective bitters. Calomel either by itself or combined with jalap to the tune of five to thirty grains for the child, gun powder on an empty stomach, red onions "beat fine" and bound to the navel, iron rust in hard cider, or steel filings in honey, all had at different times proved their merits—even once to the extent of destroying a long-standing ten and one-half foot tapeworm of an old sea captain.

Carter's book also stated that disappointment in love affairs often led to epilepsy and that restoration to normal functioning might be accomplished by swallowing the heart of a rattlesnake, sleeping over a cow stable, or being passed three times through the crotch of a forked hickory tree that had been wedged open. Otherwise, the afflicted might prefer to hang one slice of peony root for each year of his age on his right arm and left foot.

E. Maple (1972), writing about Amish superstitions, notes that an epileptic patient could regain health by swallowing the heart of a rattlesnake, an Indian symbol of life and fruitfulness.

CHANGING STATUS OF THE EPILEPTIC IN NINETEENTH-CENTURY EUROPE

By the nineteenth century, the outlook on epilepsy had definitely changed. Superstitious associations with witches, demons, and the phases of the moon were giving way to rational explanations of the disorder. It was slowly recognized that the nervous system of the epileptic differed somehow from that of the normal individual. The problem lay in explaining the difference.

Among the important steps taken early in the century to improve the lot of the epileptic and bring effective treatment closer (Temkin, 1971) was the removal of fetters from confined insane patients and epileptics housed with them. A Frenchman, P. Pinel, and an Englishman, H. Tuke, were largely responsible for providing systematic medical care for such severely afflicted epileptics. In 1815 E. Esquirol (1772–1840) of France established special hospital facilities for confined epileptics. His motive, however, was based on the misapprehension that the insane should not witness epileptic attacks lest they, too, "contagiously" acquire that disorder. "Contagion," in this context, should not be confused with communication of bacterial or virus diseases. Rather, it was used in the ancient Greek sense to suggest that mere contact with an epileptic, or even witnessing an attack, could bring on the disorder in others. Be that as it may, the results of Esquirol's efforts were fruitful. By 1860, special hospitals had been developed for epileptics in England, France, and Germany, and later at Blackwell's Island, New York, for the care of the paralyzed and the epileptic. In 1891 the first institution in the United States, solely for severe epileptics, was established at Gallipolis, Ohio (Temkin, 1971).

Segregation of epileptics facilitated daily study under supervised conditions. In the succeeding decades, there was intensified interest in the classification of attacks based on repeated observations of the same subjects. Better statistics were accumulated, and these aided in improved evaluation of the mental aspects of epilepsy.

FRENCH CLINICAL OBSERVATIONS

Esquirol spoke of severe and slight attacks as *grand* and *petit mal,* counterparts of medieval major and minor epilepsy. L. F. Calmeil (1798–1895) brought into use the term "absence"[12] to distinguish between the passing mental confusions of an epileptic and full-fledged grand mal attacks. *Status epilepticus* also became understood as an uncontrolled series of severe attacks requiring handling as a medical emergency and sometimes presenting a grave prognosis. The meaning of the aura was clarified by the careful studies of W. R. Gowers of London (see Chapter VI). Esquirol found no evidence from pathological anatomy of a seat for epilepsy. Yet J. Wenzel (1768–1808), finding abnormalities in the region of the pituitary gland, concluded that a disease of that gland was a general cause of epilepsy. In the end, this conclusion was rejected also, but a very large number of pathological changes found in the brain were linked, at least temporarily, with nervous disorders. K. F. Burdach (1776–1847), for example, compiled considerable statistical evidence concerning the pathological changes in the brain relating to various conditions, including epilepsy and general convulsions (Temkin, 1971). Of nearly 2,000 abnormalities observed, 476 derived from the epileptic group. Temkin points out, however, that the sources of statistics often were from hospital situations in which care of structural brain disorders had been especially emphasized. An interesting result of the clinical study of individual epileptics was that both somnambulism and mania, sometimes classified as symptoms of mental disorder, could occur as forms of epileptic attack.

SALAAM CONVULSIONS

These belong to a special category of infantile spasms named for their resemblance to the ceremonial low bow of obeisance seen in the Far East. However, they are truly spasms of convulsive origin. First reported in *The Lancet* of London, in 1840 by W. J. West, an English physician, they might have been overlooked as a special category for much longer had they not occurred in Dr. West's own infant son. West published a lucid description of the condition as it develops in early infancy. His child, healthy at birth, continued to thrive until 4 months of age, at which time the father first observed forward head-bobbings. In retrospect, these appeared to be the first indication of the condition. They became so frequent and powerful that they caused the head to bob forward to the knees and snap backwards to the upright position. West consulted Sir Charles Clark and Dr. Charles Locock, both of whom had large practices. Neither had seen more than a few such cases, but Sir Charles described the condition as "salaam convulsions." Of two cases he had followed, one had recovered and the other had died at age 17. Much later, a particular brain wave pattern, designated *hypsarrhythmia* (see Glossary), was linked to the salaam convulsions by F. A. and E. L. Gibbs (1952). Although the prognosis is uncertain, some children recover spontaneously and rapidly without showing residual symptoms or signs.

EPILEPSY AND ELECTRIC FISH

The use of the torpedo (ray) in the treatment of epilepsy has already been mentioned. In this work, it has been selected as a central theme for developing the concept of animal electricity. Notions concerning its mysterious force will be traced from Montaigne, through John Hunter, John Walsh, and Benjamin Franklin of the American Revolutionary period, Carlo Matteucci of Italy, Jan

Marek of France, and, finally, to its importance in developing the neurotransmitter concept of modern electrophysiology.

Among the ideas that developed out of the maturing knowledge of electricity in the early nineteenth century were analogies between the neural processes involved in epilepsy and those that occasioned the discharge of the electric fish. Schroeder van der Kolk (Moore, 1859, p. 215) spoke as follows:

> . . . perhaps, a comparison with the phenomena in electrical fishes is still better, where, likewise, a violent discharge takes place, which requires some time, especially when there is exhaustion, before it can be repeated.

In Schroeder van der Kolk's view, the electrical discharge of the fish came from the medulla oblongata, and he stressed the hindbrain forward of the spinal cord as the seat of epilepsy in man. He sought support for his theory by arranging for that part of the brain of epileptics to be sent to him for post-mortem study. Based on these examinations, he concluded that merely "to produce epilepsy no disorganization is necessary, no great change in the tissue, but only *increased excitability*" (italics supplied).

LOCOCK AND BROMIDE THERAPY

The discovery of the first drug of proved significance in lessening the frequency of epileptic attacks was reported by Sir Charles Locock (1797–1875), a prominent London physician and accoucheur to Queen Victoria. In a discussion of epilepsy read before the Royal Medical and Surgical Society, and published in 1857, Locock stated that he had tested bromides (inorganic salts of bromine) in hysterical and menstrual epilepsies of women, obtaining a cure in all but one of 14 such cases. Following his report, the use of bromides for epilepsy became widespread. Temkin (1971) reports that by the mid-1870s, 2½ tons a year were being used at the National Hospital, Queen Square, London, alone.

It is significant that J. R. Reynolds's 1861 book on epilepsy, although containing a passing reference to the use of bromides, gives no information concerning its efficacy. Yet, a statistically oriented volume, it provides a historical overview of the results of epilepsy treatment just prior to the accepted universal use of bromide as an effective medication.

COMMENT

There is a vast gap between the days when peony and mistletoe were used to treat epilepsy and the introduction of diphenylhydantoin and trimethadione. The time of gathering and, perhaps, the meticulousness of preparation of peony and mistletoe may have added to the confidence of the practitioner, who otherwise blindly followed the medical lore of his ancestors. Today, organic compounds have been developed and largely replaced inorganic ones such as bromide salts. Between the initial organic synthesis of urea by F. Wöhler (1828) and the 1950s, the number of named organic compounds has risen to three-quarters of a million (Hogben, 1970), many of them believed to be specifically useful to man and a significant number potentially useful in the treatment of epilepsy or other medical and psychiatric conditions.

Modern drugs are a by-product of the scientific revolution. Before one is used in the treatment of a patient, it must undergo scrupulous tests for chemical purity, potency as analyzed under rigidly defined experimental conditions, metabolic and toxic studies in animals, and careful trials by competent specialists on groups of selected patients not receiving other medications. Over the last two centuries, much ingenuity and inventiveness has gone into the understanding of the epileptic process and into the search for treatments effective in controlling convulsions for periods of many years and, in some cases, for life. Yet there is a great deal left for ensuing generations to accomplish.

NOTES

[1] *(From Levine, 1971, pp. 34–35):* "Air, combining throughout the body with all the blood, causes the sacred disease (epilepsy). Numerous points of congestion then develop in the veins everywhere. The impeded blood fails to pass or else irregularities are introduced which affect and reduce its free passage. Convulsions result from these irregularities, for the whole body is dragged in all directions; twisting of all kinds develops in every possible way. Throughout the duration of the seizure, those affected are insensible to every external stimulus, they are deaf to what is said, blind to what happens around them, and unaffected by pain. Such is the effect of a disturbance of air on the blood which it pollutes."

[2] *(From Clark et al.,* 1939): Whether the Tennessee goats represent an ancient breed or a comparatively recent mutation is not known. An experience of one of the discoverers suggests the former. In Egypt he observed a herd of goats from a train window. The engineer blew the whistle. Three of the goats fell over on the ground in a spasm which he recognized as due to myotonia.

[3] Harvey was the first to describe correctly the circulation of the blood, from arteries to capillaries to veins.

[4] *(From Siegel, 1968):* The four humors were black bile, yellow bile, phlegm, and blood. They occurred in the Hippocratic writings and were regarded as secretions of the body. Some spoke of observations that supported up to ten of them. When present in abnormal quantities, humors were regarded as the cause of bodily diseases. The concept of four as a mystic number dates from Pythagoras (500 B.C.). Besides four humors, there are also four seasons. Some attribute to Galen the linkage of the humors with constitutional (personality?) types—the phlegmatic, sanguine, choleric, and melancholic.

Epilepsy as due to stagnation of the cold humors within the ventricles of the brain, mostly the humor phlegm but also black bile, can be traced to the Hippocratic writings. From the modern outlook, the humors are presumptive rather than factual and are not treated in any detail in this document. However, the most intelligible account this writer has found relating to Galen's views of the humoral doctrine, of the pneuma and its delivery to the ventricles through the choroid plexuses, and of nerve conduction are to be found in Siegel.

[5] Avicenna (980–1037) was a Persian philosopher and physician. His most famous medical work is *The Canon,* a systematic encyclopedia based on the achievements of Greek physicians of the Roman imperial age. It was studied for centuries in European universities.

[6] The torpedo is also called the electric ray. It has a flattened circular body with a tapering tail, and on contact, can produce a significant shock.

[7] According to Brazeau (1970, page 898), references to ergotism date back to 600 B.C., but written descriptions first appeared during the Middle Ages. Strange epidemics occurred in which the characteristic symptom was gangrene of the feet, legs, hand, and arms, etc. A convulsive type of ergotism was also known. There is still no valid explanation as to why, in certain instances, ergotism is associated with symptoms referable to the central nervous system.

⁸ Where the medieval physician might still have believed in the possibility of miracles, his modern successor may prescribe a placebo instead.

⁹ In the Foreword to *Basic Mechanisms of the Epilepsies,* H. Houston Merritt (1969) offers a similar argument of remote origin. In speaking of the use of mistletoe as antiepileptic therapy, he cites the claim that it was effective because it clung to the tree and did not fall as did the leaves in autumn. Thus, its administration was supposed to prevent the patient from falling down during a seizure.

¹⁰ Vitriol had been used against epilepsy at least since Paracelsus.

¹¹ Marek also founded Charles University's medical school, in which both Procháska and Purkinje were trained.

¹² In modern classifications of epilepsy, the "absence" is likely to be equated with a petit mal attack.

REFERENCES AND BIBLIOGRAPHY

Blanton, W. B. *Medicine in Virginia in the Eighteenth Century.* Richmond, Va.: Garrett and Massie, Inc., 1931. 449 pp.

Brazeau, P. Oxytocin and ergot alkaloids, pp. 893–907. In L. S. Goodman and A. Gilman, eds. *The Pharmacological Basis of Therapeutics,* 4th ed. New York: The Macmillan Co., 1970.

Bullfinch's Mythology, "Druids," pp. 358–366. New York: Thomas Y. Crowell Co., n.d.

Carter, R. *Valuable Vegetable Medical Prescriptions for the Cure of All Nervous and Putrid Disorders.* Frankfort, Ky.: Gerard & Berry, 1815. 187 pp.

Clark, S. L., Luton, F. H., and Cutler, J. T. A form of congenital myotonia in goats. *J. Nerv. Ment. Dis.* 90:297–309, 1939.

Debus, A. G. *The English Paracelsians.* London: Oldbourne, 1965. 222 pp.

Fuller, J. G. *The Day of St. Anthony's Fire.* New York: The Macmillan Co., 1968. 310 pp.

Gibbs, F. A., and Gibbs, E. L. *Atlas of Electroencephalography. Vol. II, Epilepsy.* Cambridge, Mass.: Addison-Wesley Press, Inc., 1952. 422 pp.

Goodman, L. S., and Gilman, A., eds. *The Pharmacological Basis of Therapeutics,* 4th ed. New York: The Macmillan Co., 1970. 1794 pp.

Haggard, H. *The Lame, the Halt, and the Blind.* New York: Harper & Brothers, 1932. 420 pp.

Hodgkin, A. L. The method of signalling in the nervous system, pp. 11–19. In *The Conduction of the Nervous Impulse. (The Sherrington Lectures VII.)* Liverpool University Press, 1964.

Hogben, L. *The Vocabulary of Science.* New York: Stein and Day, 1970. 184 pp.

Leland, C. G. *Etruscan Magic and Occult Remedies.* New York: University Books, 1963. 385 pp.

Lennox, W. G. John of Gaddesden on epilepsy. *Ann. Med. Hist.* 1:283–307, 1939.

Lennox, W. G. Antonius Guainerius on epilepsy. *Ann. Med. Hist.* 2:482–499, 1940.

Lennox, W. G. Bernard of Gordon on epilepsy. *Ann. Med. Hist.* 3:372–383, 1941.

Levine, E. B. *Hippocrates.* New York: Twayne Publishers, Inc., 1971. 172 pp.

Lindeboom, G. A. *Herman Boerhaave; The Man and His Work.* London: Methuen and Co., Ltd., 1968. 452 pp.

Maple, E. *Superstition and the Superstitious.* Cranbury, N. J.: A. S. Barnes and Co., Inc., 1972. 152 pp.

Merritt, H. H. Foreword, pp. VII–VIII. In H. H. Jasper, A. A. Ward, Jr., and A. Pope, eds. *Basic Mechanisms of the Epilepsies.* Boston: Little, Brown and Co., 1969.

Muller, H. J. *The Loom of History.* New York: Harper & Brothers, 1958. 433 pp.

Packard, F. R. The earliest medical schools, pp. 339–488. In *History of Medicine in the United States,* Vol. 1. New York: Hafner Publishing Co., 1963.

Pickard, M. E., and Buley, R. C. *The Midwest Pioneer. His Ills, Cures, & Doctors.* Crawfordsville, Ind.: R. E. Banta, 1945. 339 pp.

Pirkner, E. H. Epilepsy in the light of history. *Ann. Med. Hist.* 1:453–480, 1929.

Reynolds, J. R. *Epilepsy: Its Symptoms, Treatment, and Relation to Other Chronic Convulsive Diseases.* London: John Churchill, 1861. 360 pp.

Rogers, L. The history of craniotomy. An account of the methods which have been practiced and the instruments used for opening the human skull during life. *Ann. Med. Hist.* 2:495–514, 1930.

Schroeder van der Kolk, J. L. C. On the nature and proximate causes of convulsive movements, pp. 215–230. In *Professor Schroeder van der Kolk on the Minute Structure and Functions of the Spinal Cord and Medulla Oblongata, and on the Proximate Cause and Rational Treatment of Epilepsy.* (Trans. by W. D. Moore.) London: The New Sydenham Society, 1859.

Servít, Z. In memory of Jan Marek (Joannes Marcus Marci, 1595–1667) who stood at the origin of Czech epileptology, pp. 5–6. In Z. Servít and R. Black, eds. *Comparative and Cellular Pathophysiology of Epilepsy. Proceedings of a Symposium Held in Liblice Near Prague, Sept. 20–24, 1965.* Excerpta Medica International Congress Series No. 124. Amsterdam: Excerpta Medica Fdn., 1966.

Sherrington, C. *The Endeavour of Jean Fernel.* London: Cambridge University Press, 1946. 223 pp.

Siegel, R. E. *Galen's System of Physiology and Medicine.* Basel: S. Karger, 1968. 419 pp.

Sieveking, E. H. Analysis of fifty-two cases of epilepsy observed by the author. *Lancet* 1:527–528, 1857.

von Storch, E. P., and von Storch, T. J. Arnold of Villanova on epilepsy. *Ann. Med. Hist.* 10:251–260, 1938.

Streeter, E. C. A note on the history of convulsive state prior to Boerhaave. *Assoc. Res. Nerv. Ment. Dis.* 7:5–29, 1922.

Taylor, J., ed. *Selected Writings of John Hughlings Jackson. Vol. I. On Epilepsy and Epileptiform Convulsions,* p. 252. London: Hodder and Stoughton, Ltd., 1931.

Temkin, O. *The Falling Sickness. A History of Epilepsy from the Greeks to the Beginnings of Modern Neurology,* 2d ed. rev. Baltimore: The Johns Hopkins Press, 1971. 467 pp.

Thompson, D. W. *A Glossary of Greek Fishes.* New York: Oxford University Press, 1947. 302 pp.

Underwood, E. A., ed. *Science, Medicine and History,* Vol. 2. London: Oxford University Press, 1953. 646 pp.

Vogel, V. J. *American Indian Medicine.* Norman, Okla.: University of Oklahoma Press, 1970. 583 pp.

West, W. J. On a peculiar form of infantile convulsions. *Lancet* 1:724–725, 1840–1841.

Chapter IV

NEUROANATOMICAL BASIS OF EPILEPSY: THE NEURON DOCTRINE

Necessarily, a book concerning science and epilepsy should have much to say about the brain and its chief appendage, the spinal cord. The left side of the brain controls the right side of the body and vice versa. For example, the left side is the dominant hemisphere in right-handed people and controls speech as well as the dexter hand. The nervous system includes the brain, spinal cord, and cranial and spinal nerves. Knowledge of it is not easy to convey and requires a vivid concept of the detailed relations between brain regions.

Epilepsy, to which this work relates, is widely distributed throughout the animal kingdom; and in science, animal brains are used as experimental models to improve our understanding of the human condition. Thus, it is fortunate that the generalities relating to the human brain are also quite applicable to small brains, such as that of the laboratory rat. The same exterior and interior parts can be identified in each. In the human brain, it is the spatial relations between regions, the expansive and convoluted pattern of the gray cover (cortex) of the cerebrum (large brain), and the large sizes of many internal nerve cell aggregates that are important. However, experimenters can be confident of the close similarities between human and animal brains whose parts have related functions that become increasingly complex as the evolutionary scale of animals is ascended.

However simple or complex the animal, its individual nerve cells—hereafter called neurons—look and behave alike. Each neuron has a body or *soma* with several receiving antennae called *dendrites* (from the Greek for "branches," as of a tree), and a single hair-thin *axon,* which conveys signals, electrical in nature, for varying—sometimes quite long—distances from the soma of origin. Thus, each neuron has both a receiving and a sending apparatus. The soma-initiated signals are conveyed along the axon at maximal rates scarcely exceeding 100 meters a second, about 10 times the speed at which an athlete runs the 100-meter dash. Messages traversing axons are phrased in a code that derives meaning from the variable spacings that separate the successive signals. Near their terminals axons arborize, as do dendrites, becoming increasingly slender as they subdivide. Axonal end-arborizations are called *telodendria* (from the Greek *telos,* "end"). The ultimate twigs form microscopic endbulbs, which make point membrane contacts with dendrites, called *synapses,* but do not fuse with dendrite surfaces. There is only one-way conduction between endbulb and dendrite, and, since the synapse traverse is ordinarily mediated chemically, there is a brief delay at the crossing amounting to half a thousandth of a second. Axons carry exclusively excitatory or inhibitory signals, no other. Thus, the effect of a coded message upon the recipient neuron must also be excitatory or inhibitory.

Some simple animalcules function neurologically through the use of a few neurons each. Complex organisms, on the other hand, require untold numbers of them, an important aspect of the brain's complexity. The number of neurons and the much larger number of synapses that are involved in human nervous activities can truly be classed among the imponderables. In arithmetic, the number 100 requires two zeros; a billion requires nine zeros. Warren Weaver (1967), in his nontechnical writings, calls anything larger than a billion a "zillion," and it is perhaps correct to say that the human nervous system contains zillions of neurons and many more zillions of synapses.

The human brain, and that of all other vertebrates as well, is made up of gray and white matter. The gray contains somata, dendrites, and the origins and terminations of axons; white matter is made up of many bundles of axons forming tracts and commissures. Often we refer to gray matter as composed of *neuron somata* and of *neuropil.* When used, the latter includes dendrites, axonal arbors, and the synaptic endbulbs, which together form a stratum filling the interstices between neuron somata. According to a rule formulated by the famed nineteenth-century neuroanatomist, R. A. Koelliker (ca. 1850), there are no axons that do not arise from neuron somata. Stated otherwise, each and every axon has a soma somewhere to which it belongs, and the endbulbs strung along its telodendria synapse with dendrites of other neurons. Further details amplifying these aspects of nervous structure will be provided in later chapters.

The neurons of simple marine organisms may be few in number, and sufficiently separated by the simple skein of axons in which they are contained to permit simultaneous recording of their electrical activities without interference by the cross-talk of other neurons. In some organisms—medusae, for example—the primitive nervous system operates through a chain of self-reexcitation. In higher invertebrates—such as the lobster—master and slave units are conjoined in predetermined working combinations (Davis and Kennedy, 1972). Among the lower forms of life, there are as many alternative arrangements as there are kinds of organisms.

In comparison, the brains of larger animals are much more compact. Their neuron somata are ordinarily too close together to record effectively from several units at a time, although computer technology may some day make such studies feasible. We do know, however, that neurons never act in isolation and that in usual behavior their linkages are complex. Yet these connections are highly flexible. Widely scattered nerve cells may be joined in action temporarily, maintaining contact through their axons. Then such an action group may disassemble, being replaced by another. Fluidity in connections is the rule. It can be presumed that a field of neighboring neurons join together in producing the brain's spontaneous rhythm, which is more characteristic of passive idling than of active functioning. Neurons drop out of the idling pattern temporarily to combine into effective working groups, returning to it later to be replaced by others.

GROSS STRUCTURE OF THE HUMAN BRAIN

Why does anatomy have relevance to epilepsy? Without an adequate knowledge of brain structure, the attempt to understand the epileptic process is a hopeless one. Early in anatomical history, when preservation of the human body was barely understood and only a few days could be allotted to a dissection, the brain and cranial nerves were ordinarily the last parts to be studied. As a result, detailed knowledge of the brain lagged behind the rest of the anatomy by a century or more. Of course, the shape of the brain and the gross relations between its parts were established during the early period of dissection. However, detailed analysis required a technology that permitted microscopic study. Invariably, the course of biological discovery proceeds from gross to fine structure.

Figure 6 illustrates left and right brain halves, drawn respectively from outer and inner surfaces. The top illustration depicts the outer surface of the left cerebral hemisphere with the convolutions labeled in the latinized terminology. Other important features are the central (Rolandic) sulcus that separates frontal from parietal lobes and the Sylvian fissure, which divides frontal and parietal lobes above from the temporal lobe below. The occipital lobe froms the posterior end of the hemisphere, seen at the far right of the drawing. The bottom illustration shows the right half of the brain drawn from the perspective of the mid-plane of the body. Besides the convolutions of the cerebral hemisphere, it reveals the centrally situated cut surfaces of the white matter commissures—corpus callosum, etc.—which connect left and right cerebral halves. The brainstem lies below and behind, and the cerebellum is wedged between the upper surface of the brainstem and the cerebral occipital lobe. Figure 7 depicts the under surface of the brain with the hemispheres separated anteriorly by the interhemispheric cleft. The brainstem extends backward and is divisible into midbrain, pons, and medulla oblongata, or, alternatively, into mid- and hindbrain. In this basal view, the bilateral symmetry of the brain is clearly illustrated.

Covering the brain is a tough protective membrane called *dura mater,* which also covers the brain's chief appendage—the spinal cord. The cranial dura consists of inner and outer layers—the outer layer also lining the inside of the cranium and the inner layer producing inwardly directed extensions that largely separate the cerebral hemispheres from each other and the cerebrum from the cerebellum. Short dural sleeves also extend outwards, enclosing the beginnings of each of the cranial and spinal nerves.

Within the protective dural coat, and separated from it by a space, is a *pia-arachnoid* membrane of delicate texture. The inner pial component covers the brain surface like a close-fitting glove, delving into the sulci that separate the convolutions of the cerebral surface. Numerous blood vessels in the pia supply nutrients to the brain substance. The arachnoid bridges the sulci. It is attached loosely to the pia by connecting tongues of similar tissue.

The pia delves into the deep transverse fissure of the brain that separates the under surface of the cerebral hemispheres from the upper brainstem. Its borders make up the choroid plexuses of the chief cerebral ventricles illustrated in Fig. 1. The cerebral ventricles form a series of cavities within the brain. The ancients believed them to be air-filled and to be the seat of epilepsy and also of the soul (see Chapter III). To the ancients, the *anterior* parts included two lateral ventricles of tripartite shape, one within each hemisphere. These ventricles communi-

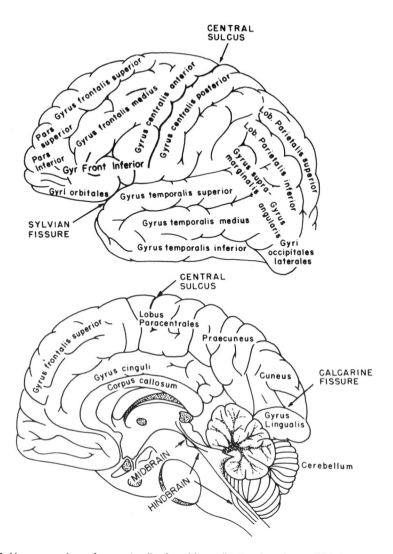

FIG. 6. Human cerebrum from outer **(top)** and inner **(bottom)** surfaces. With few exceptions, labels are in the latinized nomenclature. The exceptions include central sulcus and Sylvian fissure on the outer surface, and the midbrain and hindbrain on the inner surface. (From the author's collection.)

cate with a slit-like third ventricle situated in the midline, which, in turn, communicates via a short cerebral aqueduct with the *posterior* (fourth) ventricle, a lozenge-shaped space lying between cerebellum and brainstem. For our purposes, it is unnecessary to modernize this description, since the ventricles no longer have direct importance in understanding the mechanism of epilepsy.

The central nervous system, which includes both brain and spinal cord, connects with other parts of the body, especially muscles and sense organs, by roots

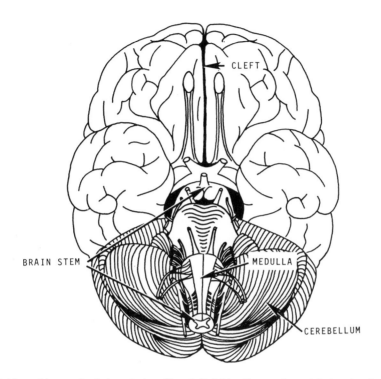

Fig. 7. View of human brain from below. The cleft divides the cerebrum into two hemispheres. (From the author's collection.)

and nerves. There are 12 cranial and 31 pairs of spinal nerves that will receive attention in this book, but which do not require detailed description. It is sufficient to say that several of the cranial nerves supply the major special sense organs of the cranium; others, special muscle groups of the head. Each of the spinal nerves connects to the spinal cord by a pair of roots, one sensory, the other motor. These are made up of axons, which, as in all other instances, derive from neuron somata.

The only simplistic approach science affords to the understanding of nervous system organization lies in tracing the steps in early embryonic development of the essentially tubular brain and spinal cord. From the moment of fertilization, specification of the future brain and cord exist in the deoxyribonucleic acid (DNA) script contained in the fertilized ovum. As it unrolls, the script provides increasing detail as development proceeds. The early cell divisions—after which there are many succeeding ones—are chiefly concerned with providing the scaffold that ensures the early embryo's survival. This includes the staking out of an oval protrusion or raised disc on which embryonic development proceeds.

Early disc cells commence to differentiate into four basic tissues—*nervous, epithelial, muscular,* and *skeletal.* The nervous system makes its first appearance as a pair of protrusions that face each other at the site on the embryonic disc that is to become the juncture of future brain and spinal cord. As the cellular divisions succeed each other—interrupted by quiet intervals devoted to cell specializations—these protrusions grow forward and backward, transforming neuraxial beginnings first into a groove and then into a tubular structure. The latter develops as a result of submergence of the embryonic nervous system beneath an enveloping layer of surface epithelial cells, which later takes in nearly all of the fully formed embryo. The growth forward from the beginning point of the embryonic neural tube proceeds rapidly in comparison to the rate of backward growth. Forward, the tube expands into the future brain; backward, it transforms into the cylindrical spinal cord. The brain part contains a continuous cavity. Through unevenness in the growth rate of its walls, the brain balloons into three primary swellings—the *forebrain, midbrain,* and *hindbrain,* respectively (Fig. 8). The hindbrain is transitional to the spinal cord.

Between the third and seventh weeks, unequal growth also establishes three flexures in the walls of the cephalic end of the tube. The first to appear is a *cephalic* one that bends the forebrain at right angles to the hindbrain. The next is the *cervical* flexure, which corresponds to the head-bend of the embryo and occurs at the transition between brainstem and spinal cord. Finally, the pontine flexure arises through a bending forward of the floor of the embryonic hindbrain, the roof remaining unaffected in the process. The last to take shape, it forms about the seventh week of fetal life.

Local thickenings and expansions in the walls of the several vesicles that now

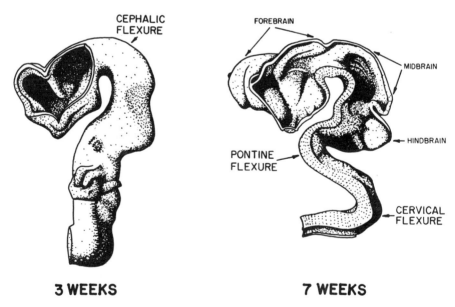

3 WEEKS   **7 WEEKS**

Fig. 8. Brain regions of nervous system of 3- and 7-week human embryos. Cephalic flexure indicated on 3-week embryo; pontine and cervical flexures, and forebrain, midbrain, and hindbrain regions on 7-week embryo. (Gray, 1973. From model by His.)

constitute the brain account for further subdivisions into the parts that produce the definitive structures of the adult brain. The forebrain, which includes the derivatives of the most forward brain vesicle, divides into the *telencephalon* and the *diencephalon*. From the former, cerebral cortex develops and from the latter, the thalamus, sensory way station to the cerebral cortex. The middle of the three vesicles (midbrain) remains undivided. The hindbrain differentiates into pons, medulla, and cerebellum.

During early development, the tubular brain and cord is of microscopic size and its parts are proportionately tiny in both their transverse and longitudinal dimensions. Growth proceeds apace with development, but the distances are still short at the time when axons commence to sprout and grow forward and backward from neuroblasts (immature neurons) situated in cord and brain. Many crossing axons pass through the cerebral commissures; other axons reach the cerebellum along its incoming paths, or extend from cerebellum to brainstem along outgoing ones. This process raises one of many puzzles of nervous organization: What directs the axonal outgrowth of a neuron to its destination? The same dilemma occurs regarding the axons of spinal motoneurons, which must reach the muscles they innervate, and the sensory axons, which invade the spinal cord along its roots. It goes without saying that once connections are established, the axons grow longer as the body and the contained nervous system lengthen until full growth is attained. Partial answers to these questions will be provided in later sections of this volume.

THE EARLY HISTORY OF ANATOMY

Efforts to understand anatomy are probably as old as man's curiosity about himself. But, as in so many other fields of knowledge, the first records of its study, as well as of epilepsy, are of Greek origin. The purposeful investigation of anatomy is said to have begun with Alcmaeon about 500 B.C., during Greece's "Golden Age." No one knows, however, whether the bodies of humans or animals were then dissected. A school of human dissection did exist in Alexandria under Ptolemy III during the third century B.C. (Rasmussen, 1947). Galen, who lived in the second century A.D., learned the structure of the brain by dissecting the heads of farm animals, although he is known to have worked extensively on apes as well. His experience with the more accessible parts of the human body could have been gained in his native Pergamum, where he was a physician to the gladiators, who were wounded frequently by lethal weapons. Later, the Jews may have dissected the human body. After the decline of Greek culture, most anatomical knowledge was available only in Arabic translations of the original Greek works.

With the help of these, anatomy had become a recognized specialty in Italy by the fourteenth century. In Bologna, Mondino (1275?–1326) brought the systematic teaching of human anatomy into the medical curriculum. His first public dissection, which included removal of the brain, was performed in 1315. A century after Mondino, the University of Bologna authorized the annual dissection of a male and a female cadaver. This practice of yearly dissections was imitated elsewhere, and knowledge of anatomy became a prerequisite to the practice of medicine.

From observations of dissections carried out by skilled professionals and from supplemental reading of treatises, students advanced to work on their own. They were not all physicians-to-be. Copernicus studied anatomy at Padua, and artists in Florence maintained an active dissection center. Leonardo da Vinci (1452–1519), perhaps the most versatile and inquisitive investigator of any age, claimed to have dissected more than 100 bodies. To be accorded scholarly fame, an anatomist had to be more than a skillful dissector. For example, Vesalius (1515–1564), who rectified many errors of Galen, wrote a textbook, profusely illustrated by a distinguished artist, that marked the beginning of the modern era of human anatomy. Then, as now, publication was recognized as essential to the progress of science.

The configuration of the brain and the relationship between brain parts eventually became superficially familiar, but the technologies available did not permit rapid progress. More detailed knowledge required a transition from the techniques of gross dissection to those of microscopic analysis, the development of methods for resolving neuron interrelationships, and, finally, the formulation and establishment of the neuron doctrine. Progress proceeded slowly until the end of the eighteenth century. Thereafter, thanks to remarkable technological discoveries, important developments emerged in rapid succession.

TRANSITION FROM GROSS TO MICROSCOPIC ANALYSIS

The cerebrum is composed of gray and white matter. Gray matter, as indicated previously, consists of neurons and neuropil. The neurons, occurring in aggregates of varying size, are enmeshed in their own arborizing dendrites, which contribute in a major way to the content of neuropil. Neuropil also contains the brush-like terminals (telodendria) through which incoming axons arborize. The endbulbs lie in close contact with the somata and dendrites of neurons. Cell aggregates may be spherical, wedge-shaped, elongated, or layered, the cortex of the cerebrum being an example of the latter.

White matter, although it appears homogeneous, consists almost exclusively of closely packed axon bundles, each having an insulating sheath of fatty material that gives to the white matter as a whole its glistening appearance. The axon bundles are of variable size, and can be separated by zealous dissection. To the naked eye, the margins of white and gray matter often appear sharp. Actually, microscopic survey of the entire nervous system reveals many gradations of infiltration of one by the other.

In the early days of medicine, the hardening of a brain, accomplished by immersing it in spirits of wine (an impure alcohol), was found to facilitate dissection. The next important innovation in dissection, leading toward fine structure analysis, was the placing of the alcohol-treated brain in a solution of sodium or potassium carbonate. These alkalis softened the components of gray matter, whereas the alcoholic spirits toughened the axons of white matter, making them resistant to breakage. Such procedures facilitated delicate work with needles to show how axons leave the cerebral cortex to converge into tracts in the upper brainstem and ultimately pass into the spinal cord. Also, certain large masses of gray matter that lie at the center of the cerebral hemispheres—called subcortical gray[1]—could be outlined by contour dissection.

The use of potassium dichromate for the fixing and hardening of the brain for dissection was introduced by J. E. Purkinje (1787–1869), a Bohemian physiologist esteemed by all neuroscientists. In France, dissection of the interior of the hardened brain was brought to its peak by A. L. Foville (1799–1878), L. P. Gratiolet (1815–1865), and J. B. Luys (1828–1897) (Rasmussen, 1947). Their meticulous handiwork did much to delineate the principal axon bundles that crisscross the interior of the cerebral hemispheres and relate cortical gray matter to that of the forward brainstem.

TECHNOLOGICAL DEVELOPMENTS AIDING FINE STRUCTURE ANALYSIS

Between 1590 and 1610, the compound microscope was developed almost simultaneously by Z. Jannsen of Holland and Galileo Galilei of Italy. However, it required considerable improvement before becoming useful in fine structure analysis. No one knows for certain who saw the first neuron, or what equipment he used.

Anthony van Leeuwenhoek (1632–1733) was known as a "globulist" (Meyer, 1971) because he reported small globules, the size of a red blood corpuscle or less, in the cortex of a turkey brain. M. Malpighi (1628–1694) described cortical "glands," which also had a globular appearance (Meyer, 1971, p. 156). Were any of these actually neurons? Van Leeuwenhoek could have seen axons within the "nerve fibers" he is reported to have studied. Apart from such precocious efforts, early microscopy was done with simple magnifying lenses, which were used to examine tissues treated with macerating agents. Small bits were compressed between transparent plates and examined by transmitted light. It took more than 200 years before pursuit of the intricate details of the human brain, visible with the aid of a light microscope, became feasible.

The first major problem in advancing light microscopy of the nervous system was to cut sections of tissue thin enough to see through. Botanists used microtomes for cutting thin sections as early as 1770, long before animal histologists. (Histologist, a general word that was coined in 1819, refers to any student of fine structure analysis, plant or animal.) Prior to 1846, B. Stilling (1810–1879) had used a razor to cut serial sections of the spinal cord and brainstem. Study of such sections, hardened in spirits of wine, permitted the publication of a detailed human brainstem atlas. Further progress, however, was necessary, since only large, densely populated cell aggregates could be identified in thick sections of unstained tissue. Staining came next.

Although van Leeuwenhoek stained animal tissues in 1714, botanists were for a time at the forefront of tissue technology; for example, they were pioneers in the use of carmine for staining plant cells. Adequate "killing" of tissues prior to staining also was important. Instead of spirits of wine, alcohol was first used by J. C. Reil (1759–1813), chromic acid by A. Hannover (1814–1894), and formaldehyde by F. Blum (in 1893).

Embedding tissues before cutting allowed sections to be cut thinner and made the stained product more transparent by transmitted light microscopy. E. Klebs (1834–1913) initiated the use of paraffin for embedding, but this process required overcoming the lack of miscibility between alcohol and paraffin. Clearing oils, which further enhanced transparency, were introduced as an intermediary. Celloidin embedding, originated by M. M. Dubal (1844–1915) in 1879, became widely used for brain sectioning because it provided good, transparent sections of quite large tissue blocks and allowed flexibility in cutting either thin or thick sections. Even before that time, Purkinje introduced the use of balsam to preserve tissue—after it had been stained, dehydrated, and cleared with oil—permanently between a glass slide and a thin glass coverslip.

Cutting thin sections of embedded material required the use of the microtome. A succession of such "cutting engines" were developed between 1770 and 1800. Basic to the design of each was a sharp knife of hard steel set at a variable angle, a rigid knife holder, and a means for advancing the tissue block by hundredths of an inch. In 1839 G. G. Valentin (1810–1883), a pupil of Purkinje, developed a double-bladed knife that permitted blade separation according to the thickness of the sections to be cut. Even before this, Purkinje had developed a true microtome, comparable in mechanical perfection to those in use for light microscopy today. By 1875, a microtome had been produced for B. A. Gudden (1824–1886) that would cut large, thin sections of brainstem. At about the same time, freezing microtomes also came into use, and an enlarged model for brain studies was built in 1888 for A. Bruce of England.

Further refinement had to be achieved before the compound microscope became truly useful in light microscopy of neurons. That advance came as the result of technological developments, about 1830. It permitted clear resolution of histological detail at magnifications of 200 to 300 times, due to the elimination of chromatic aberration from microscope lenses. The result was an achromatic microscope (Meyer, 1971).

S. G. Ehrenberg (1795–1876) is credited with the first undoubted observations of neurons, made in 1833. G. G. Valentin, working in Purkinje's laboratory, defined the neuron nucleus in 1836 and Purkinje (see Fig. 9) himself won immortality[2] by discovering neurons of cerebellar cortex in 1837. In the following years, he and Valentin characterized the cell lining of the ventricles, an important discovery in itself because all neurons differentiate embryonically and migrate to their permanent positions from the lining membrane of those cavities. At about

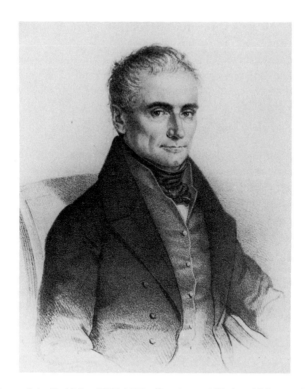

FIG. 9. Jan Evangelista Purkinje, 1787–1869. (Courtesy of National Library of Medicine, Bethesda, Md.)

the same time, the revolutionary general cell theory was being enunciated by Theodor Schwann (1810–1882). It contributed an immense momentum to the pursuit of fine structure analysis of all tissues and was the forerunner of H. W. Waldeyer's special neuron theory of 1891. Figure 10 shows drawings of neurons made by Purkinje in 1837.

The discovery of the axon evidently occurred separately from that of the neuron soma, although there were many overlaps among the workers involved. The neuron and the axon concepts were brought together at a later date. R. Remak (1815–1865) described axons in the gray rami of the autonomic nervous system in 1837. This was a remarkable feat of scientific observation, since at that time light microscopy resolution was restricted to 200 to 300 magnification, and the axons in question are among the smallest of the nervous system. It is true that he could have been preceded in seeing axons by van Leeuwenhoek, but the axons the latter is presumed to have studied were significantly larger. Remak also may have grasped the continuity between neuron somata and axons in studies of the spinal cord.

About that time, Schwann also identified a periaxial region (around or about the axon) within nerve fibers and concluded that the outside zone contained a

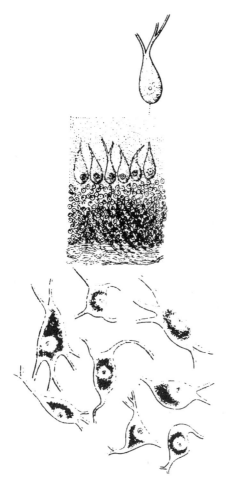

Fig. 10. Purkinje's 1837 drawing of nerve cells which antedated the cell theory (1838) of Schwann. Above, Purkinje and granule cells of cerebellar cortex. Below, ganglionic cells of the substantia nigra. Courtesy of M. A. B. Brazier, University of California, Los Angeles. (From Liddell, 1960.)

white, fat-like substance. This is known as the *myelin sheath,* which surrounds most axons of the central nervous system. It is myelin that gives white matter its glistening appearance and provides electrical insulation for the axons. A. Hannover clearly demonstrated that axons arise from neurons of the cerebrum and cerebellum. Others became aware of neurofibrillae—fibrils within axons —and M. Schultz (1825–1874) verified their existence in fresh, living giant cells of the torpedo (the electric fish) isolated in serum. In 1842 H. L. F. Helmholtz (see Chapter V) also reported the origin of axons from neurons in invertebrates.

R. A. Koelliker (1817–1905)[3] likewise saw axons emerging from neuron somata of the dorsal root ganglia and central nervous system (Meyer, 1971, p. 166). By 1850, Koelliker had propounded one of those relatively rare and highly important unifying generalizations of scientific research mentioned previously: *That there are no axons not connected with nerve cells.* Fridtjof Nansen (1861–1930), the Norwegian who later became a famed Arctic explorer, demonstrated in 1887 that the axons arising from neurons of the dorsal root ganglia divide within the spinal cord. He used the Golgi method (see page 51) and Koelliker's commendatory mention of Nansen's work helped call the attention of European scientists to the importance of the technical staining discovery of an obscure Italian scientist, Camillo Golgi (1843–1926).[4] In the hands of Santiago Ramón y Cajal (1852–1934), Golgi's method of staining was to contribute enormously to the understanding of the fine structure of the nervous system.

The anatomical difference between two classes of axons, those with and those without surrounding myelin, were by midcentury becoming clear. A. Meyer (1971) makes the quite valid point that by 1845 Koelliker had already anticipated the neuron doctrine, the crux of which was discontinuity at the synapse. If, instead, continuous, how could signals be contained within a circuit or chain without spreading chaos through neighboring chains? With all the evidence that has since accumulated, including that obtained by electron microscopy, indicating that there is discontinuity, the neuron doctrine still stands unrefuted. Because of its relevance to events leading to the neuron doctrine, O. F. K. Deiters' (1834–1863) thesis on neurons, published posthumously in 1865, requires mention (Fig. 11A). He distinguished the various processes emerging from neuron somata—the protoplasmic (i.e., dendrites), which are a branched part of the soma, and the axon, which takes on a myelin sheath a short distance away from the soma. But, he mistakenly thought that some neurons had several lesser axons as well, arising in a multiple manner from soma or dendrites. As noted by L. Barker (1899), he was not really observing axon *origins,* but instead detached fragments of the telodendria of synapsing axons, which, broken off during the processing of the tissue, adhered to dendrites. That mistake was encountered many times thereafter.

The coloring of gray and white matter by dyes markedly improved the resolution of detail. By accident, J. Gerlach (1820–1896) developed what was to become one of the most widely used early staining techniques for the nervous system. He tried a solution of ammoniacal carmine, used for quick staining by plant histologists, but found that it stained nervous tissue deeply and nondifferentially. By chance, he left some sections overnight in a much diluted solution. In those, Gerlack obtained excellent differentiation between the components of gray and white matter. In 1884 C. Weigert (1845–1904) originated a complementary method for staining the sheaths of myelinated axons in the central nervous system. Used with the Gerlach carmine method as a counterstain, it gave excellent results, coloring both gray and white substance. The combined method provided the first convincing evidence that the sheathed axons of white matter are in fact prolongation of the neurons of gray matter. For routine studies, the combined method rapidly became the most useful of the period.

In assuming that axons were extensions of the cell body of neuron, V. Hensen (1835–1924) in 1876 found it embryologically unbelievable that axon sprouts could grow away from the cell body to reach the periphery with no preexisting trace to lead them to their endings. As a result, he formulated his protoplasmic

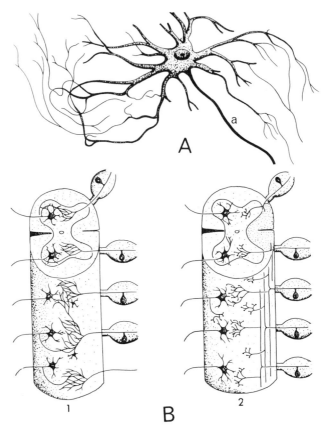

Fig. 11. A: Deiters (1865) identification of a neuron with its emerging axon (a). **B-1:** Golgi's concept of the continuous nerve net, spinal cord. Note that recurrent collaterals of motoneuron axons merge into arborizations of sensory axons entering over the dorsal roots (Golgi, 1873). **B-2:** Ramón y Cajal's concept of sensorimotor relations within the spinal cord. Note the *discontinuities* that exist between sensory terminals and motoneurons. (Ramón y Cajal, 1937.)

bridge theory that a chain of cells was laid down that later became interconnected to form a continuous axon, the cell nuclei disappearing in the process (Fig. 12). Such embryological considerations gave rise to the spurious notion that regeneration of severed nerves in animal experiments and human case material could be accomplished through similar cellular chains that grow together to replace severed axons of the central stump. This was in sharp contrast (Fig. 13) to the evidence developed later by Ramón y Cajal.

NEUROHISTOLOGICAL METHODS USED IN EXPERIMENTAL STUDIES

In the 1880s neurohistologists had commenced to follow axons from origins within the nervous system to destinations without. Their work had much earlier

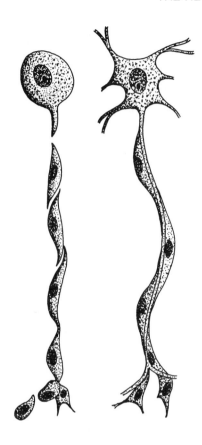

FIG. 12. Hensen's theory of protoplasmic bridges laid down as separate neuroblasts connecting immature neuroblast in centers with periphery **(left)**. Mature neuron in which bridges are fused to form a continuous axon **(right)**. [Redrawn from Ramón y Cajal's *Recollections* (1937).]

beginnings in studies of severed nerves dating back to F. C. F. Fontana (1730–1805). He had failed to find evidence for reunion of central and distal nerve stumps until he studied under J. Cruikshank (1745–1800) in 1778. The latter had reported the healing of cut human nerves while working with Monro (Secundus) (1733–1817) on nerve healing. Evidently, Fontana had both successes and failures, but he believed he could see axons bridging the tissue gaps of severed nerves. H. Nasse (1807–1892) also studied degeneration in the central and distal stumps of severed nerves of both cold- and warm-blooded animals, noting the phenomenon of degeneration of previously intact axons and their myelin sheaths, which was proved later to be a prerequisite of axon regeneration.

A. V. Waller (1816–1870) of England conducted a detailed study of degeneration within portions of nerves severed from their axons of origin, and described the degenerative process observed by Nasse in some detail. This process was thereafter named *Wallerian* degeneration in his honor. He concluded that fragmentation beyond the cut arose as a result of axons having lost their nutrient centers in the neuron somata to which each belonged. This surmise is supported by recently developed positive evidence of transport of nutrients along axons from

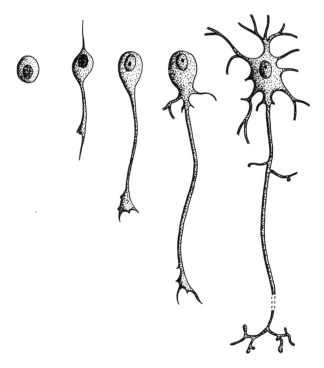

Fig. 13. Ramón y Cajal's view of an axon arising as a continuous outgrowth of a single neuro-blast. Immature ependymal cell **(left)**, and stages intervening between it **(middle)**, and a mature neuron with dendrites and terminal axonal telodendria **(right)**. (From Ramón y Cajal, 1937.)

the somata outwards, using a radioactive amino acid to tag the neurons of origin (see Chapter XII).

Ramón y Cajal, who was born more than a century after Fontana, showed that a segment of nerve severed from the somata in which its axons originated could be reestablished through axon sprouts growing outwards across the scar from the stumps of divided axons. Out of such sprouts arise hair-thin prolongations that follow the course of the severed nerves to the original termini. The rate of axon growth has been measured to be one-ninth to one-twelfth of an inch per day.

Simultaneously, neurohistologists were beginning to follow central axon paths through the white matter of brain and spinal cord from origin to telodendrial destination. Following experimental interruption of a tract composed of many such bundles, the axons degenerate when severed from their neuron somata just as is the case in peripheral nerves. A stain was devised to differentiate traces of degenerating myelin sheaths, which could be followed from the site of severance to the tract terminus. This was done in 1885 by V. Marchi (1851–1908). It permitted much more exacting deductions concerning the origin, course, and site of termination of central tracts. The use of osmic acid (osmium tetroxide) was basic to the Marchi method. Osmic acid ordinarily stains normal as well as degenerated myelin. But after the use of certain suppressor agents, normal myelin no longer stains, leaving only the trace of degenerating axons crossing the microscopic field.

In 1954, after nearly 80 years of use, the Marchi method was replaced by one based on a reduced silver method developed by Nauta and Gygax. It also uses suppressor agents to prevent the staining of normal axons intermixed with the degenerating ones. Another means of following degenerating tracts is to apply the Weigert method referred to previously. Areas that have lost many myelinated axons no longer stain, and a degenerating tract can be followed by the negative image it leaves in sections cut at successive levels of the brain and spinal cord. However large the brain and elongated the spinal cord, these methods give valuable results. They work in animals as different in size as mouse and man.

Another method of following bundles of nerve fibers through the nervous system was developed by P. F. Flechsig (1837–1929). He worked with miscarried fetuses obtained at different stages of gestation, and found that the myelination in different systems of the brain and cord occur at different times in fetal life. The results of applying such a method, compared with those obtained by the Marchi and Nauta degeneration methods, are that additional information about the courses of the various tracts is obtained.

B. A. Gudden (1820–1896), remembered because he lost his life attempting to rescue Ludwig, the Mad King of Bavaria, from drowning, has not been accorded due honor for his contributions to the knowledge of the brain. Studying the chain-link successions of neuronal organization, he found he was able to produce destruction of the entire chain composed of several synaptic links by disabling the most accessible one. This manner of following central paths inward through the nerve centers is called *transneuronal degeneration* and has recently been verified anew (see Chapter XII).

WHOLE NEURON STAINING

In 1871 Camillo Golgi, then an obscure worker in Pavia, Italy, made one of the most important contributions to the history of neurology by using a silver chromate precipitate to selectively encrust neuron somata, dendrites, and axons. Recently, electron microscopy has been used to show how the growth of opaque silver chromate crystalline deposits take the shape of a neuron and its processes by adhering to the membranes. For reasons that remain unknown, the process is a very selective one, and only a few neurons among thousands appear fully clothed with silver chromate against the pale background of their neighbors. Perhaps because he published at first in obscure Italian journals, Golgi's contribution lay neglected for 16 years until Koelliker's commentary on Nansen brought it to the attention of European workers. Meanwhile, an account of the results had also appeared in the American publication, *Alienist and Neurologist,* which regularly carried translations of studies published in European journals (Golgi, 1883).

By coincidence, Santiago Ramón y Cajal was invited to Madrid at the time of Koelliker's commentary as a judge of examinations. He heard there of the encrustation technique and saw Golgi preparations. As a result, between 1890 and 1900, a new vista opened for him. During that time, using the Golgi technique, he widely and systematically explored the nervous systems of man and animal (Ramón y Cajal, 1937). Golgi, of course, had continued his own work. He espoused the continuous net hypothesis of neural connection (to be discussed later) and engaged in extensive polemics with Ramón y Cajal. Golgi's neural studies were especially related to the spinal cord, cerebellum, hippocampus, and olfactory system. He also discovered the tendon receptors of muscle, recognized later by C. S. Sherrington (1857–1952) for their role in the mechanism of reflex action. Golgi was also first to observe the system of canals within nerve cells, later to be known to electron microscopists as *smooth endoplasmic reticulum* (see Chapter XII).

Ramón y Cajal improved the Golgi method by recycling the tissue through a second (or third) sequence of the orthodox osmic acid-potassium bichromate mixture, thus in later sequences adding to the precipitate adhering to somata, dendrites, and axons. Ultimately he was able to demonstrate, to the satisfaction of most investigators, that axons invariably make free (synaptic) contacts with somata and dendrites. In 10 short years, he revolutionized our understanding of the nervous system, making available a wealth of information about the cellular architecture of many parts of the brain. Frequently, he supplemented his animal studies with human material obtained at autopsies. For both, he paid special attention to the perinatal stage of development when myelin is just being laid down about immature axons and the dendritic branching is just reaching completeness. Beyond his mammalian studies, he investigated intensively the brain of the bee. If the human brain is likened to a clock in a watchtower, said Cajal, that of the bee is composed with the delicacy of a fine wristwatch.

To the Golgi methods, Ramón y Cajal added other silver plating techniques that he devised himself (Ramón y Cajal, 1937). He subjected tissues to silver-reducing solutions comparable to those used in the processing of photographic plates. He was an excellent photographer, a skill that not only helped him with chemistry but also enhanced his artistic ability. Often, after retiring to bed with a drawing pad on his lap, pen in hand and a bottle of ink at his side, he sketched observations he had made during the day. Among his most eminent pupils were his brother Pedro, Pio del Rio-Hortega (1882–1945), who exposed the detail of neuroglial tissue just as Ramón y Cajal had done for neurons, and Lorente de Nó, who analyzed the architectonics of the auditory and vestibular systems and the hippocampal formation of the temporal lobe. Figure 14 shows Ramón y Cajal in his laboratory.

Finally, Ramón y Cajal developed a method complementary to that of Golgi. His method, which he used effectively but not as extensively as he did Golgi's, stemmed from ideas conceived by the German genius of pharmacology and immunology, Paul Ehrlich (1854–1915). It involved staining living nerve cells

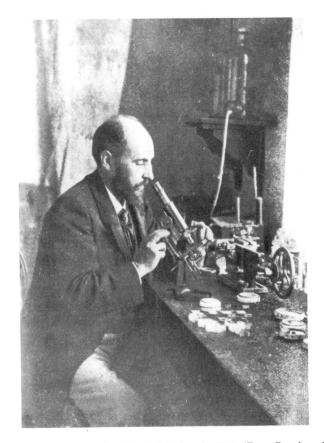

FIG. 14. Santiago Ramón y Cajal (1852–1934). Taken in 1918. (From Ramón y Cajal, 1937.)

by administering dyes. Ehrlich found, for example, that methylene blue, dissolved in saline and injected into living animals, stained many neurons, axons, and axon terminals. The method was also used extensively by A. Bethe, I. Lavdowsky, and G. Retzius.

RETICULARISTS VERSUS ANTIRETICULARISTS

J. Gerlach, who discovered the utility of dilute ammoniacal carmine in the study of nervous substrate, an undoubtedly important contribution, was also the founder of the neuron continuity (nerve net) hypothesis and the originator of the word *neuropil.* The latter term later became widely used by comparative neurologists of the early twentieth century in describing the axodendritic articulations between neurons of lower vertebrates, and by electron microscopists of the latter half in defining the fine structure characteristics of axodendritic synapsing elements (see Chapter XII).

At about the same time he developed the carmine method, Gerlach developed a gold salt method that stained the neuron's dendritic arbors to their finest branchlets. He believed the latter formed a rameous net within the spinal gray matter that extended the length of the spinal cord. He saw axons passing from the far side of the net that appeared to arise by reassembly, commencing with the finest radicals. Those, in turn, entered the dorsal roots as myelinated fibers. In contrast, Gerlach viewed motor axons of egress as deriving directly from motoneuron somata.

Shortly thereafter, Golgi developed his version of the network hypothesis based on his silver chromate preparations of the gray matter of the spinal cord. He visualized the sensory axons of the dorsal root as breaking up terminally to enter a continuous net extending lengthwise through the gray matter. Fusing with the net were the axonal arborizations of short axon cells (Fig. 15) and of recurrent

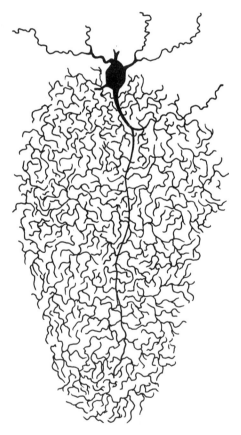

FIG. 15. Short axon arborization in cerebellum, Van Gehuchten stain. Such axon arbors joined in net formation according to reticularists. (From Barker, 1899.)

collaterals of the motoneuron axons. Figure 16A illustrates the Gerlach concept of the net; Figures 11B-1 and 16B (right) that of Golgi.

A. H. Forel (1848–1931) struck the first effective blow against the net theories. Working with the methods of Golgi and Gudden, he showed that an injury remains confined to a nerve cell and its processes and does not secondarily involve dendrites or axons of other nerve cells. W. His (1831–1904), an embryologist, proved that nerve cells are independent of each other even at their immature origins in the embryonic ependyma. He also showed that the soma is the nutritive center of the axon.

Using the Golgi method, Ramón y Cajal generalized that the collateral and terminal arborizations of each axon end freely in one of a number of ways—as pericellular and dendritic point contacts upon neurons (*boutons terminaux* or *endfeet*), as baskets, climbing terminals extending along dendrites, etc. Thus, he saw *contiguity* between the ultimate axonal branchlets and the receptive membrane of the related neuron, but not *continuity.* He also developed the concept (published in 1891 in a Spanish journal of his own) that conduction along dendrites must occur toward the soma. In 1892 he furnished added proof that impulse conduction occurred outwards along the axon.

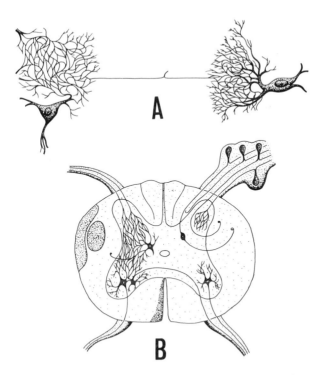

Fig. 16. A: Sketch by Gerlach (1872) of fusion of dendritic branchlets of two nerve cells to produce an axon. **B:** Pre-Golgi concept of the net **(left)**; Golgi concept **(right).** (Ramón y Cajal, 1937.)

Wilhelm von Waldeyer (1836–1921) of Germany reviewed the whole subject. He named and strongly supported the neuron doctrine in opposition to that based on a continuous net. There were objections, but Waldeyer's writing made the doctrine popular among anatomists, physiologists, pathologists, and clinicians on an international basis. He had done none of the original work, but his writing won the day by its objectivity and fairness. That has happened before and since in the history of science. Charles Sherrington, already an eminent physiologist, coined the word *synapse* (from the Greek, for "contact, point of juncture"), introducing it in 1897 in Foster's and Schaeffer's English physiology texts.

THE NET REVIVAL

Hans Held (1866–1942), a Leipzig histologist, renewed the controversy. During the year that Sherrington introduced the word synapse, Held described a zone of presumed continuity that he called *concrescence,* joining the axon terminal to the neuroplasm of the contiguous soma. To him such continuity was particularly evident in the trapezoid body of the hindbrain, a relay point upon the hearing pathway. He had deserted the silver methods for histological preparations of a more conventional type, and much of his evidence could have been interpreted differently. L. Apáthy (1863–1922) of Hungary, who worked on leeches and earthworms, believed he could distinguish neurofibrils passing from one neuron into another; and H. Bethe (1872–1954) of Germany also reported neurofibrillar continuity. According to A. T. Rasmussen, the result was that the neuron theory commenced to be discarded by many, particularly by F. Nissl (1860–1919), a world-renowned neuropathologist whose opinion carried much weight.

At first aloof, Ramón y Cajal was soon to enter the lists. Unconvinced that the preparations of Bethe and Apáthy showed the passage of neurofibrils between neurons, he adopted M. Bielschowsky's (1869–1940) reduced silver method as the one that could settle neurofibrillar continuity one way or the other. When he substituted the milder photographic silver developers for the harsher alkaline one of the original method, the neurofibrils, supposed by the revived reticularists to pass between neurons, stood out as belonging to individual neurons. No continuity could be shown. Over the next quarter century, however, the problem was resurrected from time to time, with supporting evidence always deriving from some new histological method that supposedly showed synaptic detail with more clarity than any preceding it.

THE NOBEL PRIZE

In 1906 Camillo Golgi and Ramón y Cajal, foremost members of the reticularist and antireticularist schools, shared the Nobel Prize. E. G. T. Liddell (1960) tells us that old beliefs were bared when Golgi and Ramón y Cajal gave their addresses in Stockholm. It is significant that while admitting that his theory was on the decline and that he could accept the neuron doctrine, Golgi still believed firmly in the existence of a diffuse axonal network.

TISSUE CULTURE PROOF OF AXONAL OUTGROWTH

Linked with discussion upon the nerve net versus neuronal independence was the question of axonal outgrowth or its alternative, the segmental formation of axons out of a chain of cells. Using frog tissue cultured in a drop of a tissue fluid called lymph, R. G. Harrison (1870–1959) of Yale demonstrated axonal outgrowth while at the same time proving the viability of nervous elements grown outside the body. This confirmed an important aspect of Ramón y Cajal's work and gave tissue culture technique its start. It is still used productively in ultrastructural studies of nervous tissue.

COMMENT

From the initial efforts to understand nervous organization early in the nineteenth century to the statement of the neuron doctrine near the century's end, the number of investigators participating in the total effort was not large compared with the personnel who might be required to generate a comparable breakthrough today. A. T. Rasmussen noted the names of perhaps 100 workers who played important roles in developing the knowledge that underlay the neuron doctrine; perhaps 50 relevant books were published in the last half of the century.

That does not mean that these pioneers were more intelligent or harder working than those who participate in contemporary science. It is important to emphasize that the succession of problems that were met and solved were far less complex and required much less diversified techniques than are necessary today. Modern bioscience anticipates an imminent general breakthrough into a new era of *molecular* biology, comparable to that which happened at the cellular level in the 1830s. It would be premature to speculate upon the time and effort required to extend such a breakthrough into the neuroscience area.

In the nineteenth century, space for laboratories, the provision of equipment and supplies, and the salary outlays were extraordinarily inexpensive by comparison with today's needs. Present techniques are varied, complex, and difficult to master, and technical training is sometimes prolonged. Training of the scientist is even more time-consuming because it requires the mastery of concepts, knowledge of the conduct of complex procedures, and a grasp of the voluminous current literature.

Added to today's complexity of experimentation and training, the modern creative scientist may be distracted from his research by administrative and organizational responsibilities. And in the last decades, the scientists' time has been increasingly fragmented by societal and national activities. This picture of the active contemporary scientist is in contrast to early nineteenth-century investigators who followed their science wherever their curiosity led them.

The importance of technological growth to the development of science is well illustrated in this chapter as well as in the succeeding one. It has been demonstrated by the use of chemicals to preserve and harden tissues, embedding and clearing agents to prepare them for thin sectioning, and dyes to stain them differentially. In optics, the development of achromatic lenses had to precede rapid growth of biological knowledge; and in mechanics, the perfection of microtomes for thin sectioning was also required. Such events have occurred in our own time as a result of the development of phase, ultraviolet, and electron microscopy, and the perfection of the specific procedures that permit their fullest exploitation.

NOTES

[1] Ample-size collections of neurons that lie near the center of each cerebral hemisphere. They are the *caudate nucleus, lentiform nucleus,* and *thalamus* (see Chapters VI and X).

[2] Jan Purkinje was born in Libochovice, Bohemia, in the hills of the central Bohemian highlands. His father died when he was 6 years old. O. Temkin (1971) relates that Jan had epileptic attacks in his youth. He quotes Purkinje as saying of these attacks, "I had the impression that I was being turned around with the greatest velocity in the tremendous vortex of a sea of fire and had to fight against it with all my strength. To those around me this fight appeared as a convulsion." (Temkin, 1971, p. 268.)

Educated as a child in a Piarist monastery, in 1804 he joined that order. Influenced by writings of the German romantic philosophers, he began to see in scientific endeavor the highest mission of man (Kruta, 1962). Consequently, he resigned his Piarist membership to devote himself exclusively to scientific and educational work and entered medicine. While in medical school, he undertook to study the effect of currently used medicinal drugs on himself, a normal individual. Today, the testing of drugs on normal humans is intermediary between animal testing and tests of efficacy in patients.

In 1818, Purkinje wrote his doctoral dissertation on the subjective aspects of vision, a study that gained the attention of J. W. Goethe, the immortal German poet and philosopher. By 1825, Purkinje had formulated his phenomenon of optics—fields of equal brightness but different color become unequally bright if the intensity of illumination is decreased—and had devised the first scheme for studying the retina of the eye by ophthalmoscopy. During this period of his career, he also studied the effects of gravitational stress. Also by 1825, using only a strong magnifying lens, he had discovered the germinal vesicle of the egg of the hen, which later was to prove to be the cell nucleus of the ovum. Shortly following the development of the achromatic microscope (Meyer, 1971), while reporting to the Congress of Physicians and Scientists in Prague (1836), he illustrated the Purkinje and granule cells of the cerebellum. At the same time, he was also studying plant tissue.

In addition, Purkinje discovered the specialized musculature of the heart that makes up the conducting system between the auricles and ventricles, the disease of which can be predicted by today's physicians with use of an electrocardiogram. He also provided the earliest data on the individuality of fingerprints. Finally, he wrote a section on sleep for an encyclopedia of physiology of his time, making an important contribution to sleep theory as it existed then.

Much space has been devoted to Purkinje here because of his lifelong devotion to science, to which he made very important contributions in many different areas. Importantly, his life also illustrates what can be accomplished by a scientist who was a childhood epileptic. He is said to have discovered plant and animal cells before Theodor Schwann, neurons before C. Ehrenberg, and the ophthalmoscope before H. Helmholtz. He was the most technologically innovative of the early workers, and initiated a variety of "firsts" in improving equipment and developing the facilities so necessary to successful research. His talent is well expressed by Goethe in the following witty quatrain, translated and quoted by G. W. Bartelmez (1953):

Let your delighted eye behold
All things that Plato Knew of old!
And if yourself you can't quite do it,
Purkyně'll come and help you to it.

[3] R. A. Koelliker was born in Zurich, Switzerland, in 1817. He spent most of his academic career at Würzburg, and did not retire until age 85. G. von Bonin, one of his biographers, states that Koelliker published 20 papers over the last 8 years of his life, evidence of his energy and acumen as an elder citizen. That biographer also concludes that Koelliker anticipated by almost 50 years Waldeyer's formulation of the neuron doctrine, an evaluation which should not be accepted without reservation, for it discounts the great work of Purkyně and Remak of the early period and of Ramón y Cajal, Golgi, and many others in the late period. It is important that Koelliker recognized, without hesitation, the greatness of Ramón y Cajal, who returned the compliment when he identified Koelliker as "uniting a great talent for observation—with enchanting modesty and exceptional rectitude and calmness of judgement." (von Bonin, 1970, p. 53.)

[4] Camillo Golgi was born in Corteno, Italy, the son of a medical practitioner. He studied medicine at Padua, graduating in 1865, and was attracted to psychiatry. In 1872, he took a post in the small hospital for incurables at Abbiategrasso, where he overcame many obstacles to carry on his researches and develop his silver impregnation method. He was appointed professor of anatomy at the University of Siena in 1879. In publications between 1886 and 1893, he established the cycle of development of the parasites of quartan and tertian malaria. His Nobel Prize-winning work related to the nerve endings in tendons. (Stevenson, 1953, pp. 33–36.)

[5] Santiago Ramón y Cajal was born in the Pyrenees of northern Spain. His father was a struggling physician. As a youth he was described as lazy and a dolt. His love of drawing led him first to anatomy and then to medicine. For a time he served as a regimental surgeon in Cuba, where he contracted tuberculosis, which forced his return to Spain. In 1877, two years before his marriage, he was appointed to the anatomy faculty of the University of Zaragoza. There he began his studies on the nervous system. After several academic moves, in 1892 he was assigned to the University of Madrid. He worked there the remainder of his life. Many honors came his way, including honorary degrees from Oxford and Cambridge. He received the Nobel Prize jointly with Golgi in 1906. Meanwhile, he established his own laboratory at the medical school and, in 1901, commenced to publish his own journal. He wrote many articles and monographs, a textbook, and an autobiography, and also worked in color photography. His was the soul of the scientific renaissance in Spain.

The following extract from Stevenson (1953, pp. 36–37) is indicative of his Nobel Prize work:

... morphologic dispositions which vary in form according to the nerve center one studies, attest that the nerve elements have reciprocal relations of *contiguity* and not of *continuity*, and that communications, more or less intimate, are always established not only between the nervous arborizations but between the ramifications of one part and the body and protoplasmic extensions of another part. ...

REFERENCES AND BIBLIOGRAPHY

Apáthy, S. Das leitende Element des Nervensystems und seine topographischen Beziehungen zu den Zellen. *Mitt. Zool. Station Neapel.* 12:495–748, 1897.

Barker, L. F. *The Nervous System and its Constituent Neurones.* New York: D. Appleton & Co., 1899. 1122 pp.

Bartelmez, G. W. Johannes Evangelista Purkynje (1787–1869), pp. 70–74. In W. Haymaker and K. A. Baer, eds. *The Founders of Neurology,* 1st ed. Springfield, Ill.: Charles C Thomas, 1953.

Bethe, A. Studien über das Zentralnervensystem von Carcinus Maenas nebst Angaben über ein neues Verfahren der Methylenblaufixation. *Arch. Mikro. Anat.* 44:579–622, 1894–1895.

von Bonin, G. Rudolf Albert von Kölliker (1817–1905), pp. 51–54. In W. Haymaker and F. Schiller, eds. *The Founders of Neurology,* 2d ed. Springfield, Ill.: Charles C Thomas, 1970.

Clarke, E., and O'Malley, C. D. *The Human Brain and Spinal Cord.* Berkeley: University of California Press, 1968. 1926 pp.

Da Fano, C. Camillo Golgi (1843–1926). *J. Pathol.* 29:500–514, 1926.

Davis, W. J., and Kennedy, D. Command interneurons controlling swimmeret movements in the lobster. *J. Neurophysiol.* 35:1–29, 1972.

Deiters, O. *Untersuchungen über Gehirn und Rückenmark des Menschen und der Säugethiere.* Braunschweig: Vieweg und Sohn, 1865. 318 pp.

Gerlach, J. The spinal cord, pp. 623–649. In S. Stricker, *A Manual of Histology.* (A. H. Buck, ed., American translation.) New York: William Wood & Co., 1872.

Golgi, C. Sulla struttura della sostanza grigia del cervello. *Gazz. Med. Ital.* 6:244–246, 1873.

Golgi, C. Studies on the minute anatomy of the central organs of the nervous system. *Alienist Neurol.* 4:236–269, 1883.

Goss, C. M. On anatomy of nerves by Galen of Pergamon. *Am. J. Anat.* 118:327–335, 1966.

Gray, H. *Gray's Anatomy of the Human Body,* 29th ed. rev. and ed. by C. M. Goss. Philadelphia: Lea and Febiger, 1973. 1466 pp.

Harrison, R. G. Observations on the living developing nerve fiber. *Anat. Rec.* 1:116–118, 1907.

Held, H. Beiträge zur Structur der Nervenzellen und ihrer Fortsätze (Zweite Abhandlung). *Arch. Anat. Physiol., Anat. Abth., Leipzig* pp. 204–294, 1897.

Huxley, A. *Literature and Science.* New York: Harper & Row, 1963. 118 pp.

Kruta, V. *Jan Evangelista Purkyně,* p. 143. Prague: State Medical Publishing House, 1962.

Kruta, V. J. E. Purkyně's conception of the physiological basis of wakefulness and sleep. *Scripta Med.* 40:281–290, 1967.

Kruta, V. J. E. Purkyně's contribution to the cell theory. *Clio Med.* 6:109–120, 1971.

Liddell, E. G. T. *The Discovery of Reflexes.* Oxford: Clarendon Press, 1960. 174 pp.

Marchi, V., and Algeri, G. Sulle degenerazioni discendenti. Consecutive a lesioni della corteccia cerebrale. *Riv. Sper. Freniatr. Med. Leg.* 11:492–494, 1885.

Marchi, V., and Algeri, G. Sulle degenerazioni discendenti. Consecutive a lesioni sperimentali in diverse zone della corteccia cerebrale. *Riv. Sper. Freniatr. Med. Leg.* 12:208–252, 1886.

Meyer, A. *Historical Aspects of Cerebral Anatomy.* London: Oxford University Press, 1971. 230 pp.

Nansen, F. The structure and combination of the histological elements in the central nervous system. Bergen's Museums, Aarsberetning for 1886. Bergen, 1887.

Nauta, W. J. H., and Gygax, P. A. Silver impregnation of degenerating axons in the central nervous system: A modified technic. *Stain Technol.* 29:91–93, 1954.

Ramón y Cajal, S. *Recollections of My Life.* (Trans. by E. Horne Craigie and Juan Cano.) Philadelphia: American Philosophical Society, 1937. 638 pp.

Ramón y Cajal, S. *Neuron Theory or Reticular Theory? Objective Evidence of the Anatomical Unity of Nerve Cells.* (Trans. by M. Ubeda Purkiss and C. A. Fox.) Madrid: Instituto Ramón y Cajal, 1954. 144 pp.

Ramón y Cajal, S. Degeneration of the peripheral stump, pp. 100–140. In *Degeneration and Regeneration of the Nervous System,* Vol. 1. New York: Hafner Publishing Co., 1928.

Ranson, S. W., and Clark, S. L. *The Anatomy of the Nervous System. Its Development and Function,* 10th ed. Philadelphia: W. B. Saunders Co., 1959. 622 pp.

Rasmussen, A. T. *Some Trends in Neuroanatomy.* Dubuque, Ia.: W. C. Brown Co., 1947. 93 pp.

Stevenson, L. G. *Nobel Prize Winners in Medicine and Physiology, 1901–1950.* New York: Henry Schuman, 1953. 291 pp.

Temkin, O. *The Falling Sickness. A History of Epilepsy from the Greeks to the Beginnings of Modern Neurology,* 2d ed. rev. Baltimore: The Johns Hopkins Press, 1971. 467 pp.

Waldeyer, W. Über einige neuere Forschungen im Gebiete der Anatomie des Zentralnervensystems. *Dtsch. Med. Wochenschr.* 17:1244–1246, 1267–1269, 1287–1289, 1331–1332, 1352–1356, 1891.

Weaver, W. *Science and Imagination.* New York: Basic Books, Inc., 1967. 295 pp.

Weigert, C. Über eine neue Untersuchungsmethode des Zentralnervensystems. *Zentralbl. Med. Wiss.* 20:753–757, 772–774, 1882.

Chapter V

FROM ANIMAL ELECTRICITY TO ELECTROPHYSIOLOGY

The brain, as we now know, is activated by electrical currents, albeit relatively weak ones. Thus, its functioning could not be properly comprehended by those ignorant of this ubiquitous natural phenomenon, the basis of our modern technological society. The neurosciences could not have blossomed without the discovery of electricity, especially the so-called animal electricity generated within living beings. This chapter will review the steps, some of them stumbling, leading to that discovery. It also reviews the development of methods for recording and measuring this force, which culminated in much of the promising equipment we have for pursuing contemporary brain research.

All brain activities are induced by electrochemical processes, in particular such generalized nervous phenomena as conduction, excitation, and inhibition. Generators of weak electrical currents lie in the surface membranes of the somata (bodies) of nerve cells, their dendrites, and axons. A whole cell, made up of these several parts, is called a *neuron.* The membrane coverings of somata and dendrites provide many spot contacts (synapses) with the terminal tendrils of axons arising from other cells, each such spot showing a narrow cleft at the interface between presynaptic (axonal) and postsynaptic (soma-dendritic) components. These junctures permit one-way conduction from the axon terminus to the dendritic part with which it is in touch.

When engaged in nervous activity, a neuron soma discharges clustered action potentials (also called *impulses, signals,* or *nerve spikes*). These traverse the axon at a constant rate and in a codified sequence. Such sequences, showing variable spacing between signals, pass at finite rates and without loss of signal amplitude between soma origin and the distant telodendria, where the contacting dendrite of another neuron is located. The code carries the incessant shoptalk between neurons.

Communication between neurons is achieved when signal bursts are transferred from the terminal endbulbs of an axon to the body or dendrites of a succeeding neuron. Each point of contact, of which a vast number form the synaptic scale of a single neuron, may be compared with a telephone receiver, a cleft existing between the membrane of the endbulb and that of the receiving neuron. Most synapses utilize a chemical transmitter that conveys the impact of succeeding signals of a burst across the cleft. Flow in the narrow chemical conduit is discontinuous, a packet or more of transmitter being thrown off by endbulb membrane for each signal received. Synapses divide generally into two types, excitatory and inhibitory. The latter diminishes the action of the contacted neuron rather than exciting it.

An illuminating phenomenon of animal electricity is the specialized neuromuscular mechanism found in electric organs of several fish, including both the torpedo and the electric catfish. In the better-understood torpedo, each electric organ—imagine a pipe organ—is composed of 500 columns of cells stacked on either side of the center of its body. Upon its abdominal (ventral) surface, each column has about 1,000 electroplaques (synapse equivalents). The number of cells that make up a column determines the voltage output of the organ. Electroplaques contain acetylcholine, an excitatory neurotransmitter. In the usual skeletal muscle that engages in moving the fish about, axon spikes reaching the body musculature generate only enough electricity to produce the required movement. Corresponding axon spikes reaching the electric organ musculature of the torpedo trigger a discharge of volts sufficient to stun a prey with which the fish makes contact. Comparison of the usual operations of the nervous system, powered by weak electric currents, with that of the electric organs, which require heavy currents, suggests that the bioelectric potential available to the brain should not be minimized. That which is produced normally, however, is only sufficient to meet immediate needs.

During an epileptic attack the currents produced are considerably greater than those required for normal brain activity. These stromal currents result from abnormal recruitment and timing of many unit potentials that correspond to those recorded by the extra-fine microelectrodes inserted into single neurons in the experimental laboratory. Even the current produced during a human epileptic attack does not nearly approximate the discharge of the fish's electric organ. Yet, it is sufficient to initiate the massive muscular contractions of the human body that occur during an attack and to disrupt the cerebral circuits that maintain consciousness in the waking state.

This chapter will basically cover nineteenth- and twentieth-century neuroscientific research. It will begin with the hazy concept of an imponderable agent called *nerve force, nerve fluid,* or the *active principle* of the nerves. As the effects of the electric-influence machine, which produced electricity by friction, became known, this imponderable agent was increasingly associated with, and ultimately replaced by, the concept of an animal electricity distributed along the nerves from the nerve centers.

BEGINNINGS OF ELECTRICITY

In the sixth century B.C., Thales of Miletus showed that what we now know as static electricity could be produced by rubbing resin with cat's fur or glass with silk. It was thought that these methods produced two different types of electric fluid, *resinous* and *vitreous,* respectively. About 1600, William Gilbert demonstrated the electrification of many substances. He derived the term electricity from the Greek word for amber. The first electric-friction machine was invented in 1672 by Otto von Guericke (1602–1686) of Prussia. It was a simple device consisting of a globe of sulfur mounted on a spindle and rotated by hand. By the mid-eighteenth century, such devices were common. In 1745 Ewald von

Kleist of Prussia, and the next year Pieter van Musschenbroek of Leyden, independently developed what became known as the Leyden jar for the storage and spectacular discharge of electricity. In 1756 L. Caldini of Padua found that the Leyden jar discharge caused contraction of skeletal muscle. Previously, in 1732, Stephen Hales of England and later, in 1781, F. Fontana had attributed nerve conduction to electricity.[1]

THE EXPERIMENTS OF WALSH AND HUNTER

The sixteenth-century essayist Michel Montaigne (1533–1592) provided one of the earliest descriptions of the mysterious force that emanated through the water from the torpedo.[2] In the seventeenth century Francesco Redi (1626–1698) first observed how the torpedo produces its shock. Investigation of the torpedo was renewed by John Walsh, a member of the Royal Society of London, who revealed the results of his experiments to Benjamin Franklin in letters which were published in the *Philosophical Transactions of the Royal Society* in July 1773.

Walsh's most conclusive experiment in animal electricity was conducted in the chambers of the mayor of LaRochelle, France. It is described by E. G. T. Liddell (1960, p. 32) as follows:

> Two brass wires, 13 feet long, were suspended from the ceiling by silken threads. One of these wires rested by one end on the wet napkin on which the fish lay; the other end was immersed in a basin full of water placed on a second table. Around this other table five persons stood, insulated, and were interconnected by dipping hands in basins of water. In the last basin one end of the second wire was immersed and with the other end Mr. Walsh touched the back of the Torpedo when the five persons felt a commotion which differed in nothing from that of the Leyden experiment. Mr. Walsh, who was not in the circle of conduction, received no shock. This meeting was held on 22 July 1772.

Walsh enlisted the aid of John Hunter in his studies. In addition to being an outstanding surgeon, Hunter was a comparative neurologist of some repute. His report on the dissection of the torpedo's electric organs and their nerve supply was also published in the *Philosophical Transactions*. In it Hunter describes the organs in some detail and indicates that their activation arose from the lateral and posterior portions of the brain.[3] In a later communication to the Royal Society, Hunter claimed for Walsh the honor of discovering animal electricity (Fig. 19).

GALVANI AND VOLTA

Luigi Galvani (1737–1798) was a lecturer in anatomy at the University of Bologna (Fig. 20). His studies led him to postulate animal electricity as the force producing conduction in nerve and contraction in muscle. Although he began his experiments in 1780, he did not publish an account of them until 11 years later under the title, *De Viribus Electricitatis in Moto Musculari Commentarius*.

XXXIX. *An Account of the* Gymnotus Electricus.
By John Hunter, *F. R. S.*

Redde, May 11, 1775.

TO Mr. WALSH, the first discoverer of animal electricity, the learned will be indebted for whatever the following pages may contain, either curious or useful. The specimen of the animal which they describe was procured by that Gentleman, and at his request this dissection was performed, and this account of it is communicated.

FIG. 17. Hunter's attribution of the discovery of animal electricity to John Walsh. (From Hunter, 1775.)

In this work he described (Brazier, 1959) a series of experiments that utilized a frog nerve-muscle arrangement made up of hind legs and a connecting bared sciatic nerve.[4] These experiments led him to what he believed was the inescapable conclusion that animal electricity exists. The only comparable experiments were done a century earlier, in 1678, when Jan Schwammerdam showed the Grand Duke of Tuscany how the muscle of a frog's leg contracted when it and its nerve were mounted on a copper support, and wires were twisted around the nerve and made to touch the copper support (Liddell, 1960).

According to L. A. Geddes and H. E. Hoff (1971), the first Galvani experiment (Fig. 21) consisted of dissecting a prepared (decerebrate) frog and placing it on a table at a distance from an electrostatic machine. Touching the nerve with a metal point caused a strong contraction of the musculature. The same thing happened when a spark was discharged from the conductor of the machine. Later it was observed that when using a bone-handled scalpel no contraction ensued, even though the machine produced a spark, unless the hand came in contact with the metal part of the scalpel. It is probable that in this instance Galvani did not demonstrate the phenomenon of bioelectricity, since nerve stimulation occurred by electrostatic induction in a circuit including the machine, the frog preparation, the observer, and the earth. However, this led Galvani to question whether or not atmospheric electricity would produce a similar response, just as Benjamin Franklin and others had wondered at an earlier time whether the spark of an electrostatic machine and a flash of lightning were one and the same (Geddes and Hoff, 1971). In November 1780 Galvani erected a long, insulated, iron wire antenna upon or under the roof of his house. Frogs were connected to the antenna and another wire was led to the water of a nearby well. As lightning flashed in the sky, electricity travelled along the conductor and the frog muscles contracted. Thunder was heard later. If the thunderstorms were severe, the effect could have been obtained in the lower as well as the upper rooms of the house. Electroscopes confirmed the presence of electricity.

These studies were continued in a "second experiment," reported to have taken place in September 1786. Prepared frogs, hung on iron gratings in the garden

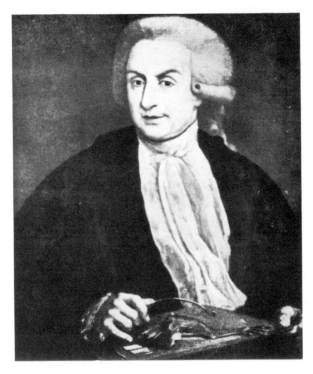

FIG. 18. Luigi Galvani (1737–1798). (From the University Library of Bologna.)

by bronze hooks that penetrated the spinal cord, went into contraction whether or not an electric storm was brewing. Liddell (1960) quotes Du Bois-Reymond as suggesting that in the initial trials Galvani used iron hooks with the iron railings. These similar metals would still have been effective in causing contraction if one contact was cleaner or warmer than the other. If the arcs were composed of two dissimilar metals joined together, they would have given stronger contractions. Glass, resin, stone, or wood used as substitutes produced no contractions.

Galvani concluded that he had discharged the animal electricity in the muscle, equating muscle and nerve as with the inner and outer conductors of a Leyden jar. He overlooked the importance of a conducting arc composed of two different metals as indispensable if contractions were to occur. These studies rate as one of the great experiments of science. Galvani's book, published in 1791, aroused intense interest. Scientists and laymen alike were avid to repeat the experiments. Volta at first accepted Galvani's results. He soon changed his mind, becoming convinced that to produce the frog contractions required the use of dissimilar metals joined at one end. He published his dissent widely.

Geddes and Hoff (1971) cite a letter written by Volta in which he stated that the same contractions could be excited by metallic contact with two parts of a

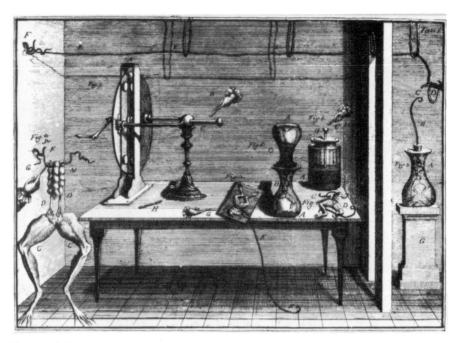

FIG. 19. Galvani's laboratory. Originally published in Vol. VII of the 1791 proceedings of the Bologna Academy, containing Galvani's original announcement of his discovery of animal electricity. (From Fulton, J. F., and Wilson, L. G., *Selected Readings in the History of Physiology*, 2d ed., 1966. Courtesy of Charles C Thomas, Publisher, Springfield, Ill.)

nerve, two parts of the same muscle, or two different muscles. Volta concluded that these results pointed not to a spontaneous animal electricity, but to a very weak artificial electricity, which did not act directly on the muscles but excited them through their nerves. After Galvani's death in 1798, Volta established the significance of dissimilarity between metals by making public the properties of his voltaic pile, which consisted of pairs of discs of dissimilar metals with acid-moistened pads between each pair; this was the first man-made electric battery (Liddell, 1960).

Earlier, in an anonymous communication filed in 1794 with the library of the University of Bologna and known as the *Trattato,* Galvani had written about "contraction without metals." Du Bois-Reymond, examining the original document, found that it presented evidence showing that when an intact nerve belonging to a nerve-muscle preparation was placed across an intact and a cut surface of another muscle, a twitch occurred in the muscle belonging to the preparation. Galvani apparently had observed the injury current of muscle.

It was Alessandro Volta (1745–1827) who made possible the utilization of electricity. Voltaic electricity, in contrast to static electricity, was a measurable force that could be transmitted by wires and turned off and on by breaking and closing the circuit through which it flowed. Volta's experiments, conducted to refute Galvani, provided the foundation of our energy-dependent economy.

OERSTED, SCHWEIGGER, AND THE EARLY APPLICATIONS OF ELECTROMAGNETISM

Electromagnetism, important for both its scientific and industrial uses, was discovered in 1820 by Hans Christian Oersted (1777–1851). He constructed a voltaic battery of sufficient size to bring a metal wire connected across it to a red heat and observed the deflection of a compass needle placed nearby. In 1821 J. S. C. Schweigger repeated this experiment and carried it further. The following quote is from Hoff and Geddes (1957, pp. 214–215.):

> Noticing that the magnetic needle was displaced in opposite directions when it was placed first above and then below the wire carrying the current, or when the polarity of the current was reversed, he deduced that the effect should be doubled if the wire looped round the compass with the needle within the plane of the coil. . . . From this observation began our knowledge of the importance of the number of turns in induction electricity. It also gave rise to the first name for the galvanometer: *the multiplier.*

Schweigger, according to Hoff and Geddes, also succeeded in developing a moving coil with a delicate mounting in which the magnetic needle was eliminated and a strong magnetic rod was held nearby. They credit Schweigger with producing the prototypes of both moving coil and moving vane galvanometers.

NOBILI'S GALVANOMETER AND ITS CALIBRATION

Another galvanometer, featuring a double coil of 72 turns, was described about this time by C. L. Nobili of Florence (Hoff and Geddes, 1957). Two magnetic needles were used, one in each opening, but they were rigidly connected on the same suspension. While mounted in parallel, the needles were of opposite polarities. As such they responded oppositely to the earth's magnetic field, mutually cancelling that force. Because the wires crossed at the waist of the "8," the needles moved in the same direction whenever current was turned on. The sensitivity of the instrument was sufficient to compare it with the Galvani frog nerve-muscle preparation, the most sensitive galvanometer then available.

In conducting his physiological studies, Nobili avoided the use of metals. A decapitated frog was positioned with its feet dipped into one beaker of fluid, its trunk in another, and a cotton thread, soaked in either water or saline solution, bridging the interiors. The frog twitched when contact was completed by means of the thread (Hoff and Geddes, 1957).

Nobili next introduced one of the more sensitive of his galvanometers into the circuit. While the frog muscle contracted, the needle did not move. He then built a still more sensitive instrument, and with it he obtained indisputable evidence of frog current. Nobili also found that frog current had a certain direction and force that could be offset by pitting the current of one frog against that of another of equal intensity. He then arranged frog preparations in series, thus producing a frog "pi₁ ." not unlike the original voltaic battery. An increase in galvanometric deflection occurred, indicating accumulation of current along the pile, and with it increasing galvanometric deflection. Intrinsic frog current had been demonstrated, yet Nobili ultimately attributed it to a thermoelectric effect (Dawson, unpublished), a misinterpretation that set back the understanding of animal electricity.

Nobili's instrument was described as an astatic galvanometer because its needles were independent of the earth's magnetism. It was refined in 1858 by William Thomson (Lord Kelvin) of England. He made it a highly sensitive device used for many years to receive telegraphic signals. According to Dawson (unpublished), this improved model was used twice in electroencephalographic (brain wave) recordings, 60 years apart.

MATTEUCCI AND MUSCLE PHYSIOLOGY

A graduate in physics from the University of Bologna, Carlo Matteucci (1811–1868) (Fig. 20) joined Nobili in Florence, where he began his electrophysiological

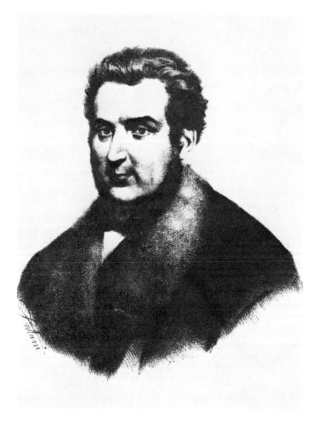

FIG. 20. Carlo Matteucci (1811–1868). (Courtesy of The Wellcome Institute.)

studies. These included investigations of electric fishes, muscle demarcation currents, and muscle action currents in the frog (Moruzzi, 1961).

In his study of the torpedo (Fig. 21), Matteucci pursued systematically what Walsh and Hunter had begun in a less scientific manner late in the eighteenth century. Matteucci showed that the discharge of the electric organ in the fish was effected from a special hindbrain area and that severing the cranial nerves arising from that area prevented the discharge of the electric organ. Yet the discharge could still be evoked if those nerves remained intact and the spinal cord was severed just behind the brain. In 1838 Matteucci also evoked a discharge of the electric organ by stimulation of the hindbrain by galvanic current. In 1844 he showed that discharge of the torpedo's electric organ could jump a spark gap. Documentation of this and other early investigations of the electric fishes can be found at the end of this chapter.[5,6]

Some of Matteucci's best work was done in trying to locate the origin of the electricity in the frog nerve-muscle preparation studied earlier by Galvani and Nobili (Brazier, 1959; Liddell, 1960; Hodgkin, 1964). Using an astatic galvanometer of his own design, he registered an electric current whenever a contact was established between a cut and an intact muscle surface. Moruzzi (1961) was convinced that this discovery of what was later to be called the demarcation potential was first made by Matteucci, not by later investigators.

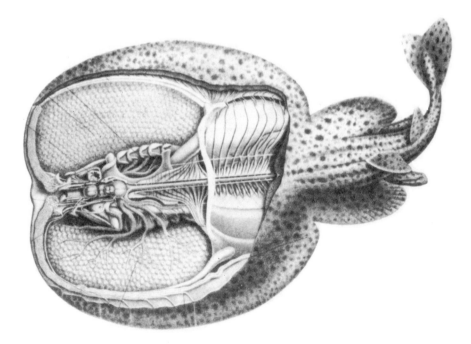

Fig. 21. *Torpedo galvani,* dorsal view, dissected on left to show the nerve supply of the electric organ. From Paolo Savi in one of Matteucci's works. (From Moruzzi, 1963.)

Setting out to determine which parts of the frog were essential to the production of the current, he found that the sciatic nerves were unnecessary and that portions of a muscle were as effective as a whole muscle. He constructed muscle piles just as Volta had made piles of alternating metals and Nobili of frogs, showing that the intensity of the demarcation current as indicated by the galvanometer increases when several muscle segments (frog half-thighs) were placed in series (Fig. 24) so that the transverse (i.e., injured) section of one touched the longitudinal (i.e., uninjured) one of the next. Leading off to his galvanometer, he got readings of 2 to 4 degrees with two half-thighs, but obtained readings of up to 60 with more of them. In 1838 Matteucci reported another basic observation, noting that the intrinsic frog current disappeared during steady muscle contraction produced by strychnine. According to Moruzzi (1961), this was the first evidence for the negative oscillation of the demarcation current, the action current of the muscle.

Matteucci's discovery of the induced twitch in 1842 was another indication of the existence of the muscle action current (Fig. 23). Quoting from Liddell (1960, p. 39):

> In his series of observations, he used a "galvanoscopic frog" which was merely a frog's nerve-muscle preparation placed inside a large-bore glass tube, with the nerve dangling out. If the muscle of another, living, frog was injured and the dangling nerve introduced into the wound, the galvanoscopic frog muscle contracted when the dangling nerve touched also the uninjured surface of the muscle.

Matteucci was at a loss to reconcile these observations of the induced twitch with his older experiment on disappearance of the demarcation current during strychnine spasm. Ultimately, he rejected his own findings and offered an interpretation of the induced twitch other than the correct one of its being a sign of the action current. Meanwhile, Johannes Müller had given a short book by Matteucci, *Essai sur les phénomènes élĕctriques des animaux,* to Du Bois-

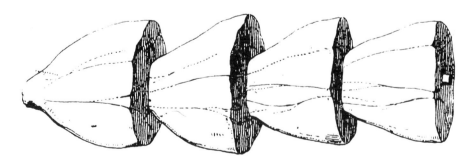

Fig. 22. Matteucci's electrophysiological pile using half-thighs of frogs. The cut surface of one muscle is in contact with the intact surface of the following one. Later investigations showed that this lead combination between cut and intact surfaces gave rise to the demarcation current. (From Moruzzi, 1963.)

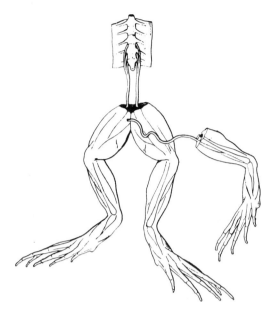

Fig. 23. The sciatic nerve of the galvanoscopic frog leg is placed upon the muscles of another frog preparation. This arrangement gave rise to Matteucci's *induced twitch.* (From Moruzzi, 1963.)

Reymond, then a student. It started him on his career as Matteucci's successor and chief competitor.

THE GERMAN SCHOOL OF ELECTROPHYSIOLOGY

Johannes Müller (1801–1858) was Germany's representative among the early physiologists. He had varied biological interests and was a very productive scientist. Many of his students became as famous as their master. Among them were Theodor Schwann and Rudolf Koelliker (neurohistology), Emil Du Bois-Reymond and Hermann Helmholtz (electrophysiology and physics), and Rudolph Virchow (pathology). Clarke and O'Malley (1968) provide detailed accounts of these scientists. Müller remains celebrated for his doctrine of specific nerve energies, which holds that although a sense organ can be activated by other than its adequate stimulus, the subjective response is the same and is not influenced by the kind of stimulus. Thus, the sensation resulting from a stimulus of a given kind depends on which nerve fibers are stimulated and not on how they are stimulated.

Du Bois-Reymond (1818–1896) succeeded Müller in the chair of physiology at the University of Berlin (Fig. 24). He had started his experimental work, as had Nobili, by building a galvanometer of increased sensitivity. It contained more than 4,000 turns (Hoff and Geddes, 1957). Du Bois-Reymond gave clear descrip-

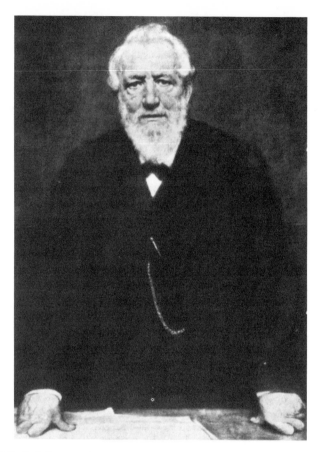

FIG. 24. Emil Du Bois-Reymond (1818–1896). (Courtesy of National Library of Medicine, Bethesda, Md.)

tions of the resting currents observed in excised nerves and muscles and postulated electromotive forces preexistent in the tissues (Gasser, 1953). He confirmed the origin of the currents of Nobili and Matteucci in muscle, and, indeed, in bits of muscle so small that the number of muscle fibers could be counted. Nevertheless, he shared the universal belief in a "frog current" existing between the outside of an uninjured muscle and its tendons (Clarke and O'Malley, 1968, p. 194).

Du Bois-Reymond resolved Matteucci's problem of the disappearance of the muscle current during spasm (Hoff and Geddes, 1957). He was able to do so because he appreciated the difference in perspective toward current detection on the part of the galvanometer and the galvanoscopic frog. He had noticed that muscle tetanus is due to an intermittent excitation producing a fused contraction, and from this made his assessment. He said that the galvanometer of his time was well adapted to detecting the presence of *continuous* electrical currents and their variations in intensity, but noted that it lost that value when instantaneous current was the focus of detection. Although disappointing in long-term detection, the frog nerve-muscle preparation is a sensitive detector of quick current variations. Better response time has been built into the modern galvanometer, but a century ago Du Bois-Reymond's remarks were quite pertinent. They recall a general observation, attributed by Hoff and Geddes (1960) to Burdon Sanderson, to the effect that "the phenomena observed are those of the instruments we employ rather than those of the organs we explore."

Du Bois-Reymond used the term *muscular current* in the case of muscle and spoke of a negative variation because he was unable to tell whether, during contraction, there was a decrease in current intensity or current direction reversal (Hoff and Geddes, 1957). Yet he was able to detect the negative variation in nerve, which Matteucci would have failed to detect because of his less sensitive instruments. Clarke and O'Malley (1968, pp. 198–202) give a lengthy account of this.

THE VELOCITY OF THE NERVE IMPULSE

The presumption of instantaneous speed in transmission along nerve routes would have been well-nigh inconceivable to the naturalists of antiquity. The thinking of practical minds did not change significantly prior to 1850. Then imagination rejected almost all inhibitions. According to Liddell (1960), the *vis nervosa, force nerveuse,* or *animal spirits* were estimated to travel at such radically different velocities as 9,000 or 32,000 feet per minute, or 57,600 feet per second. Hermann L. F. von Helmholtz (1821–1894) was the first to make accurate measurements (Fig. 25). He showed conduction rates to be definitely finite and much slower than "instantaneous." In addition to measuring the velocity of nerve propagation, he invented the ophthalmoscope (see Purkinje, Chapter IV), and performed important studies on vision, hearing, and in physics. His measurement of nerve conduction rates are best described by Hoff and Geddes (1957). An extract of Helmholtz's writings on the subject is also to be found in Clarke and O'Malley (1968, p. 207).

By then the galvanometer was 20 years old, and its defects for electrophysiology were well known. To obtain the high sensitivity required for dealing with nerve and muscle currents, a long response time—10 seconds per minute—was needed. Helmholtz employed another method of measurement, one analogous to that which was then used to determine the velocity of a bullet shot from a gun. On the whole, his results are in good agreement with those obtained by present-day methods.

The work of Eduard Pflüger (1829–1910) alerted other scientists against careless use of jerry-built electrodes. Proper nonpolarizable electrodes were developed by Du Bois-Reymond. They were used by the generation of investigators commencing with Caton, who laid open the field of electroencephalography (see Chapter IX). Had the electrodes used on exposed brain not possessed the required stability, it is very possible that true responses to stimulation could have been confused with polarization artifact.

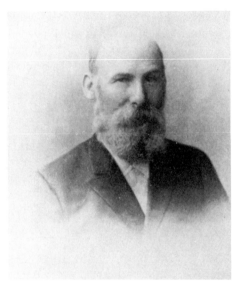 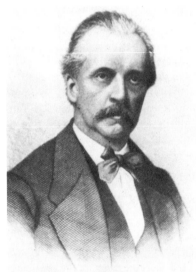

Fig. 25. Portraits of **(left)** Julius Bernstein (1839–1917) and **(right)** Hermann L. F. von Helmholtz (1821–1894), who were among the masters of German electrophysiology. (From H. Grundfest, 1957.)

THE ACTION CURRENT

L. Hermann (1838–1914) began his research activities at Du Bois-Reymond's Institute of Physiology, but eventually disagreed with his mentor's theories. He doubted the existence of resting currents. Observed differences, he held, revealed contrasts between normal and injured tissue. His great work lay in examining the details of Du Bois-Reymond's negative variation, which he called the *action current.* He showed this to be a wave of excitation, of a self-propagating state, conveyed from one section of nerve to the next (Clarke and O'Malley, 1968, p. 212).

BERNSTEIN AND THE MEMBRANE THEORY

The outlines of the membrane theory were first visualized by Du Bois-Reymond, but J. Bernstein (1839–1917) receives credit for its formulation (Fig. 25). Bernstein (Grundfest, 1965) accepted Hermann's notion that propagation depends on the flow of the electric current in a cable-like structure,[7] but suggested ways in which the "resting" and "action" currents originate. He based his theory on observations that all living animal tissues contain the ions of salt solutions. He supposed that "action" current involved a neutralization of membrane current but not an actual reversal, as evidence now indicates. In 1868 he showed that the "action" current of nerve was opposite in direction to the demarcation current, exceeding the latter by more than twofold at the peak of the spike. But he finally rejected this finding, leaving the "overshoot" to become a "new" discovery when reported in 1939–1945 by A. L. Hodgkin and A. F. Huxley and in 1942 by H. J. Curtis and K. J. Cole. Its rediscovery raised a challenge to Bernstein's ionic explanation of the membrane theory, which Hodgkin and Huxley (Grundfest, 1965) were able to explain by developing the "sodium hypothesis," followed by their more elaborate ionic theory. The latter has become a general theory applicable to most, if not all, known forms of bioelectric activity.

EIGHTEENTH- AND NINETEENTH-CENTURY LABORATORY INSTRUMENTS

Stimulators so far have been largely ignored. The innovator of the simplest of these has been lost to posterity, but the tool had its origin in the Galvani-Volta controversy. It was a bimetallic forceps for applying minute stimuli to excitable parts during dissection; Claude Bernard was one of the early users (Brazier, 1959).

The inductorium, once almost universally used as a stimulator in physiology laboratories, was a derivative of Du Bois-Reymond's sliding secondary induction coil that he used for stimulation in nerve experiments on the demarcation currents. Basic to the equipment is a primary coil made up of several turns of heavy wire, a slideable concentric secondary consisting of many turns of fine wire, and a battery (or several) as the power input. Current starting to flow in the primary sets up an electromagnetic field that induces a pulse of electricity in the secondary. Depending upon the power input and the number of wire turns in each coil, an intense shock can be produced, reducible toward a threshold by moving the secondary coil outward on a long slide. An oscillatory make-break provided rapid-fire repetitive or faradic stimulation.

Other coils, some meticulously built, became available for a variety of electrotherapeutic uses, just as static machines had been used by past generations. In the United States the most commonly available inductorium for student laboratories was developed by H. P. Bowditch (1840–1895), who studied under Carl Ludwig (1816–1895) of Germany and was founder and first head of the Department of Physiology at Harvard Medical School. Bowditch's instrument was further modified in 1902 by W. T. Porter to provide an instrument that would put out very low currents without requiring a long slide. In Porter's instrument (the coil of the Harvard Instrument Company), the apparatus was elevated high enough to permit the secondary to be tipped from horizontal to vertical after being slid outward past the primary. It allowed a finely graded reduction in current strength down to zero. Modern stimulators are discussed in Chapter VII.

The rheotome of Bernstein consisted of a commutating switch controlled by an inductorium stimulator that shocked the nerve periodically (Hoff and Geddes, 1957). Later, and at an adjustable time, a circuit between the nerve and a sensitive slow-speed galvanometer was completed for a brief interval. After several rotations of the rheotome, the galvanometer attained a steady reading. By varying the time after the stimulus when the galvanometer was connected to the nerve, a series of readings could be made that, when plotted, reconstructed the form of the nerve action current.

Other developments at the turn of the century foreshadowed events to come (Dawson, unpublished). In 1883 Thomas A. Edison discovered the phenomenon of electron emission. This was followed in 1905 by J. A. Fleming's discovery of the diode and two years later by Lee De Forest's discovery of the triode, which paved the way for the construction of electronic amplifying circuits. An important technical contribution was the *Braun tube,* named for Carl Braun (1850–1918), the innovator of the cathode ray oscillograph and television tube. Its phosphor-coated internal face fluoresced when struck by electrons. Bernstein was the first to entertain the notion of using it for nerve recording, but the voltages required for its operation seemed impossible to manage. Nothing further came of the idea until the H. S. Gasser–J. Erlanger developments of the early 1920s.

MODERN CURRENT-VOLTAGE MEASURING INSTRUMENTS

Two late nineteenth-century recording instruments met well the needs of the twentieth century, the *A. d'Arsonval galvanometer* and the *Gabriel Lippmann–Jan Marey capillary electrometer.*

The d'Arsonval galvanometer involved a mirror mounted on a movable coil. A light beam was focused on this mirror, and when a current passed through the coil, it rotated, deflecting the light beam.

The capillary electrometer was a product of the combined skills of two scientists having different training and interests that coincided in the development of the instrument. Its influence upon the basic concepts of electrophysiological recording long outlasted its popularity. It could record briefer transients than was hitherto possible. Gabriel Lippmann (1845–1921) was a physicist. Early in his training he came under the influence of G. R. Kirchowoff, a pioneer in the theoretical aspects of electrical circuitry. At that time Lippmann's chief interest lay with electrocapillarity. Later he was to be awarded a Nobel Prize for developing a revolutionary theory of color photography. Lippmann died in the service of France near the end of a tour of duty that outlasted World War I.

H. J. Marey (1830–1894) had a multiplicity of interests. Geddes and Hoff (1961), to whom we are indebted for an account of the development and use of the capillary electrometer, credit him with knowledge of mechanics, electricity, and photography, which he used in wide-ranging studies of the phenomena of living organisms. His records, photographic and otherwise, of the gaits of men and animals and the flight of birds are of great importance in the history of cinematography; and to this day a selection from his works remains on display in Paris.[8]

Even before Lippmann and Marey, it was known that the shape of a drop of mercury was altered when it carried a current. Lippmann noted that if a current was passed through an interface between mercury and weak sulfuric acid, the crescent-shaped mercury meniscus would change in proportion to the current. By enclosing the interface in a capillary tube, the meniscus could be made to obscure part of a ray of light. Using a proper light source and suitable lenses, it was possible to obtain a shadow image of the mercury surface. The passage of current across the mercury-sulfuric acid interface would change the meniscus contour in response to variation in intensity of the current. By introducing a narrow slit between the electrometer and a moving photographic plate, the electric signal was convertible to a shadowgraph of a height that varied with current change. Figure 26 provides a sketch of the capillary system of the electrometer.

The earliest records made by Marey were of the turtle electrocardiogram in 1876 and the electrical organ of the torpedo in 1877. Geddes and Hoff (1961) indicate that with the use of the instrument two camps arose, one supporting and the other opposing its use. These judgments, based on technical considerations, referred to the operation and the interpretation of results. Until 1890, the records were used even though they involved a recognizably small error in response time. Thereafter, corrections were made.

Among the uses of the instrument were V. Burdon-Sanderson's repetition of Du Bois-Reymond's work on muscle currents and his proof of action potentials associated with the contraction of fly-catching plant leaves. In 1887 A. D. Waller

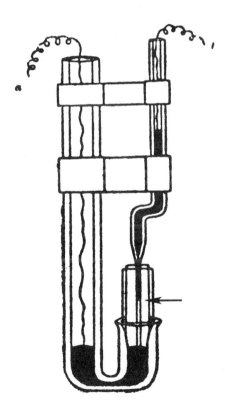

Fig. 26. The essential element of the capillary electrometer of Lippmann and Marey which operated according to the laws of static electricity. When a potential difference is applied to a tiny meniscus of mercury *(arrow)* in a glass capillary tube, it changes in shape. The meniscal change can be photographed with a shadowgraph moving film camera. (Drawing from Geddes and Hoff, 1961, p. 284.)

also concluded a classical study of the human electrocardiogram using the instrument. Even W. Einthoven, leader of the opposition, published work accomplished using the instrument (Rasmussen, 1947). With it, F. Gotch and V. Horsley recorded the first action potentials of nerve and described the action potentials of the spinal cord during cortically induced seizures.

E. D. Adrian was among the last to use the instrument in conjunction with a vacuum tube amplifier. He achieved an overall sensitivity of 10 microvolts and a response time of a few milliseconds. His classical papers on sensation obtained with the instrument won him his share of the Nobel Prize.[9]

The string galvanometer developed by Einthoven in 1903 became the standard electrocardiograph and was used for electrophysiological recording until the 1930s. It, too, had its difficulties. Records had to be made photographically and the metal-plated quartz fibers were difficult to prepare and broke easily. These hazards were less evident in electrocardiography, where the potentials recorded are of much higher voltage and thus require less sensitivity.

ELECTRONIC AMPLIFYING EQUIPMENT

The need for improved radio equipment and recognition that the triode vacuum tube could be used as an amplifier led to mass production of these tubes and a government effort during World War I to improve amplifying equipment. Alexander Forbes of Harvard (Eccles, 1970), while in the military service, came to know amplifying equipment and those who understood its use. In 1920 he and C. Thacher, using vacuum tube equipment, were able to amplify the nerve impulse displayed by an Einthoven (Hindle) string galvanometer from which permanent records could be made. Of the three possible techniques for interconnecting the amplifier and the string galvanometer, they selected the coupled condenser as best suited to recording voltage changes. This was a significant turning point in instrumentation, establishing a new electronic era for electrophysiology.

CATHODE RAY OSCILLOGRAPHY

By 1921 Herbert Gasser (Fig. 27) and H. S. Newcomer of Washington University had also developed an amplifier (triode tubes) suited to the purposes of physiology. They had succeeded in amplifying nerve action potentials to a point whereby they could be recorded with accuracy on the Einthoven string galvanometer[10] (Erlanger and Gasser, 1937). They soon realized, however, that neither the string galvanometer nor the capillary electrometer was quick enough to record accurately the form of the briefer nerve currents. They settled on the Braun tube to overcome these limitations (see Bishop, Chapter IX).

The moving part in such a tube is the electron beam, which, in the contemplated equipment, would be deflected by the action of the amplified potential derived from the nerve so that the changes would appear on the screen as an

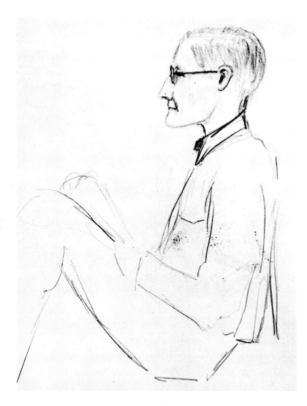

FIG. 27. Impromptu sketch of Herbert S. Gasser made by an unknown person at the time when the cathode ray tube was first used for nerve recordings.

illuminated deflected spot of light. This had the immeasurable importance of being photographable as it was viewed. Since the mass of the electron, the moving part in the system, is negligible, the recording instrument is without inertia. Out of this came accurate measurements of the duration of the action potential and of the refractory period and the resolution after conduction of the compound action potential into several fiber groups, each with differing conduction velocity and other characteristics. The last component to be discovered was the slowly conducting C wave, derived from the high-threshold nonmyelinated axons discovered by Remak long before by use of the light microscope.

COMMENT

Successful implementation of the knowledge of electricity during the eighteenth and nineteenth centuries contributed largely to the understanding of both its industrial and its biological potential. From random beginnings—including the development of friction machines to produce and the Leyden jar to store the mysterious force, Benjamin Franklin's proof that the lightning of thunderstorms and friction-generated electricity were the same, and the study of fish that exerted the mysterious force—man came upon one of the most important developments of modern technology. In particular, the disagreement between Galvani and Volta over the former's frog experiments led to the development of the principal fountainheads of animal and industrial electricity.

Innumerable lessons arise from a survey of the development of knowledge of animal electricity. They show how the scientific mind probes for the solutions of specific problems. They also reflect the periods of elation and dejection that occur as the pendulum swings between success and failure. Early in the nineteenth century, the physiologists were more successful than the physicists. They could devise their own equipment and prove its sensitivity through experimentation on frogs, both processes congenial with their temperament. Until 1850, the calibration of equipment was largely on a "does or does not" basis. By the century's end, the situation had reversed. Many of the physicist's devices were being adopted by the physiologist to improve recording accuracy and versatility.

Pursuing the trace of animal electricity as it leads into electrophysiology, problems that from our retrospect may appear to have been solved continued to nag the innovator. Solutions sometimes were rejected to be rediscovered by a successor. This happened to Nobili who, having shown the existence of the intrinsic frog current, later rejected the correct findings in favor of a thermoelectric effect. Matteucci, who strove to bring order to animal electricity studies, met his own paradox in seeking to resolve the inconsistency between the disappearance of intrinsic frog current during strychnine-induced muscle spasm and the ease of producing an induced twitch from another type of frog preparation. Seemingly contradictory, both actually contributed evidence for the existence of the still undiscovered action currents of nerve and muscle. Finally, Bernstein, who discovered the overshoot of the axon spike only to reject it later, missed the solution of a basic problem of his own membrane theory, which was later solved by Hodgkin and Huxley.

Much of the neuroscientific knowledge and technology used successfully in the twentieth century to explore the nervous system and analyze its activities is traceable directly to those who in the early nineteenth century developed the basic knowledge discoverable from nerve-muscle preparations. In the late nineteenth century, the improvement of stimulators for clinical use in electrotherapy and of galvanometers for recording purposes both aided the uncovering of the plan of cerebral localization and initiated the embryonic efforts to record brain potentials. Yet the effort to explore the brain more comprehensively had to await electronic amplification, the development of the cathode ray oscillograph, and effective "on-line" recorders with satisfactory frequency responses. The recorders could operate successfully over long time intervals as adjuncts to the oscillograph. Such developments have done more to advance our understanding of the epileptic process than any other line of investigation.

NOTES

[1] Gentlemen scientists of that period were as fascinated by electricity as Sir Henry Wotton (1568–1639), Izaak Walton's fishing companion and King James' ambassador to Venice, had been by optics the century before.

[2] The following extract is from Montaigne's essays:

And, in proof, the torpedo has this quality, not only to benumb all the members that touch her, but even through the nets to transmit a heavy dullness to the hands of those that move and handle them; nay, it is further said that, if one pour water upon her he will feel the numbness mount up the water to his hand and stupefy the feeling through the water. This is a miraculous force but 'tis not useless to the torpedo; she knows it and makes use of it; for to catch the prey she desires she will bury herself in the mud that other fishes, swimming over her, struck and benumbed with this coldness of hers, may fall into her power. (Hazlett, 1952, pp. 223–224.)

[3] John Hunter said in part:

The magnitude of the number of nerves bestowed on these organs in proportion to their size, must on reflection appear as extraordinary as the phenomena they afford. . . . If it then be probable that those nerves are not necessary for the purposes of sensation and action, may we not conclude that they are subservient to the formation, collection, or management of the electric fluid? Especially as it appears evident, from Mr. Walsh's experiments, that the will of the animal does absolutely control the electric powers of the body, which must depend on the energy of the nerves. How far this may be connected with the powers of the nerves in general, or how far it may lead to an explanation of their operations, time and future discoveries alone can fully determine. (*Works,* Vol. IV, pp. 409–410.)

In a later communication, Hunter claimed for John Walsh the honor of discovering animal electricity (Fig. 19).

[4] Unconfirmed stories circulate that Signora Galvani's physician ordered frog soup for her and that the cook had a batch of cleaned frogs on the kitchen table with an electrostatic machine nearby. Inadvertently the action of the machine set the frog legs to twitching.

[5] H. J. Marey of Paris wrote a science classic of the late nineteenth century entitled *Animal Mechanism: A Treatise on Terrestrial and Aerial Locomotion* (1874, pp. 52–53). It includes the following history of the investigation on the torpedo:

Musschenbroeck, in the last century, ascertained the electrical nature of the torpedo's discharge. Walsh, in 1778, saw plainly that the numbness produced by this animal differs in no respect from that which is caused by the discharge of an electrical machine. At a later period Davy obtained with the current of the torpedo the deflection of the galvanometer, the magnetization of steel needles placed within a spiral of brass wire traversed by the discharge, and the decomposition of saline solutions. Becquerel and Breschet verified the same facts in the wire of the galvanometer, the current passing from the back to the belly of the animal. The demonstration of the spark came still later. Father Linari and Matteucci obtained this spark by breaking in various ways a metallic circuit through which the current of the torpedo was passing. The most ingenious process is that of Matteucci who made use of a file in the following manner: A metallic plate attached to a brass wire is fixed under the belly of the torpedo; on its back is placed a file on which the end of a metallic wire rubs. The animal is then irritated and one or even several sparks are seen in the dark to pass between the wire and the file. The production of the spark is probably effected when the circuit is broken at the precise moment of passage of the torpedo's current. The use of the file is clearly seen, since the friction causing the circuit to be closed and broken at very short intervals, some of them will necessarily coincide with the discharge, as it has but a short duration . . . the production of two sparks during the discharge of the torpedo, shows very clearly that it has an appreciable duration, measured at least by the time which has elapsed during the passage of the wire across two successive teeth of the file.

[6] Finally, the reader should note that the electric fish played an important role in both bioelectricity and therapy. Kellaway (1946) states that the earliest man-made records of electric fish are represented in fishing scenes depicted on the walls of certain Egyptian tombs (ca. 2750 B.C.). The fish in those scenes is *Malopterus electricus,* the Nile electric catfish, which, due to the arrangement of the piles in series, is capable of producing a shock exceeding 450 volts!

[7] Cable theory views nerve and muscle fibers as cylindrical conductors surrounded by surface membranes that insulate them from the external electrolyte solution, endowing the fibers with properties analogous to those of a submarine cable. This is an analogy that cannot be pursued too far (Katz, 1966).

[8] The Marey Institute in Paris grew out of his "Commission internationale de contrôle des instruments enrégistreurs et l'unification des méthodes en physiologie." (Fenn, 1968.)

[9] E. D. Adrian (1889–   ) shared the Nobel Prize in Medicine for 1932 with C. S. Sherrington (1857–1952). He used the capillary electrometer with amplifier in his work on sensory nerve fibers.

[10] In an autobiographical sketch in *Perspectives in Biology and Medicine,* Paul C. Hodges writes of his experiences in 1916 with H. S. Gasser (then an instructor in physiology) in St. Louis, where they lived together in a rented room and worked together in the physiology laboratory. About Gasser's work with the Einthoven galvanometer, Hodges notes the following:

> Having learned from Walter Meek (of the University of Wisconsin) how to draw fine quartz fibers, silver them, and mount them as strings in the Einthoven galvanometer, H. S. hoped to be able to mount an unusually fine string with so little tension that it would respond to the action currents of nerves, much smaller than those produced by contracting cardiac muscle. He failed invariably because if the string was fine enough and lax enough to deflect with feeble currents, it would stick to the poles of the electro-magnets, and if tight enough not to stick to the magnets, would be too insensitive. What was needed, we concluded, was a string possessed of electrical sign but devoid of mass, but how to get it we could not guess. At length, groping for an answer but with nothing definite in mind, I neglected school work and jobs for a full day in the university library, located several miles away from the medical school campus. There, by good fortune, I found, among texts ordered by Arthur Compton in advance of his coming to the Department of Physics, a book by the Englishman, G. W. C. Kaye, and was introduced to the cathode ray tube. Its 'string' of electrons did, indeed, have electrical sign with no appreciable mass, but at the time neither H. S. nor I could figure out how it could be put to work recording the action currents of nerves. Four years later, after I had reached Peking, there came from H. S. a letter saying, 'The string with sign but no mass is at work.' And work it did for Herbert Gasser and Joseph Erlanger, bringing them the Nobel Prize (Hodges, 1973, pp. 28–29).

The reference to G. W. C. Kaye (1916) on X-rays was sought out to locate the pertinent passage. It occurs on page 15 of the second edition, under the heading "Braun Tube" and is very informative as well as having strong historical implications:

> A practical application, due to Braun, of the bending of cathode rays under magnetic or electric force has come into use in electrical engineering for the purpose of studying the wave-form of rapidly changing alternating currents. In the Braun tube, a narrow pencil of cathode rays is received on a fluorescent screen, and is subjected *en route* to both a magnetic and an electric field. The two fields are at right angles, and are both actuated by the alternating current. The cathode rays, having practically no inertia, are able to follow the most rapid vagaries of the fields, and so trace out on the screen a pattern, from which the wave-form can be deduced.

REFERENCES AND BIBLIOGRAPHY

Brazier, M. A. B. The historical development of neurophysiology, pp. 1–58. In J. Field, H. W. Magoun, and V. E. Hall, eds. *Handbook of Physiology, Section 1: Neurophysiology,* Vol. 1. Washington, D.C.: American Physiological Society, 1959.

Clarke, E., and O'Malley, C. D. *The Human Brain and Spinal Cord.* Berkeley: University of California Press, 1968. 926 pp.

Curtis, H. J., and Cole, K. S. Membrane resting and action potentials from the squid giant axon. *J. Cell. Physiol.* 19:135–144, 1942.

Dawson, A. S. The Evolution of Instrumentation for Neural Electrophysiology. M.S. thesis, Cornell University Graduate School (unpublished).

Du Bois-Reymond, E. *Untersuchungen über thierische Elektricität.* Berlin: Riemer, Vol. I, 1848, 743 pp; Vol. II, Pt. 1, 1849, 608 pp; Vol. II, Pt. 2, 1860, 579 pp.

Eccles, J. C. Alexander Forbes and his achievement in electrophysiology. *Perspect. Biol. Med.* 13(3):388–404, 1970.

Erlanger, J., and Gasser, H. S. *Electrical Signs of Nervous Activity.* Philadelphia: University of Pennsylvania Press, 1937. 221 pp.

Fenn, W. O., ed. *History of the International Congresses of Physiological Sciences, 1889–1968.* Bethesda, Md.: American Physiological Society, 1968. 100 pp.

Forbes, A., and Thacher, C. Amplification of action currents with the electron tube in recording with the string galvanometer. *Am. J. Physiol.* 52:409–471, 1920.

Fulton, J. F., and Wilson, L. G. *Selected Readings in the History of Physiology,* 2d ed. Springfield, Ill.: Charles C Thomas, 1966. 492 pp.

Gasser, H. S.   Emil Du Bois-Reymond (1818–1896), pp. 178–181. In W. Haymaker and F. Schiller, eds. *The Founders of Neurology,* 2d ed. Springfield, Ill.: Charles C Thomas, 1970.

Geddes, L. A., and Hoff, H. E. The capillary electrometer. The first graphic recorder of bioelectric signals. *Arch. Int. Hist. Sci.* 56–57:275–290, 1961.

Geddes, L. A., and Hoff, H. E. The discovery of bioelectricity and current electricity. The Galvani-Volta controversy. *IEEE Spectrum* 8(12):38–46, 1971.

Gotch, F., and Horsley, V.   Croonian Lecture VI. On the mammalian nervous system, its functions, and their localisation determined by an electrical method. *Philos. Trans. R. Soc. Lond.* [Biol.] 182:267–526, 1891.

Grundfest, H. Excitation at synapses. *J. Neurophysiol.* 20:316–327, 1957.

Grundfest, H.   Julius Bernstein, Ludimar Hermann and the discovery of the overshoot of the axon spike. *Arch. Ital. Biol.* 103:483–509, 1965.

Hazlett, W. C., ed. Essay 12, pp. 223–224. (Trans. by C. Colton.) In R. M. Hutchins, ed.-in-chief. *Great Books of the Western World,* Vol. II. Chicago: Encyclopaedia Britannica, Inc., 1952.

Hodges, P. C. An autobiographical sketch. *Perspect. Biol. Med.* 17:16–66, 1973.

Hodgkin, A. L. *The Conduction of the Nervous Impulse. (The Sherrington Lectures VII.)* Liverpool University Press, 1964. 108 pp.

Hodgkin, A. L., and Huxley, A. F. Action potentials recorded from inside a nerve fibre. *Nature* 144:710–711, 1939.

Hodgkin, A. L., and Huxley, A. F. Resting and action potentials in single nerve fibres. *J. Physiol.* 104:176–195, 1945.

Hoff, H. E., and Geddes, L. A. The rheotome and its prehistory: A study in the historical interrelation of electrophysiology and electromechanics. *Bull. Hist. Med.* 31:212–234, 327–347, 1957.

Hoff, H. E., and Geddes, L. A. Ballistics and the instrumentation of physiology. The velocity of the projectile and of the nerve impulse. *J. Hist. Med.* 15:133–146, 1960.

Hunter, J. Anatomical observations on the torpedo. *Philos. Trans. R. Soc. Lond.* [*Biol.*] 63:481–487, 1773.

Hunter, J. An account of the Gymnotus Electricus. *Philos. Trans. R. Soc. Lond.* [*Biol.*] 65:395–407, 1775.

Katz, B. *Nerve, Muscle, and Synapse.* New York: McGraw-Hill Book Co., 1966. 193 pp.

Kaye, G. W. C. *X-Rays,* 2d ed. London: Longmans, Green, and Co., 1917. 285 pp.

Kellaway, P. The part played by the electric fish in the early history of bioelectricity and electrotherapy. *Bull. Hist. Med.* 20:112–137, 1946.

Liddell, E. G. T. *The Discovery of Reflexes.* Oxford: The Clarendon Press, 1960. 174 pp.

Marey, H. J. *Animal Mechanism: A Treatise on Terrestrial and Aerial Locomotion.* New York: D. Appleton Co., 1874. 283 pp.

Matteucci, C. Sur le courant électrique ou propre de la grenouille. *Bibl. Univ. Genève* 7:156–168, 1838.

Matteucci, C. *Essai sur les Phénomènes Electriques des Animaux.* Paris: Carilian-Goeury and Dalmont, 1840. 88 pp.

Moruzzi, G. Electrophysiological work of Carlo Matteucci, pp. 139–147. In L. Belloni, ed. Per la storia della neurologia italiana. Atti del simposio internazionale di storia della neurologia. Varenna—30. VIII/1.IX, 1961. Milan: Istituto di Storia della Medicina Università degli Studi, 1963.

Pflüger, E. F. *Untersuchungen über die Physiologie des Electrotonus.* Berlin: August Hirschwald, 1859, 500 pp.

Rasmussen, A. T. *Some Trends in Neuroanatomy.* Dubuque, Ia.: W. C. Brown Co., 1947. 93 pp.

Walsh, J. On the electric property of the torpedo. In a letter from John Walsh to Benjamin Franklin (July 1, 1773). *Philos. Trans. R. Soc. Lond.* [*Biol.*] 63:461–462, 1773.

Walsh, J. Extracts of a letter from Mr. Walsh to Dr. Franklin dated Paris, 27th of August, 1772. *Philos. Trans. R. Soc. Lond.* [*Biol.*] 63:464–466, 1773.

Walsh, J. Extract of a letter from the Sieur Seignette, Mayor of la Rochelle, and second perpetual secretary of the academy of that city, to the publisher of the French Gazette. *Philos. Trans. R. Soc. Lond.* [*Biol.*] 63:466–477, 1773.

Chapter VI

NINETEENTH-CENTURY PHYSIOLOGISTS AND NEUROLOGISTS

There seems to be an insuperable objection to the notion that cerebral hemispheres are for movements . . . the reason, I suppose, is that the convolutions are considered to be not for movements but for ideas. (Taylor, 1931, p. 81.)

V. Hughlings Jackson

Some ancient writers placed the seat of motion and sensation in the cavities of the brain instead of in its substance, and Galen attributed epilepsy to sludginess of the phlegm lying within those cavities. Even after Vesalius, knowledge of the brain's interior developed slowly. According to Georg Procháska (1747–1820), Casper Bauhin (1560–1624) was among the first to deny that the cavities of the brain contained a laboratory for animal spirits and taught instead that sensation and motion were generated in brain substance. Thomas Willis (1621–1675) and others shared similar views. Yet, as some erroneous concepts were discredited, others just as wrong were accepted. For example, the seat of insanity was declared to be in the gray matter of the brain, epilepsy in the white. Combinations of epilepsy and insanity were explained by continuity.

The budding French school of experimental physiology played an important role in the clarification of thought (Clarke and O'Malley, 1968). J. J. C. Legallois (1770–1814), earliest of that school, demonstrated segmentation of the spinal cord and proved its sensory and motor properties. He also is credited with correctly placing the control of inspiratory breathing within the hindbrain just above the spinal cord. This was the first instance of the localization of any function within the brain. François Magendie (1783–1855) became well known for his controversies with Sir Charles Bell (1774–1842) over credit for restricting the spinal sensory inflow to dorsal spinal roots and motor outflow to ventral ones.

The work of Pierre Flourens (1794–1867) (Fig. 30) on the higher levels of nervous action was firmly nonlocalizationist in emphasis and supported cerebral nonexcitability. He discovered the *noeud vital* (respiratory center) of the hindbrain, loss of which results in cessation of breathing and death. Flourens also divided other brain functions between cerebrum and cerebellum, the former receiving and controlling sensation and the latter coordinating voluntary bodily movements. J. M. D. Olmstead (1953, pp. 290–291) may be quoted briefly on Flourens: "Suppression of the first (i.e., functions of the cerebrum) destroyed intelligence and will without abolishing the power to move—all spontaneity of movement was lost, though if movements were evoked they were still co-ordinated." Destruction of the second (function of the cerebellum) led to distur-

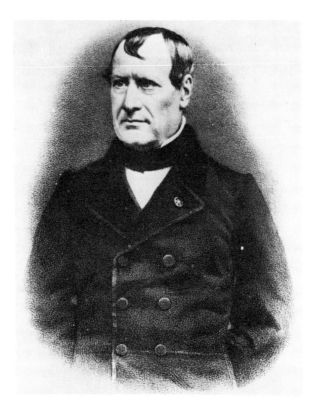

Fɪɢ. 28. Pierre Flourens (1794–1867). (Courtesy of National Library of Medicine, Bethesda, Md.)

bances in equilibrium of movement without altering intelligence. Such studies, however, provided only a temporary scaffold for the assembly of facts. They required radical revision by future investigators.

REFLEX MECHANISMS OF BRAINSTEM AND SPINAL CORD

Although not documented experimentally, G. Procháska's dissertation, translated into English in 1851 by T. Laycock for the Sydenham Society, was important in laying the groundwork for reflexology. He conceived of the "reflexive" system as coextensive lengthwise with the origins of sequentially arranged spinal and cranial nerves. He referred to his *sensorium commune* as the instrument that the soul directly uses for performing its own "animal" actions. For Procháska, the sensory components of cranial and spinal nerves met centrally and mingled with the complementary motor nerves, providing a "reflexion" of activity by which externally derived impressions were carried rapidly inward over sensory nerves, there to cross over into motor nerves for return to the corresponding muscles, thus occasioning movements. His sensorium commune included the spinal cord, the fullest extent of the brainstem, and the peduncles of cerebrum and cerebellum.

Marshall Hall (1790–1857), who followed Procháska, believed that the nervous system contained a special reflex system independent of the conventional motor outflow and sensory inflow. His concept of the spinal cord was that of an organ that might live an independent life separated from the brain. In this he could have been influenced by observations of spinal reflexes of beheaded criminals made by Francesco Redi (1626–1698), Robert Boyle (1627–1691), and Robert Whytt (1714–1766).

Hall's experiments were simple. They were performed on amphibians and reptiles. According to G. Jefferson (1953), only the interpretations, not the evidence on which they were based, were new. Hall believed the spinal cord could function independently after the overriding influence of the brain was withdrawn; the brain might sleep, the cord never did. It was when the brain nodded that the cord came into its own.

Hall saw that it would be impossible for a stimulus to reach the spinal cord without having an effect above or below the cord level at which the exciting nerve entered. Earlier it had been believed that switching from sensation to movement (as from one set of tracks to another) could actually occur within the outlying nerve plexuses that intervene between the spinal roots leaving the cord and the nerves supplying arms and legs. Jefferson (1953) remarks that by Hall's time the notion of the plexuses as switching yards had become outworn among the dissectors; and Hall's view, which advanced switching operations to the cord's interior, was a welcomed substitute. We are now certain that all such spinal reflex events occur within the gray interior of cord and brainstem.

Hall's theory of epilepsy, as outlined by Jefferson (1953), is especially interesting. He supposed that the reflexes of the high cervical cord became exaggerated and that the neck muscles were thrown into spasm as the result of an irritation arising anywhere in the body. The result was compression of the jugular veins within the neck, leading to congestion of the brain, which set off a violent convulsion. He explained the epileptic cry as a cause, not a warning, of an impending attack. Hall reached the conclusion that epilepsy was to be cured by performing a tracheotomy and thus ensuring proper oxygenation of the brain. Four cases were deemed cured on the basis of short-term observation, but there was only sparse, if any, evidence to support surgical intervention during an epileptic attack.

CONTRIBUTIONS OF BROWN-SÉQUARD TO EPILEPSY

Charles Eduoard Brown-Séquard (1817–1894) (Fig. 29) was a French physiologist of the line beginning with Legallois and Magendie. (See Olmsted [1946] for an excellent biography of Brown-Séquard, and Olmsted [1943] for additional material.) Brown-Séquard was also a clinical neurologist and a preceptor of Hughlings Jackson. Born on the island of Mauritius of an American father and

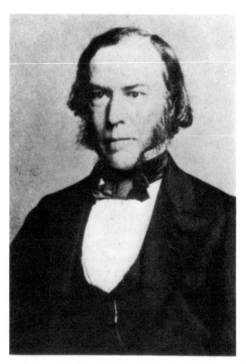

Fig. 29. Charles Edouard Brown-Séquard (1817–1894). (From Fulton, J. F., and Wilson, L.G., *Selected Readings in the History of Physiology,* 2d ed., 1966. Courtesy of Charles C Thomas, Publisher, Springfield, Ill.)

a French mother, he went to Paris for his medical education and thereafter turned to research, making the nervous system his principal interest.

Soon he became involved in a controversy with Sir Charles Bell of England (1771–1842) and F. A. Longet of France (1811–1871) over the crossing or noncrossing of sensory paths in the spinal cord (Olmsted, 1943). At the time he was an unknown who signed his communications C. E. Brown.

The polemics of the controversy were protracted by the vigorous objections of his distinguished opponents that the cord of the guinea pig, or even the rabbit, was too small to ascertain that the nerve tracts in the dorsal column, by which the noncrossed sensory impulses were transmitted, were included in the experimental half-sectioning of the spinal cord. A committee consisting of Pierre-Paul Broca[1] (1824–1880) as chairman, Claude Bernard (1813–1878), premier physiologist of the period, E. F. A. Vulpian[2] (1826–1887), and two veterinary professors carried out hemisections of the spinal cord both on a sheep and a horse at the veterinary school of Paris. The operations were successful and so were the dissections confirming the completeness of the experimental lesions. Broca wrote the committee's opinion supporting Brown-Séquard's claim that sensory pathways cross in the spinal cord over the claim of Bell and Longet. The report was read before the Société de Biologie, in Paris, on July 21, 1855. Broca, 7 years

Brown-Séquard's junior at the time, became the latter's enduring champion. (About this time Brown added his mother's to his father's name and became Charles Edouard Brown-Séquard.) Later he was to have an opportunity to confirm the condition known as Broca's syndrome (since studied by many generations of medical students) in a sea captain he examined in San Francisco. The captain had a paralysis on one side of the body and a loss of pain and temperature sensations on the other as a result of a lesion that half-severed the spinal cord at the cervical level.

Besides his absorbing interest in the nervous system, Brown-Séquard was an indefatigable worker and traveller. He taught and practiced medicine in Philadelphia, Richmond, New York, Boston, London, and, of course, Paris. He always valued his French origin. Ultimately, he was appointed to the Distinguished Professorship of Physiology at the Collège de France, succeeding Claude Bernard (1813–1878). His epilepsy research, however, does not show him at his best. He published his introductory paper on experimental epilepsy in 1851. The work began as an offshoot of his studies on spinal hemisection. As in those studies, he used guinea pigs as his principal experimental model. Mild attacks commenced 8 days postoperatively and increased in strength for 4 or 5 weeks. Then the animals went into what Brown-Séquard described as convulsions, characterized by violent jerking of the muscles of the face and front and hind legs. The convulsions lasted a quarter of an hour, when the animals supposedly became unconscious, and would not recur for several hours. A fit could be induced by pinching the face and neck on the side of the cord lesion, an area Brown-Séquard designated as the *epileptogenic zone.* Later he showed that the zone could be bilateral if the cord had been completely transected. Even later he noted that if his animals were kept within a restricted space and fed well, the convulsions were stronger and more frequent. If the animals were given open space and a less abundant diet, it became difficult to induce the attacks. Removal of the fore part of the brain did not affect their occurrence.

During such studies the experimental animals continued to bear and wean progeny. As they did so, Brown-Séquard observed signs of epilepsy in some of the offspring, which had not been operated on. Not all of the parents suffering from artificial epilepsy bore epileptic young, but in the many guinea pigs used in his experiments he claimed never to have seen spontaneous epilepsy in the young of parents that had not had spinal cord operations. He believed that the offspring had inherited some general alteration of the nervous system.

In 1869 Brown-Séquard reported that the unilateral section of a sciatic nerve could create an epileptogenic focus over the face and neck of the opposite side. Lice might accumulate in the zone, he said, even though the animal could scratch the site. T. Graham Brown (1909), an English physiologist, contended that what had been set off in the guinea pigs was not a convulsion at all but a vigorous scratch reflex, analyzed by Sherrington and others. This was a crushing blow to the idea of cutaneous epileptogenic zones, but by that time the theory had already been abandoned.

Brown-Séquard's start in the practice of neurology, which owed much to the efforts of a close friend, Charles Rayer (1793–1867), provided him with added income. Rayer referred to him patients who might benefit from the application of galvanic currents. This was a new treatment, also espoused enthusiastically by Magendie. The faradic current of Du Bois-Reymond (1847), however, proved more adaptable for therapeutic purposes, and Rayer lent Brown-Séquard one of the latter new machines for his use.

Brown-Séquard carried his experimental ideas over into his clinical neurological work. His practice, wherever he went, was composed largely of epileptics. In lectures given in Boston, in 1856, he especially stressed his concept of *aura epileptica,* by which he meant a portion of the body skin, differing in location from one individual to another, that seemed to activate seizures. In one person, he found a spot on one arm, and in another on the neck where applications of electric current incited convulsions of the whole body. He suggested that nerve centers of the spinal cord, rather than of the brain, were extremely sensitive to carbon dioxide in the local blood flow, setting off neural processes culminating in generalized convulsions. He called this theory of activation "action at a distance." It seems curiously reminiscent of Hall's theory.

By 1858, Brown-Séquard's influence was felt as strongly in England as in France, and he was appointed a physician at the National Hospital for the Paralyzed and the Epileptic in London. When Hughlings Jackson (1835–1911) arrived there as a young man, Brown-Séquard, who was in attendance, persuaded him to take up neurology. Eventually, Hughlings Jackson (Fig. 30) far overshadowed his former chief in epilepsy research.

During the London period, Brown-Séquard was sometimes credited with the introduction of bromides in the treatment of epilepsy (Olmsted, 1946), a priority that belongs to Locock (see Chapter III). In winning Jackson over to neurology, Brown-Séquard accomplished more for epilepsy than had anyone else of his period, for it was unquestionably Jackson who laid the foundations for our current clinical understanding of the epileptic process.

The relationship between the two men gives added importance to Jackson's several references to Brown-Séquard in his *Selected Papers* (Taylor, 1931). Jackson credits Brown-Séquard with a precise knowledge of the relation between external irritation and the production of convulsive paroxysms. This presumably refers to the "action at a distance" hypothesis and to the studies on guinea pigs with spinal lesions (Taylor, 1931, p. 16). Later he speaks somewhat plaintively of a difference between his views and those of Brown-Séquard, as follows (p. 231): "I am trying to show that diseases like epilepsy are not hereditary. But Brown-Séquard finds that epilepsy artificially produced in guinea pigs is hereditary." Finally, Jackson (pp. 362–365) describes in a patient a case of fits resembling those induced artificially in guinea pigs. Whatever their interpretation, those cases, involving "action at a distance," resemble what was described by Galen and his followers as "epilepsy by sympathy."

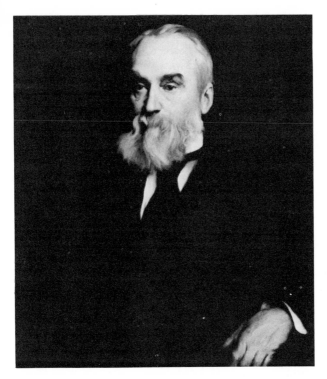

FIG. 30. John Hughlings Jackson (1835–1911). (By permission of the Royal College of Physicians of London.)

BEGINNING OF MODERN IDEAS ON EPILEPSY

Unquestionably, Jackson was the trailblazer necessary to the development of definitive techniques in neurology. In his lifetime the neuron doctrine came to fruition, and the significant work of the German school of electrophysiology was accomplished. Neuropathology and neurological surgery were born. No doubt Jackson relied most heavily upon his own observations, analyses, and syntheses. Yet his inquiring mind with its flair for detached, objective comprehension was broadened by the contributions of his predecessors and his contemporaries, some of whom could justly claim priority in the presentation of material similar to that from which Jackson's generalizations were drawn.

In 1827 L. F. Bravais gave much attention to a variety of epilepsy in which the seizures involved but one side of the body. He distinguished attacks that began in a side of the head, an arm or foot, or that were signalled by an aura referable to abdominal or thoracic viscera. He noted a subsequent paralysis of the affected side (Temkin, 1971).

R. Bright (1789–1858) combined a clinical and an anatomical approach to similar material. He detected lesions of the side of the brain (or covering membranes) opposite the body side affected. He studied speech involvement related to lesions on the left side and observed the retention of consciousness during seizures (Temkin, 1971).

R. B. Todd (1809–1860) described cases in which an arm or an arm and leg on the same side showed paroxysmally recurring seizures that began with sensation or motion or both, in which consciousness also was impaired, and which were followed by weakness or paralysis of the convulsed parts. He, too, traced such seizures to lesions at the surface of the brain on the side opposite the convulsed parts. Through the intervention of W. B. Carpenter (1813–1885), a popular physiological writer of the period, Todd's work became the basis for a theory holding that the two divisions of the basal ganglia (thalamus and corpus striatum) of the forebrain were the organs of cutaneous sensibility and automatized motion, respectively. Sensory impressions relayed from thalamus to striatum activated the latter (Temkin, 1971).

JOHN HUGHLINGS JACKSON (1835–1911)

An authoritative yet brief account of the spread of Jacksonian seizures is provided in a 13-page summary by F. M. R. Walshe (1961) and especially in his Section II, "On Movements and their Organization." Commenting on the state of neuroanatomical knowledge in the 1860s, Walshe reported that the pyramidal tract that courses between cerebral cortex and spinal cord was not recognized before 1875. Previously, the motor tract was presumed to emerge from the corpus striatum. Jackson himself speaks at times of an origin from the cerebral cortex and at others of a striatal origin. Both areas, in fact, are composed of gray matter, cortical and subcortical, respectively, and both lie within the distribution of the middle cerebral artery, which is one of the most stroke-prone regions of the brain. Describing convulsions commencing unilaterally, Walshe (1961, p. 122), paraphrased here for brevity, says:

> Jackson found them to develop from three foci in the order of frequency of thumb-index finger, face, and great toe. Such a convulsion could remain within the area in which it commenced, or it could spread, according to site of onset. As such a convulsion spreads up a limb, it does not do so like a wave leaving relaxed muscle in its wake, but intensifies in the muscles affected in their order of involvement.
>
> When spread occurs it follows a characteristic order of march, and exhibits a compound quality. For example, commencing in the foot it travels up the leg, then appears in the proximal upper limb, thereafter spreading to the hand. Beginning in the hand, it passes to the base of the upper limb and then involves face or hip girdle. When the spread from the initially involved parts crosses the midline, the convulsion appears first in the trunk musculature of the other side and then in the limbs of that side. At that time, if not earlier in the occupation of all three members of the side of origin, consciousness is lost. Brief loss of speech could accompany a convulsion occupying the right side of the face.

Jackson (Taylor, 1931) spoke of convulsions as expressions of discharging lesions, meaning that they are caused by excessive discharges of nerve cells. He also contrasted the results of discharging and destroying lesions, the latter resulting from a stroke or tumor that immobilized body parts in the supply of affected cortical areas.

The following is Jackson's most lucid description of what some current electro-physiologists would call the *epileptic neuron:*

> . . . The discharging lesion is of a few cells which have got far above the rest of the cortical cells in degree of tension and instability of equilibrium. The lesion is made up of cells of nervous arrangements which represent some special movements of a particular muscular region; the sudden and excessive development of these movements from the discharge of those cells is the convulsion incipient ("signal symptom" of Séguin) or if there be no spreading of the spasm, it is the convulsion total. (Taylor, 1931, Vol. I, p. 430.)

WILLIAM R. GOWERS, EPILEPTOLOGIST

A star of first magnitude at London's National Hospital, Queen Square, where Jackson also practiced, was William R. Gowers (1845–1915). He acquired a special following among neurologists whose primary interest relates to an understanding of what is going on in the rest of the patient as well as in his brain. A noted generalizer from clinical data, he spoke, in his *Epilepsy and Other Chronic Convulsive Diseases* (1885), of chronic convulsions as of "functional" origin and as divisible into two classes—epileptic and hysterical attacks. His characterizations of types of attacks were crisp, and his matter-of-fact generalizations suggested distillations from vast clinical experience. They were presented in a small reference work and covered every imaginable detail of academic importance—the predisposing and exciting causes, severe attacks, minor attacks, hysteroid fits, pathology, and treatment. His Hughlings Jackson lecture (1910) was a discourse on sensory discharge in epilepsy replete with exacting detail not to be found elsewhere.

Pathologically, Gowers (1885, p. 176) saw every neuron as a storehouse of latent energy, much like a charged Leyden jar or a bent spring. He thought the latter analogy more apt, saying that the energy of the spring is due to the force that bends it and depends on the resistance that keeps it bent. He also recognized a resistance to action by neurons and spoke of the role this plays in nervous activity. Today we ask, instead, "What keeps a neuron quiet?" Nevertheless, it is a fact that, collectively, the energy requirement of neurons is high, and many modern neurophysiologists might agree with the proposition that the power resources available within the brain, nascent or restrained, could be far greater than is ordinarily used. Indeed, the brain contains a powerhouse of potential energy. Yet, according to W. Weaver (1967), it uses only 10 watts in its moment-to-moment activity, less than what is required to keep a very dim light bulb lit.

WILLIAM ALDREN TURNER (1864–1945)

It may be said that Jackson and Gowers, in their writings, gave an illusion of detachment in time and place from their reading audience. Jackson, events proved, wrote also with a prescience of the future; Gowers wrote for those who would not underestimate the importance of the details of his experiences; whereas Turner, in *Epilepsy, a Study of the Idiopathic Disease* (1907), wrote of the realities of his time as they related to the problem of epilepsy. His opening statement defined epilepsy as "a chronic progressive disease of the brain characterized by the periodic occurrences of seizures in which loss of consciousness is an essential feature." He spoke of the apparent complacency of the Greek and Roman physicians who described the disorder. In today's view, the average epileptologist's attitude is not complacent but rather optimistic concerning outcome given a fair therapeutic break. The opinion is held that cases of severe manifestations with an ominous outcome are much outweighed in number by those having a reasonable chance of cessation of seizures due to a combination of modern antiepileptic drugs.

To those familiar with psychiatric history, the excessive emphasis of Turner on stigmata of degeneration in epilepsy is reminiscent of Augustin Morel (1809–1873). In all, Turner probably was more representative of the commonly held views than was any other writer of late Victorian England. His work is a valuable source for comparison with more recent collations of clinical experience.

COMMENT

Undue emphasis may have been given to Brown-Séquard's studies on epilepsy. Certainly, they left no lasting imprint on the research ledgers of his period. Other experimental studies, concerning cerebral anemia and trauma as causative factors, were equally unproductive. Collectively, their only value was the impetus they gave experimental research in epilepsy, which moved very sluggishly at the start. Brown-Séquard's conversion of Hughlings Jackson to neurology was, in fact, his major contribution to epilepsy.

The grouping of relevant aspects of nineteenth-century neurology and physiology in the same chapter emphasizes the singular value of the contributions of such neurologists as Jackson and Gowers to clinical knowledge of cerebral functioning. Today, the communications media, through lack of critical screening of science information, often obscure the firm line the professional draws between clinical research relating to neurological disorders involving speech, epilepsy, and the like in man and that generated in the animal experimental laboratory and later carried over to the human subject. The ethics of applying these results might be open to question at times. A noteworthy exception lies in the cerebral localization studies of Ferrier, outlined in the next chapter.

With respect to the clinical research approach, F. M. R. Walshe (1961) remarked that nature conducts the experiments and not the neurologist. In the clinical domain, animal experimentation, however sophisticated it becomes, cannot challenge the neurologist's advantage. He works within the well-defined boundaries of patient care in the exercise of his diagnostic abilities and analyzes his findings inductively and deductively. To the contrary, the physiologist, even one who works with higher apes, is handicapped in not being able to communicate with his subjects. Any successful clinical research endeavor related to the highest nervous functions must include such communication, and that is where the neurologist runs far ahead of the laboratory scientist in developing knowledge of psychoneural manifestations.

NOTES

[1] Pierre-Paul Broca was the discoverer of the motor speech center in the posterior part of the left inferior frontal convolution. His main work was in the field of anthropology, although he held the chair of *pathologie externe* in the School of Medicine in Paris.

[2] E. R. A. Vulpian was professor of pathologic anatomy at the School of Medicine in Paris after 1867. From internship days at the Salpêtrière, he was a close friend and collaborator of J. M. Charcot, who gave the following eulogy upon his death: "Alone durable and alone equitable in posterity; it piously cultivates the name of the scientist and preserves it as a 'glorious souvenir.' " From P. Bailey's translation (Guillain, 1959, p. 182).

REFERENCES AND BIBLIOGRAPHY

Brown, T. Graham. Studies in the reflexes of the guinea pig. The scratch-reflex in relation to "Brown-Séquard's epilepsy." *Q. J. Exp. Physiol.* 2:243–275, 1909.

Clarke, E., and O'Malley, C. D. *The Human Brain and Spinal Cord.* Berkeley: The University of California Press, 1968. 1926 pp.

Dawson, A. S. The Evolution of Instrumentation for Neural Electrophysiology. M.S. thesis, Cornell University Graduate School (unpublished).

Flourens, P. (Recherches Expérimentales sur les Propriétés et les Fonctions du Système Nerveux dans les Animaux Vertébrés. Paris: Chez Crevot, pp. 85–122, 1824.) Investigations of the properties and the functions of the various parts which compose the cerebral mass, pp. 3–21. In W. W. Nowinski, ed. *Some Papers on the Cerebral Cortex.* (Trans. from the French and German by G. von Bonin.) Springfield, Ill.: Charles C Thomas, 1960.

Fulton, J. F., and Wilson, L. G. *Selected Readings in the History of Physiology,* 2d ed. Springfield, Ill.: Charles C Thomas, 1966. 492 pp.

Gowers, W. R. The Hughlings Jackson lecture on special sense discharges from organic disease. *Brain* 32:303–326, 1909.

Gowers W. R. *Epilepsy and Other Chronic Convulsive Diseases: Their Causes, Symptoms and Treatment,* 1885. Reprinted. New York: Dover Publications, 1964. 255 pp.

Guillain, G. *Charcot, 1825–1893; His Life—His Work.* (Edited and translated by P. Bailey.) New York: Paul B. Hoeber, Inc., 1959. 202 pp.

Jefferson, G. Marshall Hall, the grasp reflex and the diastaltic spinal cord, pp. 304–320. In E. A. Underwood, ed. *Science, Medicine and History,* Vol. 2. London: Oxford University Press, 1953.

Olmsted, J. M. D. The aftermath of Charles Bell's famous "Idea." *Bull. Hist. Med.* 14:341–351, 1943.

Olmsted, J. M. D. *Charles Edouard Brown-Séquard.* Baltimore: The Johns Hopkins Press, 1946. 253 pp.

Olmsted, J. M. D. Pierre Flourens, pp. 290–302. In E. A. Underwood, ed. *Science, Medicine and History,* Vol. 2. London: Oxford University Press, 1953. 646 pp.

Prochárska, G. *A Dissertation on the Functions of the Nervous System,* pp. 363–450. Translation by T. Laycock for the Sydenham Society, 1851.

Rasmussen, A. T. *Some Trends in Neuroanatomy.* Dubuque, Ia.: W. C. Brown Co., 1947. 93 pp.

Taylor, J., ed. *Selected Writings of John Hughlings Jackson, Vol. 1. On Epilepsy and Epileptiform Convulsions.* London: Hodder and Stoughton, Ltd., 1931. 500 pp.

Temkin, O. *The Falling Sickness. A History of Epilepsy from the Greeks to the Beginnings of Modern Neurology,* 2d ed. rev. Baltimore: The Johns Hopkins Press, 1971. 467 pp.

Turner, W. A. *Epilepsy—A Study of the Idiopathic Disease.* London: Macmillan & Co., Ltd., 1907. 272 pp.

Walshe, F. M. R. Contributions of John Hughlings Jackson to neurology. *Arch. Neurol.* 5:119–131, 1961.

Weaver, W. *Science and Imagination. Selected Papers of Warren Weaver.* New York: Basic Books, Inc., 1967. 295 pp.

Chapter VII

CEREBRAL LOCALIZATION

Many persons, mocking, ask—What has Mind to do with brain substance, white and grey?

Alexander Bain
(1882, p. 1)

The thrust of neurological research during the last two centuries has led to the judgment that the human cerebral cortex is at the top of a neuraxial hierarchy in the same way that man's behavior surpasses that of his closest relatives among the apes. In the recent past the frontier at which man emerged from primate stock has been pushed back from 100,000 to several million or more years, and the slow evolutionary trek is recognized to have been much longer than once supposed. Civilized man may have existed before the Sumerians, who had a flourishing civilization in 4000 B.C. The evolution of the brain as the base of human intelligence could have been a much longer process than was heretofore thought.

Much of the validity of behavioral theory depends on whether the cerebral cortex is an organ of itself or whether it is composed of many organs. The former view is traceable to P. Flourens (1824), the latter to F. J. Gall (1758–1828) and G. Spurzheim (1776–1832). Flourens held that the parts of the nervous system have specific properties, but that all in effect belong to a single system. He did not accept the view that localization exists within the cerebrum; special senses and the intellectual faculties, in his belief, are represented throughout.

J. M. D. Olmsted (1953), in discussing Flourens' book *Examen de la Phrénologie,* credits him with a major service to neurology by overthrowing the pseudoscience of phrenology. As long as Gall adhered to anatomical facts, he was on sound ground, but he went too far in attempting to localize 30 or more faculties in various regions of the brain and in theorizing that any well-developed character trait would require a corresponding local growth of nervous structure and be reflected in a protuberance of overlying bone (Olmsted, 1953). In the process of refuting the phrenologists, Flourens swung the pendulum of localization back too far. Not until 1870 did G. Fritsch and E. Hitzig return it again.

Localization was furthered by the clinical studies of P. Broca (1824–1880) on aphasia in 1861. He reported a clear-cut case in which a patient with a chronic loss of speech (aphasia) was shown to have a localized frontal lobe lesion. His report of the autopsy findings, translated by G. von Bonin in *Some Papers on the Cerebral Cortex* (Nowinski, 1960, p. 66), follows:

> On the lateral side of the left hemisphere, at the level of the Sylvian fissure, the pia mater is lifted up by a collection of transparent serum which lies in a large and profound depression of the cerebral substance. When this fluid was evacuated by a puncture, the pia mater became profoundly depressed, and there

resulted a long cavity about as large as a hen's egg, which corresponded to the Sylvian fissure, hence separated the frontal and the temporal lobes. . . .

Broca noted that the original seat of the lesion was in the second or third frontal convolution, more likely in the latter. Hughlings Jackson in 1864 reported the case of a girl who at age 17 developed loss of speech with right-sided hemiplegia. She married and died some years later during labor without having regained her power of speech (Clarke and O'Malley, 1968, pp. 500–501), substantiating Broca's claim of a localized speech center.

EVIDENCE CONCERNING CEREBRAL STIMULATION

One of the persistent questions of the nineteenth-century controversy over cerebral localization was whether or not the cerebrum was excitable. Before the voltaic cell, galvanic stimulation was not possible, and faradic stimulation by the Du Bois-Reymond induction coil did not become available until 1847. Hence, the earliest studies of excitability depended on pinching, pricking, or rubbing the cortex and looking for muscular contractions. Zinn and Haller (1760) reported convulsive movements after lesions of the white matter of the brain, but these statements were not believed later. Among those who reported negative results were F. Magendie (1783–1855), P. Flourens, C. Matteucci, using electrical currents, E. H. Weber (1795–1878), F. A. Longet (1811–1871), and M. Schiff (1823–1890). Longet summarized the data thus:

> On dogs, rabbits and some kids we have irritated with a knife the white substance of the cerebral lobes, we have cauterized them with potash, nitric acid, etc.; we have run galvanic currents through them in all directions without succeeding in evoking involuntary muscular contractions. The same negative results were found in directing these agents to either grey or white matter. (Walker, 1957, p. 438)

THE CORTICAL STIMULATION EXPERIMENTS OF FRITSCH AND HITZIG

A. E. Walker (1957) indicates that the birth of modern cortical stimulation occurred on the dressing table of a small Berlin home, used because the university laboratories were overcrowded and had no space for more research. Both investigators, G. Fritsch (1838–1927) and Eduard Hitzig (1838–1907), were somewhat over 30; perhaps more experienced scientists would have been influenced unduly by the many earlier negative results. Fritsch had pursued a varied, often adventuresome, career as a physician and explorer. While dressing a head wound during the Prusso-Danish War in 1864, he provoked muscular contractions upon the opposite side of his patient. He regarded this not as a mere accident but as a phenomenon demanding explanation.

Hitzig (1871) had prior experience of a different sort. He had noticed that when a current was applied across the human head with electrodes situated on the temporal area, the subject's eyes moved. Since this occurred in even the sightless, Hitzig reasoned that it was directly elicited rather than a secondary result of induced vertigo. Thus, both men had cause to believe that the human brain was electrically excitable. Hitzig also had conducted experiments indicating that a current applied at the back of the skull caused rotation of the eyes. The further experiments, undertaken together, proved to be of significant historic value for their positive results, for the methods used, and for the research avenues opened up to neurophysiology.

In appraising the achievements of Fritsch and Hitzig, another historic investigator has been overlooked too often. L. N. Simonoff first used implanted electrodes to stimulate the brainstem of unanesthetized animals (Simonoff, 1866; Doty, 1969). His experiments were largely forgotten until W. R. Hess (1928) undertook the experimental sleep studies in the 1920s, for which he was later awarded the Nobel Prize.

The Fritsch-Hitzig studies (Nowinski, 1960) were conducted on dogs under ether anesthesia, exposing but one hemisphere, minimizing blood loss, and leaving a bony bridge to protect the midline venous sinus. Nonpolarizable, platinum stimulating electrodes were used, minimizing damage due to application of current. The electrodes were made with pinpoint terminals to lessen the chance of damage to tissue or its blood supply. They were bipolar, insulated with guttapercha, and their paired tips lay close together. A galvanic current provided the stimulus. The investigators' own tongues determined its threshold tingle, which was then applied to the brain. With a maximum stimulus of 11 volts and 1 milliampere of current, the entire convexity of dog cerebral cortex was explored. Only the anterior region produced motor responses. Frontal stimulation on one side caused muscular contraction of the opposite limbs. With weak stimuli the responses were quite specific; an excessive stimulus caused a convulsion. Ablations of corresponding frontal areas resulted in contralateral motor deficits. These experiments opened the higher brain centers to physiological study. The future of cortical localization depended on their success.

Charcot (Guillain, 1959) had said that up until 1860 the Flourens doctrine (von Bonin, 1952) was not debated and that the brain was generally conceded to be a homogeneous organ in which all parts were equivalent. In different words C. S. Sherrington (1928) made a similar remark in an obituary on Ferrier: "Current scientific opinion, physiological and medical, at that time," he said, "held that the cerebrum was the 'organ of mind' and, being a unity, presented as regards its mode of functioning no detectable spatial difference."

Fritsch is a fine example of the kind of versatile mind that is so valuable in science. As a man of means, he was able to follow at least three distinctive life interests in addition to the work on cerebral localization that made his lasting reputation. He visited South Africa to study the electric fish. As an anthropologist, he utilized his photographic skill to display the beauty of the human body in opposition to the prudery of his time. The human retina was his third interest, and he toured the world seeking support for a theory that there were racial differences in visual acuity. To prove his point, he carried out physiological tests and also gathered retinal specimens fixed within the hour of death. Yet he had won immortality on his first throw of the dice, realizing his avid desire to prove a single important point, the excitability of cerebral cortex.

Next on the scene was David Ferrier (1843–1928). He was a pupil of A. Bain (1818–1903), a Scottish logician and psychologist. Using a model of the human brain that he kept on his classroom desk, Bain described the nervous system, stressing the union of physical and psychological mechanisms. The quotation at the head of this chapter is the first sentence of his classical work, *Mind and Body* (Bain, 1882).

After graduating in medicine, Ferrier acted temporarily as assistant to T. Laycock, who translated the Procháska dissertation referred to in the last chapter. Later he worked as assistant to a physician in Suffolk. There he used his spare time to study the comparative anatomy of the brain. In 1870 Ferrier was appointed Lecturer on Physiology at the Middlesex Hospital, London. He and his friend, Crichton Brown, Director of the West Riding Asylum, discussed the questions raised by the recent reports from Germany by Fritsch and Hitzig. Brown willingly provided space, animals, and equipment, and Ferrier's memorable career began in earnest. His plan was an ambitious one—to explore by faradic stimulation all parts of the nervous systems in all vertebrates, high and low. In Sherrington's opinion, his choice of faradic over galvanic stimuli was an important advance past earlier work, making possible the elicitation of sustained and deliberate, instead of twitch-like, movements without causing tissue damage.

A grant from the Royal Society helped him to include observations of the brain of the ape, an organ much closer to the human brain than that of any other animal. It seems that he was the first person since Galen to explore an ape's brain. Ferrier put cerebral localization of function on the basis of proven experimental fact (Ferrier and Yeo, 1884). He located the motor cortex as lying in front of the Rolandic sulcus and extending on to the mesial aspect of the brain. Its area was shown to be greater and its character of opposite-side response more complex than that of species lower on the animal scale. Furthermore, he showed that the results of stimulation of a given motor area could be predicted.

Destruction of limited portions of motor cortex had more serious effects in apes than in dogs, paralyzing the whole of the opposite side of the body. At a showing of his hemiplegic apes to a European neurological conference in 1881, Charcot (1825–1893), premier neurologist of France in his period and a keen observer, was heard to exclaim, "It is a patient!" For those days that was an important pronouncement, as Ferrier was then contending against F. L. Goltz (1834–1902), another physiologist, who had done large cerebrectomies in dogs and denied evidence of localization of cortical function.

After his operative successes in monkeys, Ferrier (Fig. 31) asserted that man's brain offered no prohibitive surgical difficulty save that of antisepsis. In 1883 a Glasgow surgeon operated for the second time for intracranial disease; and in the next year the pioneer operation for removing a cerebral tumor was carried

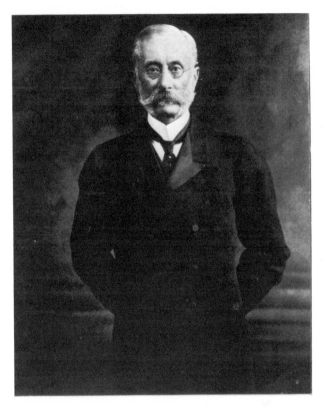

Fig. 31. Sir David Ferrier (1843–1928). (From Haymaker, W., and Schiller, F., eds., *The Founders of Neurology,* 1953. Courtesy of Charles C Thomas, Publisher, Springfield, Ill. Photo from Dr. John F. Fulton; Photographer: Maull & Fox, London.)

out, correctly localized by knowledge gained initially through animal experiments (Ferrier and Yeo, 1884). Ferrier became the target of persecution by antivivisectionists, but the publicity led to the rapid growth of his consulting practice.

Like Fritsch and Hitzig, Ferrier, with little prior knowledge, had entered a field about which few knew anything. He used an animal species closer to man and probed more profoundly and successfully than did his predecessors. Thus, he linked the details of localization to the human brain.

According to A. E. Walker (1957), confirmation of the studies of Fritsch and Hitzig in humans occurred during the year following their work. An American woman of Cincinnati, Ohio, granted her surgeon, R. Bartholow (1874), permission to insert wires through the granulation tissue overlying the crater of a cerebral abscess. Needles were inserted to the dura, which covered the left posterior convolutions, and current was applied with resulting muscular contractions in the right arm and leg. Figure 32 shows a 1908 map of localization in the human cortex which originated with Harvey Cushing. Later O. Foerster (1936) of Germany and W. Penfield and H. Jasper (1954) of Montreal became adept at stimu-

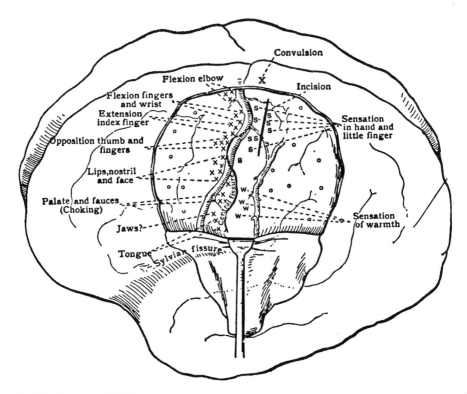

Fig. 32. Early map (1908) of cortical localization in man compiled by Harvey Cushing, who founded U.S. neurological surgery. (From Fulton, J. F., and Wilson, L. G., *Selected Readings in the History of Physiology,* 2d ed., 1966. Courtesy of Charles C Thomas, Publisher, Springfield, Ill.)

lating the human cerebral cortex electrically to determine the sites of epileptogenic involvement in cases of incurable epilepsy of focal origin. In the process they confirmed and extended preceding work, using the normal responses to stimulation of surrounding cortex to guide their assessments of the borders of the epileptogenic cortex that required removal (Fig. 35).

Different investigators obtained varying motor maps using galvanic stimulation, showing the postcentral as well as the precentral gyrus to contain motor points. V. Horsley and A. E. Schafer (1888), for example, explored the cortex of monkey and orangutan. However, A. S. F. Leyton (1869–1921) and C. S. Sherrington (1857–1952), employing unipolar faradization (by an induction coil) to explore the cortex of 16 anthropoids, including orangutan, chimpanzee, and gorilla, reported (1903) that the excitable areas that activate movement were confined to the pre-Rolandic cortex.[1] This was long the authoritative position, although it was challenged occasionally.

E. G. T. Liddell and C. G. Phillips (1950) became especially cognizant of the importance of depth of anesthesia and form and duration of stimulus to studies

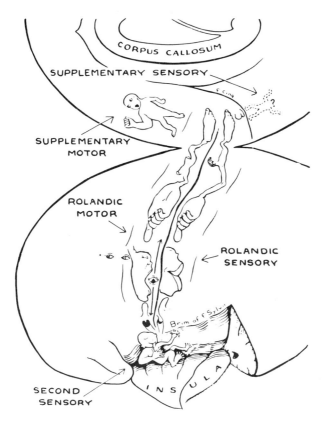

FIG. 33. Somatic figurines drawn upon the pre- and postcentral areas of the left human cerebral hemisphere. (From Penfield and Jasper, 1954.)

such as those discussed here. Using a square-wave stimulus activated from a thyratron stimulator giving pulses of five-thousandths of a second duration, they showed that movements could be elicited from the opposite side of the face, the thumb-index finger of the hand, and the great toe over much wider areas of motor cortex than those that excited larger body parts. This indicates that what F. M. R. Walshe (1961) called the "leading parts" of the Jacksonian seizure have the widest distribution within the cell arrangement of cortex. The Liddell-Phillips team indicated that sufficiently intense stimulation of cortical surface can spread downwards to activate directly the pyramidal cell axons as they plunge into the white matter. Thus, they short-circuited the complex of excitatory and inhibitory effects that activate discrete movements upon threshold stimulation of the overlying gray matter.

In comparing the results of modern cortical stimulation with earlier work, it should be remembered that the technology of stimulation has come a long way since the galvanic make-and-break of the early nineteenth century and the induced tetanizing currents of Du Bois-Reymond. Today's stimulators are quite versatile as to frequency output, wave shape, duration, and current and voltage parameters, a multivibrator circuit being at the heart of each unit.

Over the last quarter century, maps based on surface stimulation have been supplemented by others produced through adaptation of electrophysiological techniques that utilize potentials evoked in special and general sensory cortex after stimulation of eye, ear, and body surface. The evoked potential method has shown that the pre-Rolandic motor cortex has a sensory input as well as a motor output to lower centers. General sensory cortex is also said to have a well-organized, although subordinate, motor outflow. These motor points lie in back of the central Rolandic fissure.

The latest developments have been the delineation of maps of sensory and motor cortices for each body part (foot, leg, torso, arm, hand, and face) to show an areal representation proportionate to the sensory reception and the diversity of the movements it controls. With leg and foot at the upper midline and face next to the Sylvian fissure, the other body parts lying between, corresponding motor and sensory maps meet along the axis of the Rolandic sulcus. Foot, hand, and face representations lie closest to the sulcus with the back farthest away. Such mapping of the human brain was first undertaken by W. Penfield and H. Jasper (1954) (Fig. 33), the resulting figurines being called *homunculi*. In monkeys, C. N. Woolsey and associates (1958) named the maps *simunculi* (Fig. 34). Corresponding schemata have also been worked out for lesser mammals. The body shape disproportion inherent in such mapping shows how the allotments of brain organization oversee the body parts controlled, ludicrous as the size and shape distortions may seem.

Historically, other writers espoused seats for epilepsy at several levels of the nervous system, including spinal cord, medulla, and midbrain. The designation of any such "seat of functioning" is capricious, be it related to a normal process such as sleep or consciousness or to an abnormal one such as the spread of an epileptic attack. The cerebral cortex should be recognized as an extensive sheet-

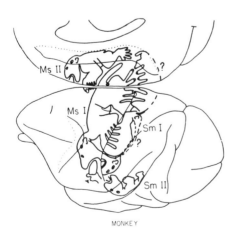

MONKEY

Fig. 34. Motor and sensory figurines, macaque monkey. (From Schaltenbrand and Woolsey, 1964.)

like reservoir of closely spaced and richly interconnected neurons. Thus, it provides abundant opportunity for the direct spread of a hyperexcitable process across the cortex as well as by downward-directed pyramidal cell discharges passing via axons that provide tandem linkages with the brainstem and spinal centers.

In an essay on normal brain functioning, R. W. Gerard and B. Libet (1939) emphasized the slow, sinelike potentials that arise from neuron masses beating in unison (like the human alpha rhythm) as an expression of slow cyclic changes that occur in neuronal activity. The same rhythm as that of the masses also can be recorded from single neurons through microelectrodes, leading to the presumption that the beat of neurons over wide areas is synchronized. It seems possible that the massive synchronization of neurons in an epileptic seizure could arise in such manner.

STEREOTAXIC TECHNOLOGY FOR EXPLORING THE CEREBRAL INTERIOR

Cerebral localization is not only concerned with the allocation of functions to parts of the exposed cerebral cortex, but also with the deep-lying neuron aggregates of the subcortex, such as hippocampus, striatum, thalamus, and brainstem. Imagine using skull landmarks to construct a tridimensional grid of the cerebral interior and a stereotaxic technology that permits placement of an electrode tip within any millimeter cube of the brain's interior. With the use of such a rig, electrical currents could be used to activate selected neuronal aggregates. If connected through amplifiers to an ink-writer or cathode ray oscilloscope, records of electrical activity generated by the cells in contact with the tip also could be obtained. By replacing needle electrodes with microelectrodes and directing them to known points in depth, even single neurons could be heard from. Finally, such equipment could make possible painless implantation of electrodes for recording on a chronic basis in freely moving, unrestrained animals, or such electrodes could be used to produce behavioral alterations by threshold or higher stimulation. Many if not all these objectives have been accomplished using Clarke-Horsley stereotaxic equipment.

R. H. Clarke (1850–1926) (Fig. 35), a physician with engineering ability, envisioned and designed such a technology, calling it at first *rectolinear cranioencephalic topography*. The first account of its development was provided in 1906 by Sir Victor Horsley in the proceedings of a meeting of the British Medical Association at Toronto. Almost half a century elapsed before the initial use of a revision of Clarke's equipment to aid the neurosurgical treatment of patients with intractable epilepsy and Parkinson's disease. Its range of values in the conduct of clinical procedures had been considered by Clarke and Horsley early in the equipment's development.

Clarke is a fascinating example of the future-oriented scientist. His boyhood spanned the 1850s (Davis, 1964). Those were the years of which G. M. Young

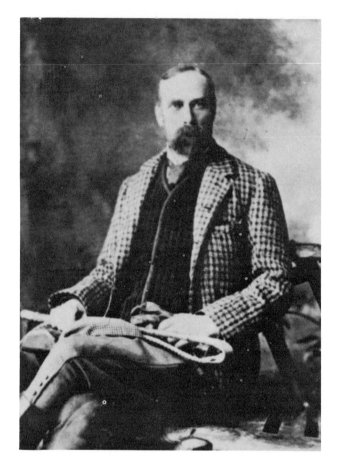

Fɪɢ. 35. Robert Henry Clarke, 1850–1926. (From Davis, 1964, by permission of *Surgery, Gynecology & Obstetrics.*)

(1953, p. 77) wrote in *Victorian England:* "Of all decades of our history, a wise man would choose the eighteen fifties to be young in." In London, then the world's center, medicine and scientific research were making giant strides. Britain had been free of war for several decades and was enjoying unparalleled economic prosperity. For epilepsy, it was the decade of Locock, who found the first effective treatment for the disorder.

Clarke attended Queens College, Cambridge, and began the study of medicine at St. George's Hospital, London, in 1872. An accomplished athlete, he represented his school in cricket and football and rowed in the Queen's boat. At medical school he participated in rugby.

In the 1890s, Ferrier and Horsley were bright on the scientific horizon and Clarke eventually joined Horsley in research at the Brown Institute, London. Sometime thereafter, to hasten recovery from a pneumonia that developed from

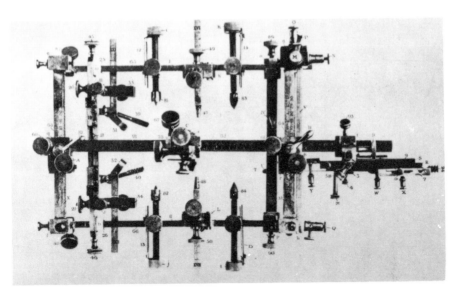

Fig. 36. Clarke-Horsley stereotaxic apparatus. (From Davis, 1964, by permission of *Surgery, Gynecology & Obstetrics.*)

aspiration of an aspirin tablet, he travelled to Egypt. On that trip he developed the basic ideas for the stereotaxic instrument; on his return he presented them to his colleague, Horsley.

The scheme was a revolutionary one, but Horsley received it cordially. Under contract, James Swift of London built the first instrument for them in 1905. In those days the original machine cost only 300 pounds (Fig. 36). A patent was not obtained until 1914. Between 1905 and 1910, Clarke and Horsley did a tremendous amount of work together, including the exact placement of the first minute lesions in the animal nervous system. They also published a definitive paper on use of the technology (Horsley and Clarke, 1908).

Unhappily, Clarke came to believe that Horsley, who had meanwhile attained world fame as a surgeon and scientist, had not given him due credit for his part in their joint accomplishment. He also vented his frustration on the Royal Society, blaming it for not supporting stereotaxic research when it failed to grant 20 pounds requested by another of his collaborators, Henderson. Considering the ultimate importance of those pioneer studies, Clarke's feelings are understandable. He practiced medicine for much of the remainder of his life and died in 1926. Horsley had died in 1916, while serving with the King's army in Mesopotamia.

Richard A. Davis (1964), who became Clarke's biographer, praised the contribution for sheer brilliance of imagination and originality in achieving a specific goal. He stressed Clarke's mechanical ability and concentration on detail. Certainly, the man deserved much more recognition than he received, a reminder in these days of public relations that prizes may result sometimes more from promotion than from merit.

GENERAL BASIS OF CEREBRAL CORTICAL STRUCTURE

The ultimate depth of neurobiological understanding of nervous mechanisms will depend on the precision with which fine structure interpretation can be related to knowledge of function. Architectonics, once a popular work among neuroanatomists, covers cellular arrangements common to all cortex. The term also implies diversification to suit different functions. Out of such specializations the features arise that identify regions of different architecture.

A review of the simpler facts that concern the cerebral cortex will both aid in the understanding of its structure and emphasize its extent and complexity. Measurements have established that the cortex is a continuous sheet of gray matter some 770 square centimeters in extent. It comprises a little less than half the weight of the brain, and its surface is furrowed by convolutions, some of which are 2 to 3 centimeters in depth and branch at their base. The thickness of the cortex may be less than 1.3 millimeters at the bases of the sulci and 4 millimeters at the crowns of the convolutions.

Some estimate that the entire brain has a population of 10 billion nerve cells; others say that there are that many in the cortex alone. Individual cortical neurons vary upward in size from that of a red blood corpuscle, smallest of the body's cells, to just under naked-eye visibility. About half of all cortical cells are glia (the brain's own supportive and nutritive tissue). Those play an indirect role in normal nervous operations, but possibly a substantial one in the prevention of epileptic seizures.

The chief cells of the cortical circuits have bodies in the shape of truncated cones and tapering dendritic shafts that reach terminal arborizations within the subsurface cortical layer (Fig. 37). They are called pyramidal cells by microscopists. Because of their generally larger size and prominent dendritic shafts, they lend a dimension of verticality to the microscopic appearance of the cortex.

In another type of tissue preparation, however, the cell bodies also give the appearance of being packed into transverse layers, like a multilayered cake. Pyramids of even the deepest layers send dendritic shafts to the cortical subsurface, and since cortical thickness is a maximum of 4 millimeters, the dendrite shafts of the lowest layers are unusually long, in fact, the longest of the nervous system. Estimates of 60,000 terminal contacts by multibranched axons have been made for individual pyramids, and Lorente de Nó (1953) estimates that only 6% of those occur on the membrane of the cell body, the remainder being made on the dendritic arborizations. Thus, the fictional Hercule Poirot's "little gray cells" are in reality a maze of branching dendrites of neurocellular origin, and the principal component of cortical neuropil. Figure 38 illustrates the dendritic components of the cortical plexus (left) and the axonal components (right). Electron microscopy reveals axons and dendrites of the plexuses in close contact, forming axodendritic synapses by the thousands. Such complexity might give pause even to M. Poirot.

The vertical as compared with the horizontal (transverse) dimension of the

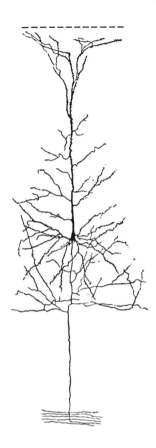

FIG. 37. Pyramidal neuron, cerebral cortex, surface of cortex up. Note subsurface dendritic arbor and axon with recurrent collaterals. Axon stem directed downwards. *Broken line* above, cortical surface. (From Ramón y Cajal, 1955*b*, p. 535.)

cortical cell layers has workaday, as well as historical, significance. In the study of cortical cytoarchitectonics, still to be discussed, the emphasis on parcellation of fields is chiefly connected with differences in makeup of the transverse cellular layers. Some physiologists of an earlier era believed one could incapacitate the surface layers in animal experiments and record electrically from the deeper ones alone. To them the cortex was truly a cake of separate layers. They forgot the magnificent illustrations of whole cortical pyramids by Rámon y Cajal and Golgi. By clipping away the subsurface arbors, they left dead cell bodies and their dendrite shafts behind.

Aided by electron microscopy and carrying out unit electrophysiological recordings serially from surface to depth, more recent students again have brought the vertical arrangement of the cortical pyramids into true perspective. Pyramids extending through all layers have been shown to be arranged in vertical columns, forming a mosaic of several interrelated elements that work, as well as live, together.

Like other cellular elements of the brain, those of the cerebral cortex require outgoing and incoming axons, for cortical activity must have its tie-ins with other

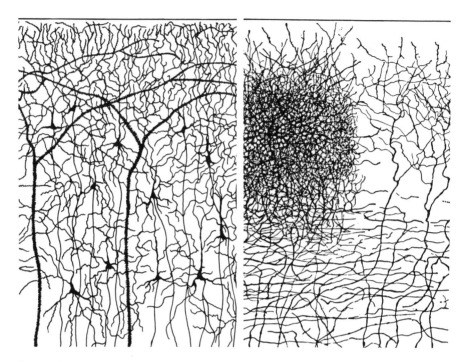

Fɪɢ. 38. Subsurface sector of the pre-Rolandic motor cortex. Dendritic plexus **(left)** contains dendrites arising from cells in the deeper half, arborizing between corresponding cells and thinner dendrites of superficial neurons. Corresponding axonal plexuses **(right)** show, toward the center left, the fine branching plexus of thalamocortical axons; toward the right, the dichotomizing coarser branchings of the same entering axons. (From Ramón y Cajal, 1955*b*, pp. 534 and 641.)

cortical areas and with the brainstem and spinal cord. The neuron masses of the thalamus serve as the principal relay points for impulses ascending from the lower levels of the nervous system, their cortically directed axons arborizing in a restricted cortical zone of intermediate depth. Commissural axons from the opposite cerebral hemisphere and association axons from the same side produce terminal axonal arbors, confined in the transverse but spread out in the vertical plane. The axons leaving the cerebral cortex derive in their entirety from pyramidal cells. They reach destinations in cortical areas of the same and the opposite hemisphere and also are directed to cell aggregates in the lower levels of the nervous system, chiefly the brainstem and spinal cord.

Finally, each level of cortical depth is provided with an assortment of nerve cells whose axons arborize entirely within the cortex (i.e., intrinsically). Collectively, they are called *short axon cells.* The axons of such cells ramify in their neighborhood and do not send extensions outside the cortex. Their local arborizations weave the pyramids together into a variety of working groups.

From the viewpoint of its fine structural organization, the brain is the most highly organized product of biological evolution. Implications of a hierarchical rise in structural complexity from spinal cord to cerebral cortex should be avoided, however, until there is more evidence. It is presumed, but has not been proved, that the higher levels are more intricately structured than the lower. This is suggested by the existence of an overwhelmingly large neuron and synapse population in the cerebral cortex. However, the cerebellum, too, has a large cell population, yet insofar as can be determined, its actions are entirely automatic.

ARCHITECTONIC VIEW OF CEREBRAL CORTEX

The principle of a six-layer cortex (Fulton, 1937; von Bonin, 1952) was initially formulated by J. G. Baillarger (1809–1890). Only a few years earlier others had reported no structure whatever; and Baillarger's observations related only to a distinction between alternating zones of white and gray matter traversing the cortical thickness. At the time, cellular and axonal detail was not resolved. Examining free-hand sections placed between plates of glass (Fig. 39), Baillarger counted six alternating gray and white layers. The white ones later were found to consist principally of accumulations of sheathed axons and the gray ones to contain neurons and their surrounding neuropil. Even earlier than Baillarger, Francesco Gennari (1752–1797), an Italian medical student, had identified a white streak of exaggerated clarity as occurring at the posterior pole of the human brain. His observation was made too early in neuroscientific development to recognize the white streak as a unique feature of the structure of the human visual cortex. G. Elliott Smith (1871–1937) was to confirm Baillarger's findings two generations later and to identify some 40 cortical areas, based on the examination of similar crude sections with a hand lens.

The contemporary opinion on distinctions of structural significance between areas of cerebral cortex began to take form with almost simultaneous studies by Korbinian Brodmann (1868–1937), A. W. Campbell (1868–1937), and C. and O. Vogt (1875–1952 and 1870–1959, respectively). Much of their analyses was based on large, thin sections of human, ape, and other brains. The cell bodies were stained deeply in aniline dyes. Little dendritic or other detail was visible. Low-power photomicrographs of such sections were made, enlarged, and subjected to examination from a distance of 6 feet or more. The observer marked the limits of fields appearing to have a homogeneous structure. Several criteria were employed, including density of cells, change in cell arrangement, and occurrence of cells of large size (Fig. 40). Such plotting of fields, based on inspection of cellular size, distribution, and arrangement, became known as *cytoarchitectonics.* Other workers specialized in the use of a complementary method that colored myelin sheaths and left cells unstained. That branch of structural analysis was called *myeloarchitectonics.*

Brodmann (Nowinski, 1960) carried on his studies at the Institut für Hirnför-schung in Berlin. There he compiled his well-known 1908 map of the human brain

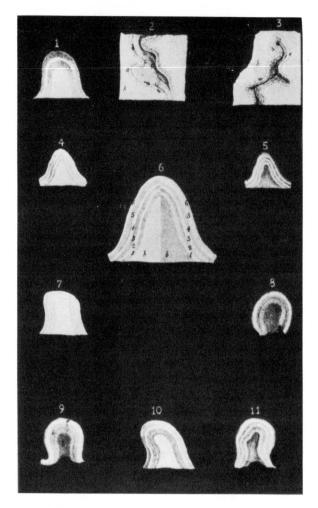

FIG. 39. Early sketches of human cerebral cortex, six-layer plan, by J. Baillarger (1840). (From von Bonin, G., *The Cerebral Cortex,* 1960. Courtesy of Charles C Thomas, Publisher, Springfield, Ill.)

(Fig. 41) and wrote his book (1909) on comparative cytoarchitectonics of cerebral cortex. Essentially, he concluded that the cortex was organized anatomically on the same principles throughout the mammalian series from rat to man. In man he recognized 52 different fields, each a modification of a basic six-layer cortical plan found in all mammalian species.

Campbell was Brodmann's English contemporary. His classification was more functionally oriented. It was derived from parcellations of three normal human hemispheres and those of chimpanzee and an orangutan. He correlated cyto- with myeloarchitectonic patterns. The Vogts carried out myeloarchitectonic studies comparable with those of Brodmann. They were firm believers in the possibility

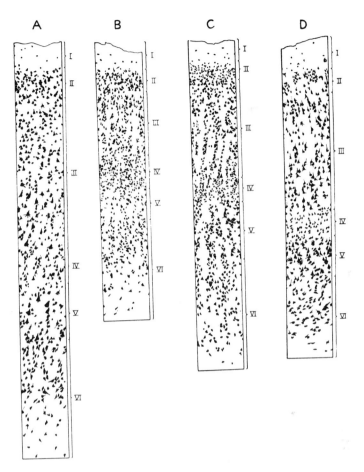

FIG. 40. Six-layer plan, human cerebral cortex. Left to right, pre-Rolandic motor cortex, post-Rolandic sensory cortex, association cortex at junction of parietal, temporal and occipital lobes, and temporal cortex adjoining the hippocampus. (From Bailey and von Bonin, 1951.)

that unequivocal correlations between function and structure could be established between fields, based on cortical ablation, on stimulation studies in animals, on clinical appraisal of the effects of destructive lesions in man, and on anatomical criteria.

C. von Economo and G. N. Koskinas (1929) produced an extensive cytoarchitectonic analysis of human cortex that generally followed Brodmann's analysis but used a different nomenclature. They distinguished 107 fields. In the hands of other workers, the minutiae of parcellation became a fetish and the number of fields distinguished went still higher. Most of these minutely designated fields proved to have no anatomical correlates with experimental animal or clinical studies. In recent times von Bonin (1952) distinguished 20 principal cortical areas. In fact, he observed that human cortex is remarkably homogeneous.

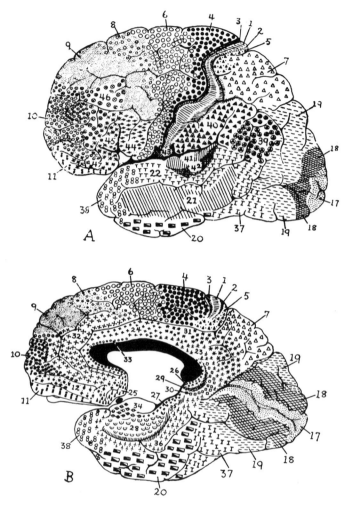

Fig. 41. Brodmann map showing cytoarchitectonic fields of the lateral and medial surfaces, human cerebral cortex. (From Brock and Krieger, 1963.)

The most critical study of the principles underlying cytoarchitectonic parcellation was conducted by K. S. Lashley (1890–1958) and G. Clark, who in 1946 compared the cortices of new- and old-world monkeys. They were able to identify only seven cortical regions in which structural differences in cell size, density, and arrangement superceded the field variations between one animal and another of the same species. They concluded that many localized structural differences between animals are not related to the functions of the areas. This dampened the ardor for further laborious studies of cytoarchitectonics. It made Brodmann's goal of developing a comparative organology of cerebral cortex an unrealistic one.

Yet, it is possible to distinguish a limited number of regions. The door is still open for those who would establish truly objective criteria of parcellation.

COMMENT

The Flourens view that cerebral localization did not exist was held until 1870, bolstered by the apparent inexcitability of both gray and white matter. Then, in well-designed experiments on dogs using galvanic current, Fritsch and Hitzig found proof of both excitability and localization. Ferrier, who followed them within a decade, advanced the subject materially by selecting the monkey as his principal experimental animal and by using faradic stimulation instead of galvanic. He proved beyond doubt that the pre-Rolandic convolution, homologous to that of man, was both electrically excitable for opposite-side musculature and showed a spatial pattern of body representation reproducible from animal to animal of a species. Ablating portions of monkey cortex produced weakness of the opposite half of the body, comparable to that resulting from a stroke. Visual and auditory fields within the cerebral cortex were also identified. Leyton and Sherrington, pursuing similar studies on higher apes, demonstrated the motor eye fields. Cortical mapping, related to body surface stimulation, confirmed earlier clinical studies indicating that the post-Rolandic gyrus is the principal cortical site for reception of body sensibility, the spatial representation being a mirror image of the motor map of pre-Rolandic cortex.

The earliest evidence that cerebral cortex was anything other than a structureless gray layer investing the hemisphere was discovered before the close of the eighteenth century by Gennari. Baillarger in 1840 had recognized six cortical layers of alternating gray and white. From that beginning, the complexity of the cortical substrate and its connections was gradually disclosed. Nevertheless, we are still far from understanding the full significance of field differences in cortical complexity, the criteria for parcellation of fields being less exacting than was thought earlier. The need for precise criteria has become increasingly apparent.

In modern electrophysiological mapping studies, each of the major sensory fields has been shown to be surrounded by satellite fields having a constant bearing with respect to the major one, and presumably having a subsidiary function. The primary visual field, for example, has no less than six such lesser fields related to it. Since anatomical mapping has come largely to a standstill, the establishment of reliable structural and electrophysiological correlates is probably a task for the distant future.

NOTES

[1] "Pre-Rolandic cortex" is a term that came into clinical usage for the latinized *gyrus centralis* anterior of Ferrier's time and is also called *'precentral cortex.'* If the reader will compare Cushing's map of the human motor cortex (Fig. 32) with that of Woolsey (Fig. 34) for the macaque, as recently explored, he will note that in both instances the digits correspond exactly to the line of the central sulcus.

REFERENCES AND BIBLIOGRAPHY

Bailey, P., and von Bonin, G. *The Isocortex of Man.* Urbana, Ill.: University of Illinois Press, 1951. 301 pp.

Bain, A. *Mind and Body. The Theories of Their Relation.* New York: D. Appleton & Co., 1882, 200 pp.

Bartholow, R. Experimental investigations into the functions of the human brain. *Am. J. Med. Sci.* 67:305–313, 1874.

von Bonin, G. Symposium on Brain and Mind. Notes on cortical evolution. *Arch. Neurol. Psychiatry* 67:135–144, 1952.

Broca, P. Remarks on the seat of the faculty of articulate language, followed by an observation of aphemia, pp. 49–72. (Remarques sur le siège de la faculté du langage articulé; suivies d'une observation d'aphemie. *Bull. Soc. Anat.* [*Paris*], 36th year 2ème serie, tome 6:330–357, 1861.) In W. W. Nowinski, ed. *Some Papers on the Cerebral Cortex.* (Trans. from the French and German by G. von Bonin.) Springfield, Ill.: Charles C Thomas, 1960.

Brock, S., and Krieger, H. P. *The Basis of Clinical Neurology,* 4th ed. Baltimore: Williams & Wilkins Co., 1963. 616 pp.

Brodmann, K. On the comparative localization of the cortex, pp. 201–230. (Kapitel IX, Vergleichende Lokalisationslehre. Leipzig: J. A. Barth, 1909.) In W. W. Nowinski, ed. *Some Papers on the Cerebral Cortex.* (Trans. from the French and German by G. von Bonin.) Springfield, Ill.: Charles C Thomas, 1960.

Clarke, E., and O'Malley, C. D. *The Human Brain and Spinal Cord.* Berkeley: The University of California Press, 1968. 1926 pp.

Davis, R. A. Victorian physician-scholar and pioneer physiologist. *Surg. Gynecol. Obstet.* 119:1333–1340, 1964.

Dawson, A. S. The Evolution of Instrumentation for Neural Electrophysiology. M.S. thesis, Cornell University Graduate School (unpublished).

Doty, R. W. Electrical stimulation of the brain in behavioral context. *Annu. Rev. Psychol.* 20:289–320, 1969.

von Economo, C., and Koskinas, G. N. *The Cytoarchitectonics of Human Cerebral Cortex.* London: Oxford University Press, 1929. 186 pp.

Ferrier, D., and Yeo, G. F. A record of experiments on the effect of lesions of the different regions of the cerebral hemispheres. *Philos. Trans. R. Soc. Lond.* [*Biol.*] 175:479–564, 1884.

Flourens, P. (Recherches Expérimentales sur les Propriétés et les Fonctions du Système Nerveux dans les Animaux Vertébrés. Paris: Chez Crevot, pp. 85–122, 1824). In W. W. Nowinski, ed. *Some Papers on the Cerebral Cortex.* (Trans. from the French and German by G. von Bonin.) Springfield, Ill.: Charles C Thomas, 1960.

Foerster, O. The Motor cortex in man in the light of Hughlings Jackson's doctrines. *Brain* 59:135–159, 1936.

Fritsch, G., and Hitzig, E. On the electrical excitability of the cerebrum, pp. 73–96. (Über die elektrische Erregbarkeit des Grosshirns. *Arch Anat. Physiol.* 1870, pp. 300–332.) In W. W. Nowinski, ed. *Some Papers on the Cerebral Cortex.* (Trans. from the French and German by G. von Bonin.) Springfield, Ill.: Charles C Thomas, 1960.

Fulton, J. F. A note on Francesco Gennari and the early history of cytoarchitectural studies of the cerebral cortex. *Bull. Hist. Med.* 5:895–913, 1937.

Fulton, J. F. Alfred Walter Campbell, M.D. Ch.M., 1868–1937. *Arch. Neurol. Psychiatry* 40:566–568, 1938.

Fulton, J. F. Jules Baillarger and the discovery of the six layers of the cerebral cortex. *Gesnerus* 8:85–91, 1950.

Fulton, J. F., and Wilson, L. G., eds. *Selected Readings in the History of Physiology,* 2d ed. Springfield, Ill.: Charles C Thomas, 1966. 492 pp.

Gerard, R. W., and Libet, B. On the unison of neural beats, pp. 288–294. In *Livro de Homenagem aos Professores Albaro e Miguel Ozorio de Almeida.* Rio de Janeiro: Atlantica Editora, 1939.

Goltz, F. L. On the functions of the hemispheres, pp. 118–158. (Über die Verrichtungen der Grosshirns. *Pflügers Arch. Ges. Physiol.* 42:419–467, 1888.) In W. W. Nowinski, ed. *Some Papers on the Cerebral Cortex.* (Trans. from the French and German by G. von Bonin.) Springfield, Ill.: Charles C Thomas, 1960.

Grundfest, H. The different careers of Gustav Fritsch (1838–1927). *J. Hist. Med.* 18:125–129, 1963.

Guillain, G. *Charcot, 1825–1893; His Life—His Work.* (Edited and translated by P. Bailey.) New York: Paul B. Hoeber, Inc., 1959. 202 pp.

Haymaker, W., and Schiller, F., eds. *The Founders of Neurology.* Springfield, Ill.: Charles C Thomas, 1970. 616 pp.

Hess, W. R. Hirnreizversuche über den Mechanismus des Schlafes. *Arch. Psychol. (Frankf.)* 86: 287–292, 1928.

Hitzig, E. Über die beim Galvanisiren des Kopfes entstehenden Ströngen der Muskelinnervation und der Vorstellungen vom Verhalten im Raume. *Arch. Anat. Physiol. Wiss. Med.* 716–770, 1871.

Horsley, V., and Clarke, R. H. The structure and functions of the cerebellum examined by a new method. *Brain* 31:45–124, 1908.

Horsley, V., and Schäfer, E. A. A record of experiments upon the functions of the cerebral cortex. *Philos. Trans. R. Soc. Lond. [Biol.]* 179:1–45, 1888.

Lashley, K. S., and Clark, G. The cytoarchitecture of the cerebral cortex of Ateles: A critical examination of architectonic studies. *J. Comp. Neurol.* 85:223–305, 1946.

Leyton, A. S. F., and Sherrington, C. S. Observations on the physiology of the cerebral cortex of the anthropoid apes. *Proc. R. Soc. Med.* 72:152–155, 1903.

Liddell, E. G. T., and Phillips, C. G. Thresholds of cortical representation. *Brain* 73:125–140, 1950.

Lorente de Nó, R. General discussion, pp. 40–41. (G. J. Romanes. The motor cell groupings of the spinal cord, pp. 24–38.) In G. E. W. Wolstenholme, ed. *A Ciba Foundation Symposium. The Spinal Cord.* Boston: Little, Brown and Co., 1953.

Nowinski, W. W., ed. *Some Papers on the Cerebral Cortex.* (Trans. from the French and German by G. von Bonin.) Springfield, Ill.: Charles C Thomas, 1960. 396 pp.

Olmsted, J. M. D. Pierre Flourens, pp. 290–302. In E. A. Underwood, ed. *Science, Medicine and History.* Vol. II. London: Oxford University Press, 1953.

Penfield, W., and Jasper, H. *Epilepsy and the Functional Anatomy of the Human Brain.* Boston: Little, Brown and Co., 1954. 896 pp.

Ramón y Cajal, S. *Studies on the Cerebral Cortex, Limbic Structures.* (Trans. by L. M. Kraft.) London: Lloyd-Luke, Ltd., 1955a. 179 pp.

Ramón y Cajal, S. *Histologie du Système Nerveux.* Vol. 2. Madrid: Instituto Ramón y Cajal, 1955b.

Schaltenbrand, G., and Woolsey, C. N., eds. *Cerebral Localization and Organization.* Madison, Wis.: The University of Wisconsin Press, 1964. 164 pp.

Sherrington, C. S. Sir David Ferrier, 1928. *Proc. R. Soc. Lond. [Biol.]* 103:viii–xvi, 1928.

Simonoff, L. N. Die Hemmungsmechanismen der Säugethiere experimentell bewiesen. *Arch. Anat. Physiol. (Leipzig)* 33:545–564, 1866.

Vogt, C., and Vogt, O. Allgemeinere Ergebnisse unserer Hirnforschung. *J. Psychol. Neurol. (Leipzig)* 25:279–461, 1919–1920.

Walker, A. E. Stimulation and ablation. Their role in the history of cerebral physiology. *J. Neurophysiol.* 20:435–449, 1957.

Walshe, F. M. R. Contributions of John Hughlings Jackson to Neurology. *Arch. Neurol.* 5:119–131, 1961.

Woolsey, C. N. Organization of somatic sensory and motor areas of the cerebral cortex, pp. 63–81. In H. F. Harlow and C. N. Woolsey, eds. *Biological and Biochemical Bases of Behavior.* Madison, Wis.: The University of Wisconsin Press, 1958.

Young, G. M. *Victorian England: Portrait of an Age,* 2d ed. Gloucester, Mass.: Peter Smith, 1953. 219 pp.

Zinn, J., and Haller, A. *Memoires sur les parties sensibles et irritable du corps animal.* Lausanne: C. d'Aunay, 1760. 500 pp.

Chapter VIII

ORIGINS OF ELECTROENCEPHALOGRAPHY

The discovery that the brain is electrically active and that it produces rhythmic waves led to one of the great breakthroughs in the long history of epilepsy. The currents thus generated can now be amplified electronically to permit recording through skull and scalp. At the beginning of electroencephalography, only the galvanometer was available for recording. The capillary electrometer was just coming into use. The galvanometer, modified and improved during the century following its development by J. Schweigger and L. Nobili, could detect the pulse of brain waves, but amplification and recording were exclusively dependent on deflection of a light beam. In the late nineteenth century, it became possible to record that beam photographically. The capillary electrometer had response characteristics that could cope with the faster transients of brain activity, but it, too, was dependent on light beam amplification.

Both galvanometer and capillary electrometer were improved by the introduction of electronic amplification. The development of ink-writing electromagnetic recording devices with broad frequency response characteristics made possible the construction of the electroencephalograph, an amplifying and recording system made up of multiple noninterfering channels that draw brain currents from many equally spaced electrodes attached to scalp areas overlying the brain. The recorder provides on-line traces in ink. The amplified wave patterns derived from the multiple channels are written side by side on a paper strip moving continuously at 1½ to 6 centimeters (2.5 centimeters equals 1 inch). That range is an arbitrary but convenient one that permits recording of the principal frequencies of both normal and convulsive brain activity. The slower brain waves distribute over a spectrum covering 1 to 40 or more cycles per second. On the other hand, the recording of fast transients of brain activity, such as the responses of single neurons recorded by microelectrodes, requires a cathode ray oscillograph as a recorder.

Electroencephalographs require several channels because the brain itself is large; and some wave-forms, especially the abnormal waves of convulsive activity, may emanate from regions instead of from the brain as a whole, or even from quite discrete cortical loci. Furthermore, the cerebral cortex—from which the chief pick-up occurs—is deeply furrowed and has a much larger surface area than the enclosing cranium would indicate. The cortex also presents an intricate pattern of localization of the general and special senses and of movements. Those, too, are discrete in their distributions. The brain, like the overlying cranium and scalp, has symmetrical left and right halves, corresponding loci that presumably carry on comparable functions within a master plan of localization.

Each electroencephalograph channel has two inputs. If these derive from neighboring scalp electrodes, both overlying active brain but separated by an inch or more, the record is an algebraic sum of what is picked up from each input. Otherwise, an input from an individual scalp electrode may be combined with an inactive lead attached to one or both of the relatively silent ear lobes. In that case the brain wave pattern is chiefly referable to the scalp electrode that overlies the brain, the other serving to complete the amplifier input circuit. Either way, it is possible to impute a local origin to any extraordinary activity that derives consistently from either a single electrode or a group of neighboring ones and at the same time is absent or recorded at reduced amplitude from electrodes remote from the apparent source of activity. That is the basis for detection of focal abnormalities within the brain.

In the relaxed normal subject with eyes closed, the posterior region of the normal human brain produces a sine-like rhythm of 8 to 13 pulsations per second, called *alpha rhythm*. If the subject of recording is activated behaviorally, either by opening the eyes or solving a problem, this rhythm disappears and is replaced by an irregularly fast tracing of low amplitude having no dominant frequency (Fig. 42). Hereafter, such an activation trace will be referred to as composed of *low-voltage fast* activity. With the subject relaxed and the eyes closed, the little gray cells become synchronized to produce a regular sine-like rhythm at the alpha frequency.

We have indicated that the cortical gray matter, were it spread out like a sheet instead of being deeply convoluted, would cover a much greater expanse. As in a computer, there is always a considerable premium on compactness, and the cells and their associated connections in gray matter take up much more of the interior than do the tightly packaged axon bundles that make up the white matter and serve as the communication channels between the parts of the nervous system. Compared with peripheral nerves, where there is a premium on fast conduction because of the long distances to be traversed, brain axons span shorter distances and can be quite small because speed of conduction is of negligible importance. If all central axons had a thickness comparable with those of peripheral ones,

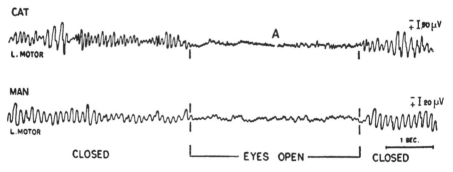

FIG. 42. Effect of opening the eyes upon the alpha rhythm of cat and man. Beta rhythm is also evident in the tracing from the cat. (From Rempel and Gibbs, 1936.)

we would require brains twice the size of those we have. (See Fig. 6 for illustrations of the shape and relations of the human brain.)

The feasibility of localizing the sites of origin of abnormal brain rhythms has already been indicated. These rhythms include both the high-voltage epileptic spike and spike-wave patterns as well as other abnormally fast or slow patterns recorded from the epileptic brain during the waking state. Location is indicated by a significant drop in amplitude over the scalp, increasing with remoteness from the source of potentials. The procedure now in use was devised in 1936 by W. Grey Walter.

Compared with the simple difference which exists in the electroencephalogram (EEG) of the waking subject, eyes open and eyes closed, the brain shows rather complex rhythmic differences during sleep (Fig. 43). The waking-sleep transition is not abrupt; sequences of waves are slower than the four-per-second shuttling in and out of the tracing during gradual suppression of the alpha rhythm of the waking trace. Fourteen-per-second sleep spindles identify an early stage of sleep, but they, too, disappear as sleep deepens. There are several other intervals during a night's sleep during which all rhythmic activity is lost, being replaced temporarily by the pattern hitherto described as *low-voltage fast*. This is identical to

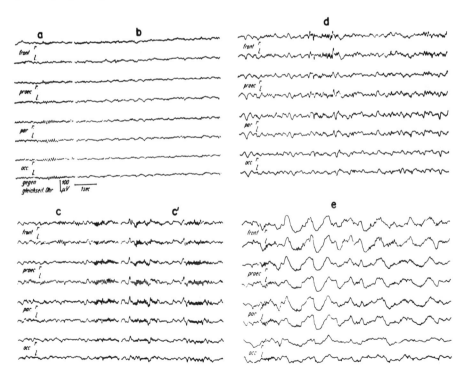

FIG. 43. EEG sleep stages in a healthy human; (a) Waking, alpha waves; (b) drifting, alpha waves suppressed; (c) sleep spindles; (d) increasing slow activity; (e) slow-wave sleep. (From Jung, 1968.)

the *eyes-open* pattern of the waking trace. Each such nocturnal epoch may last from 15 to 30 minutes before it disappears again into the slow-wave activity of usual deep sleep. During such interludes, eye jerks occur, and those neck muscles that hold the head erect relax almost completely. The entirety, *low-voltage fast brain activity,* eye jerks, and relaxed neck muscles is called REM (rapid eye movement) sleep.

While the EEG is used regularly for a variety of nonclinical studies of trained normal subjects, it is most important clinically in the appraisal of epilepsy and other neurological conditions. The uniquely abnormal signal of the epileptic brain is called a *spike* because of its resemblance to the conducted spike of axons in peripheral nerve. Rather than indicating axonal conduction, however, the epileptic spike signifies a highly synchronized cell discharge. The other distinctly abnormal occurrence in the waking EEG is the *slow-wave,* which has a variety of shapes and amplitudes. Some of these wave-forms are combined with spikes to produce unique electrical events in the record of epileptic brain activity. These are called *spike-waves.*

During clinically observed seizures in grand mal or petit mal epilepsy, the EEG trace may consist largely of repetitive spikes (grand mal) or spike-waves (petit mal). Both patterns are of extraordinarily high voltage compared with the much lower alpha rhythm of the normal brain.

During recordings of petit mal epilepsy, paroxysmal bursts lasting a few seconds may occur without the subject losing consciousness or showing other evidence that an attack has occurred. Thus, it is not necessary to record during an obvious seizure in order to identify a seizure state. Herein lies a considerable value of the method—its use for detecting epilepsy from evidence collected during recordings made between seizures.

Not infrequently, the seizure on which a presumptive diagnosis of epilepsy rests may have been witnessed only by family members, perhaps not even by them. Apart from continuing hospital observation, physicians of the pre-EEG era rarely had the opportunity to witness an attack and may have had serious doubts about second-hand reports. The EEG has changed that. Support of a diagnosis now may be derived from brain wave traces recorded on an outpatient. Also important is the chance of obtaining EEGs of the sequence of events that precede a typical seizure. From these it is possible to locate the site of origin.

The entire pool of recordings of seizures of focal origin is studied in selecting those cases in which surgical treatment offers the possibility of relief from attacks that persist unabated in spite of adequate trials on antiepileptic medication.

ORIGINS OF ELECTROENCEPHALOGRAPHY

The "feeble currents of the brain"—as they were called by Richard Caton (1842–1926) (Fig. 44), who discovered them in 1875—were first observed as fluctuations in the galvanometric traces from the cerebral cortex of experimental animals. He recorded these currents directly from the brain, so they were not

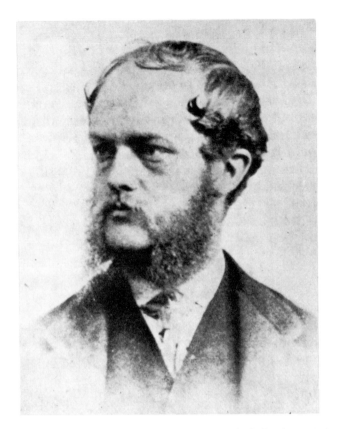

Fig. 44. Richard Caton (1842–1926). (From M. A. B. Brazier, 1961.)

attenuated by passage through the skull and scalp as they are in the modern human EEG. This should be remembered because it makes a difference in interpreting the apparently low sensitivity of Caton's equipment in comparison with that of modern instruments, which instead record brain activity from scalp electrodes.

As reported by M. A. B. Brazier (1961) in her very readable account of this admirable man and his momentous research, Caton started his scientific career with a thesis on the formation of blood cells with respect to the origin of pus. This gained him both the M.D. degree and a gold medal. In the following year he was appointed a lecturer in physiology at the Royal Infirmary School of Medicine, Liverpool, and there began investigating the electrical activity of the nervous system. By February 1874, he had locally presented his nerve and muscle studies. Essentially, these repeated the earlier work of Matteucci and Du Bois-Reymond (see Chapter V). He had used nonpolarizable electrodes for picking up nerve and muscle potentials and a Thomson galvanometer as his recording instrument. To illustrate his findings for an audience, he reflected a beam of light from the galvanometer mirror onto a wall screen, showing muscle currents activated by a nerve stimulus compared with those that resulted from direct muscle stimulation.

On the basis of that modest success, in 1875 he applied to the British Medical Association for a grant to support an investigation of similar phenomena that might occur within the central nervous system. He obtained the grant, and by August 1875 he had used his earlier equipment to record directly from the brain, a truly pioneering endeavor. It was also a salutary demonstration of the potential efficacy of a small grant.

In brief summary, Caton's galvanometer indicated the existence of electrical currents in the brains of living animals, the external cerebral gray matter being positive to a wall of a cut extending into the interior. His premise was not too different from that of the frog experiments of Nobili and Matteucci and later variants of these. When any part of the gray matter was in a state of functional activity, its electrical record presented a "negative variation," using the Du Bois-Reymond equivalent of action potential. He realized the importance of using nonpolarizable electrodes in such experiments. With ordinary electrodes, polarization of the metal through the passage of currents could vitiate proof that the currents in question were of brain origin.

Two years later, Caton published a much fuller account, reporting experiments on 40 rabbits, cats, and monkeys. He noted a steady difference of potential between cortical surface and the sidewall of a section through it. From the sidewall, a constant minor oscillation (brain waves?) was recorded. Caton also attempted to localize cortical areas responsive to the various sensory modalities. For example, he demonstrated the visual cortex area by a current variation resulting from shining a bright light upon the retina.

As further evidence of functional activity, he noted that the electrical currents of the cerebral cortex also fluctuated significantly when the recording electrodes were placed next to a cortical region that was shown earlier by Ferrier to have a masticatory function. The electrical response started before mastication, indicating that it truly arose from the brain and was not due to pick-up from jaw movement. Caton thought it related to the perception of an odor of food, but cautiously regarded his findings as provisional until confirmed by others. Further work showed that he had indeed made important discoveries.

Had Caton reported his finished study before the Royal Society, his results would have been quickly known to scientists over the world. But as Brazier (1961) notes, he decided instead to publish them in the journal of the association that had given him the supporting grant. So in 1887, more than a decade later, when he attended the Ninth International Medical Congress in Washington, D.C., his discoveries were new to attending scientists. By then he had added to his earlier work the search for electrical changes occurring during voluntary acts.

Caton resigned the chair of physiology at Liverpool in 1891.[1] In 1897 Caton visited Russia to attend the International Medical Congress in Moscow. There, Brazier remarks, he might have met Sechenov, an outstanding Russian neurophysiologist. Still later he became active in the civic affairs of Liverpool. He was elected mayor in 1907. A much revered scientist and civic leader, Caton died in 1926.

V. Y. DANILEVSKY (1852–1939)

Educated in medicine at the University of Kharkov, Danilevsky graduated in 1874 and published his first writing on the brain less than 3 years later. In the progress of his studies, he first observed changes in the brain's electrical activity evoked by sensory stimulation. Later he obtained evidence that the brain showed spontaneous activity apart from that engendered by stimulation of a sense organ. His own studies, comparable with those of Caton, were conducted on dogs, using a Du Bois-Reymond galvanometer and nonpolarizable electrodes. In 1891 he gave credit to Caton, saying that his own studies were corroborative. Besides his interest in brain activity, Danilevsky engaged in research in protozoology and parasitology, including, as did Golgi, the study of the malarial parasite.

A. BECK (1863–1942) AND N. CYBULSKI (1854–1919)

I. M. Sechenov, who trained with Du Bois-Reymond in Berlin and became one of the greatest of the Russian physiologists, introduced electrical recordings from the nervous systems of animals into Russian science. Beck, who began his medical studies in Krakow, Poland, in 1886, was encouraged by Sechenov's successes to turn his attention to what today would be called *steady potentials.* He recorded them at the medullary and spinal levels of the frog, in both the presence and absence of cord damage, and following removal of the cerebral hemispheres. The physiologists of his day found slow potentials easier to record than oscillatory activity using a galvanometer and nonpolarizable electrodes. However, it was the oscillatory phenomena that proved of prime significance in the early development of knowledge of the EEG.

Beck then moved on to mammals (rabbit and dog) for more detailed examination of brain responses. He began by stimulating the retina by using bright light, the auditory system by sound, and the skin by faradic current. Early in those studies, he observed a difference in oscillatory currents picked up by electrodes placed on visual cortex. The steady potential underlying the oscillations of visual cortex showed shifts during light stimulation, an effect also observable using modern electronic methods of direct current recording. The oscillatory activity, however, was "blocked" by the effect of the stimulus. Such "blocking" also was produced by a sound but with no accompanying evidence of response. Faradic stimulation of the skin over a hind leg also produced "blocking" of what are now known as intrinsic (spontaneous) cortical rhythms.

Beck added desynchronization of cortical activity to Caton's initial observations on evoked effects, a phenomenon to be described later with respect to the development of knowledge of the ascending reticular activating system (see Chapter X). Beck also provided more detail than did Caton. His 1890 publication in *Centralblatt für Physiologie* was a critical one, for that journal was very widely read. Somewhat later (Brazier, 1961) Beck, with his chief, Cybulski, undertook studies of cortical activity in the monkey. Their results were reported in 1895 to the Third International Physiological Congress in Berne. Shortly thereafter, Beck was appointed professor of physiology at the University of Lwow, where he continued to investigate electrical activity of the brain, emphasizing its role in sensory functioning, especially as related to pain. In his work with Cybulski and at Lwow, he continued to emphasize blocking of the intrinsic cortical rhythms by sensory stimulation.

In 1908 Beck began his study of cerebrocerebellar relationships. This work was of double significance; it was the first instance, we believe, of the use of the Einthoven string galvanometer to record brain activity (without preceding electronic amplification) and the earliest study of the cerebrocerebellar relationships. Lately, return to such efforts has excited workers in epilepsy research by yielding evidence of the suppression of the electrical manifestations of cerebral convulsive activity by cerebellar stimulation. Cybulski's work after Beck left Krakow is recounted in Chapter XIV. During World War II, rather than succumb to the Nazis, Beck committed suicide by swallowing a capsule of potassium cyanide. He was then almost 80 years old.

E. FLEISCHL VON MARXOW (1846–1891)

Beck's paper, *Die Strömme der Nervencentren* (1890), published in *Centralblatt für Physiologie,* drew letters to the editor contesting priorities from, among others, Fleischl von Marxow, professor of physiology at Vienna. In 1883 Fleischl had deposited a sealed envelope containing an account of his results, as was then the custom, with the Imperial Academy of Science of Vienna.[2] Fleischl had described and claimed priority for what seems a bit of trivia from the perspective of today's complex research on perceptual phenomena. He wrote that, using different species of animals, he had placed his paired electrodes symmetrically over the left and right visual areas and had noted that on stimulation of one eye and then the other, the needle deflected oppositely. Evidently, he had only recorded the underlying steady state change and not the oscillatory currents or their "blocking" as described by Beck. Thus, the research results Fleischl so carefully deposited in the sealed envelope had not even the exactness of that done 8 years earlier by Caton.

V. V. PRAVDICH-NEMINSKY (1879–1952)

Born in Kiev in the Ukraine, Neminsky received his early medical training there and later transferred to the University of Kazan to continue his scientific education. After writing his dissertation in chemistry, he returned to Kiev in 1903 and turned to physiology, a subject he taught with zest. Becoming interested in electrical activity of the brain, he began, as Beck had, with studies on the frog. By 1913, he was working on the dog brain, using an Einthoven string galvanometer and a camera. He was one of the first investigators, if not the first, to make photographic records of brain activity.

Recording through the intact skull, as well as from the dura and the brain surface, Neminsky found evidence of a 12 to 14-per-second frequency range in dogs and a faster one of about 35 per second. He also saw "blocking" of such frequencies by sensory stimulation, as discovered by Beck. The slower and faster frequencies were perhaps comparable with the alpha and beta waves, discovered later in the human brain by Hans Berger.

Neminsky's pioneer studies were published in 1913 in German and in Russian. He returned briefly to electroencephalography after World War I.

HANS BERGER (1873–1941), ORIGINATOR OF ELECTROENCEPHALOGRAPHY

Hans Berger (Fig. 45) of Jena in 1929 was the first to describe the human EEG. He was trained in medicine and neuropsychiatry. After military service, in 1897

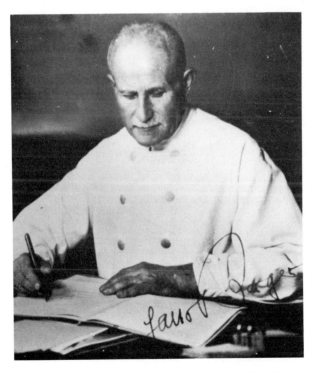

FIG. 45. Hans Berger (1873–1941). (From Haymaker, W., and Schiller, F., eds., *The Founders of Neurology,* 1953. Courtesy of Charles C Thomas, publisher, Springfield, Ill.)

he became a junior staff member in psychiatry at the University of Jena. There he remained, save for another military interlude, until his retirement.

Berger's consuming interest in the electrical expressions of brain activity dated from 1902, at which time he was attempting to record from the dog's brain and to measure temperature changes in cerebral cortex in response to a variety of stimuli. Many of Berger's animal experiments were unsuccessful, though he was evidently able to detect the spontaneous oscillations reported earlier by Caton, Beck, and Neminsky. He failed, however, to evoke specific responses to sensory stimulation.

Perhaps this failure, together with his keen interest in possible psychic manifestation in brain functioning, led him to attempt human electroencephalography. By 1924, he had made a successful recording from a youth with a cranial defect. He repeated this success through scalp recordings on other subjects.

After World War I, he was appointed head of the department of psychiatry and director of the clinic, positions he continued to hold until 1938. His retirement in that year was due, probably, to his refusal to adapt to the Nazi regime rather than to his age. Thus, shortly after reaching the pinnacle of his productivity and acclaim, Berger was enveloped in an obscurity that largely deprived him of the fruits of his research and the opportunity to develop the rich lode his persistence had opened up. He died in 1941. P. Gloor (1969) has translated his major works.

Berger, a shy man, hid a humane personality behind a facade of sternness and self-discipline. His clinic was run in a quasi-military manner, his colleagues regarded him as unimaginative, and he never spoke during clinic hours of what interested him most—the human EEG. His EEG studies were carried out in the seclusion of his research quarters after a full day's work. In those after-dinner hours, he also dictated his correspondence.

At Jena, Berger's contacts with those in the field of electrophysiology—defined as the study of nerve processes associated with excitation, inhibition, and conduction—were tenuous. In 1910 he had aid from an assistant of Professor Wilhelm Biedermann, head of the Department of Physiology, but he evidently had no contacts with Biedermann himself, a foremost electrophysiologist and author of one of the classic works on excitation processes in nerve.

Although primarily a psychiatrist, Berger was evidently an excellent neurologist, whose knowledge of cerebral localization greatly facilitated his EEG studies. He drew on this knowledge when he identified the site of origin of an epileptic discharge in a case of Jacksonian epilepsy as in the opposite motor cortical area. He was the first to show that the oscillations of potential during seizures appearing in EEG traces, recorded through skull defects, represented discharges arising in the same region from which the records were taken, preceding in time the clonic jerks of the opposite extremity.

His attention to the cerebral origin of the waves that he was recording was commendable, even in modern electroencephalography, a field in which insufficient attention is paid to volume-conductor considerations. By systematically eliminating every biological and mechanical source of outside stimulation, Berger was able to record the uncontaminated brain rhythms from the surface of the human brain through the dura and the thin tissue overlying skull defects. Measured by today's standards, the early recording equipment he used to produce his often excellent tracings was quite crude; that he succeeded at all is evidence of his remarkable tenacity.

The EEG studies Berger undertook in 1924 were conducted with a minimum of technical aid. His first subjects were patients with skull defects, such as trephine holes; later he undertook scalp tracings from subjects with intact crania. On these he used zinc-plated needle electrodes inserted to the periosteum and, alternatively, electrodes placed upon the skin. His first instruments were Edelman galvanometers designed to record electrocardiograms. Later he used a Siemens' coil galvanometer, and still later (1932), an electronic amplifier oscillograph, a voltage-measuring device. His favorite arrangement of electrodes connected points high on the forehead and on the back of the head above the inion. Figure 46 illustrates an original tracing Berger recorded in 1931 from an epileptic. It shows undoubted spike-wave activity. Professor Richard Jung of Freiburg permitted its use here to illustrate the excellence of Berger's records.

Berger's publication of his electroencephalographic studies in 1929 was greeted with universal skepticism. To quote from the Gibbs' dedication to him in their *Atlas of Electroencephalography* (1941):

> Berger's studies, like most works of genius, were at first disparaged and later praised. Fortunately the praise came quickly, so that though beyond middle age when he published his first article on electroencephalography, he lived to hear himself acclaimed.

The earliest confirmation of Berger's work came in 1934 from E. D. Adrian and B. H. C. Matthews in England. They proved beyond doubt that rhythmic activity can be recorded from the surface of the human brain. Subsequently, more and more supporting evidence poured in. Today, Berger is universally acknowledged as the originator of electroencephalography.

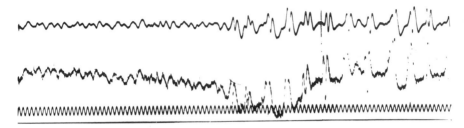

Fig. 46. An original trace taken by Berger on August 26, 1931, showing epileptic-type activity. Upper record was obtained directly on a Siemens' galvanometer. Lower record was taken with another amplifier and galvanometer. (From Jung, 1975.)

THE BERLIN INVESTIGATORS

Initially, many physiologists and neurologists in Germany, as elsewhere, were skeptical of Berger's results. The published results of the Berlin group appear to have given Berger encouragement, and their tracings of seizures in experimental animals could have caused him to reconsider his recordings from epileptic subjects. In retrospect, it would seem that, exercising undue caution, in some instances he attributed valid spike-wave sequences to extraneous or movement artifacts.

The electrophysiological group in Berlin developed as a result of a planned expansion of space and staff at the Institut für Hirnforschung, now called the Max-Planck-Institut, headed at that time by C. Vogt. J. F. Tönnies (1902–1970) joined the institute after an engineering education and 2 years spent with Siemens' Industries, which earlier had given important technological aid to Berger's research. Tönnies had a keen interest in development and research and became active in both at Berlin. M. H. Fischer also joined the staff as professor and head of physiology. At first he undertook the recording of visual-evoked potentials, publishing in 1932. Later, with H. Löwenbach, he studied picrotoxin convulsions in animals.

Tönnies developed the first ink-writing electroencephalograph in 1932 and 3 years later constructed an improved model called Neurograph II. It was a five-pen unit with independent channels. He also devised and built a differential amplifier that permitted multiple recordings independent of ground effects. With A. E. Kornmüller (1905–1965), a graduate of the University of Prague, Tönnies in 1934 undertook correlative studies between architectonic field boundaries and those of spontaneous and evoked potential phenomena. Tönnies also started human brain recording, aided by R. Jung. In 1950 he published with Jung a concept of epilepsy that held that the ordered neuronal coordination of the brain resists the spread of abnormally synchronized epileptic discharges. It emphasized the inhibitory mechanisms contained in the ordered brain rhythms as the restraining mechanism that prevents seizure propagation (see Chapter XIV). Jung, who retained an enduring interest in electroencephalography, also developed the methodology of the polygraph, which records simultaneously a number of other bioelectric phenomena, as well as those of electroencephalogram and electromyogram.

ENGLISH, FRENCH, AND BELGIAN CONTRIBUTIONS

The confirmation of Berger's key studies by Adrian and Matthews, noted previously, was the most important early encouragement that Berger received and his first token of worldwide acceptance. Beyond his work, W. G. Walter was the first to establish the value of electroencephalography in localizing cerebral tumors, his 1936 observations being quickly confirmed by the American school. Walter (1943) also was the first to build a wave analyzer to provide a measure of the time percentage of the different frequency band of the EEG. With V. J. Dovey and H. Shipton, Walter (1946) also initiated the recording of the response of human cortex to photic stimulation.

A. Baudouin and H. Fischgold were contemporaries in French neuroscience. Baudouin established the EEG in French clinical neurology; Fischgold was his collaborator. A. Fessard, an outstanding French electrophysiologist of the modern period, abstracted Berger's original papers in French. With G. Durup as collaborator, in 1936 he followed Adrian and Matthews in confirming Berger's results. F. Bremer (1938) introduced electroencephalography into Belgium by confirming Berger. He was a leader in applying electronic technology to studies of the nervous system. He distinguished the *cerveau isolé* from the *encéphale isolé* preparation—the former converting the animal's normal waking pattern to that of permanent sleep through a midbrain transection of the neuraxis; the latter leaving the usual rhythms undisturbed after a corresponding transection between brainstem and spinal cord. That discovery established the basic premise from which many succeeding studies of the electrophysiological changes during sleep in experimental animals took their departure.

COMMENT

A biomedical discovery such as Berger's can radically alter patient care, thus affecting large numbers of people; at the same time, it can show up a previously undiscerned gap in knowledge and technology. The discovery of insulin by Banting and Best is an example. It revolutionized the care of innumerable diabetics and it reopened a clinical research area in which medical investigation had reached a stalemate.

Berger's discovery was not weighed fully until the end of World War II. It made slow progress, despite early impacts at some of the world's great medical centers. Recording equipment satisfactory for clinical purposes was developed slowly. Lack of trained personnel to conduct the tests and interpret the tracings was another problem. There was no government support for training in the United States, for example; and, as is all too often the case, patient income was insufficient to support large-scale effort.

Much of the recording equipment was suitable only for research. The simple Berger recordings, based on symmetrically placed electrode couplets spanning the length of the head, would not suffice for neurological purposes. Rather, a grid of electrodes was required, the spacings of which provided a map corresponding to knowledge of cerebral localization. Such recordings required multichannel amplifying equipment with minimal cross-interference through the necessary grounding system. Electromagnetic ink-writers soon became the obvious solution to the recording dilemma; but they, too, offered problems of mechanical interference between pen channels. There also was the problem of a sufficient pen excursion and a broad enough frequency response to record the fastest and the slowest waves of the EEG without diminution in amplitude or distortion in shape.

In considering frequency response, it must be kept in mind that both the older capillary electrometer and the newer cathode ray oscillograph were geared to record the faster transients of nerve activity, those which were axonal responses to stimulation. On the other hand, the galvanometers of Thomson and Du Bois-Reymond were principally effective for detecting current flow when used with nonpolarizable electrodes in bioelectric situations. Such was the equipment the pioneers of brain research in animals had to rely on.

Besides training and technological gaps, there was also a knowledge gap to contend with in interpreting brain waves. Axonologists of the pre-World War II era were chiefly knowledgeable about the fast-conducting axon potentials. A few, like Gerard and Heinbecker, saw the possibility of unit cell potentials of spontaneous origin that were enduring enough to sum into the slower brain waves and arose from an amalgam of excitatory and inhibitory postsynaptic potentials. Thus, with the erudite axonologists unable to explain brain wave origins, could early electroencephalographers be blamed for treating them as a class of phenomena to be examined by the analysis of wave spectrum while in search of electrical correlates for epileptic phenomena?

NOTES

[1] He was succeeded by F. Gotch, who later became a collaborator of Horsley in important early studies of the activity of the nervous system. The chair at Liverpool was occupied after Gotch by Charles Sherrington, the undisputed pioneer of English neurophysiology.

[2] Much earlier Galvani had followed the same custom, but for a different reason, and had deposited with the library in Bologna a letter summarizing his last animal electricity studies, which was opened posthumously.

REFERENCES AND BIBLIOGRAPHY

Adrian, E. D., and Matthews, B. H. C. The Berger rhythm: Potential changes from the occipital lobes in man. *Brain* 57:355–385, 1934.

Baudouin, A., and Fischgold, H. Les phénomènes bio-électriques du système nerveux et leurs applications possibles à la médecine. *J. Radiol. Electrol. Med. Nucl.* 22:401–428, 1938.

Baudouin, A., Fischgold, H., and Lerique, J. L'électroencéphalogramme multiple de l'homme normal. *Bull. Acad. Med. (Paris)* 121:89–100, 1939.

Beck, A. Die Ströme der Nervencentren. *Zentralbl. Physiol.* 4:572–573, 1890.

Berger, H. Über das Elektrencephalogramm des Menschen. *Arch. Psychiatr. Nervenkr.* 87:527–570, 1929.

Brazier, M. A. B. *A History of the Electrical Activity of the Brain. The First Half-Century.* London: Pitman Medical Publishing Co., 1961.

Bremer, F. Effets de la déafférentation complète d'une région de l'écorce cérébrale sur son activité électrique spontanée. *C. R. Soc. Biol. (Paris)* 127:355–359, 1938.

Caton, R. The electric currents of the brain. *Br. Med. J.* 2:278, 1875.

Caton, R. Interim report on investigation of the electric currents of the brain. *Br. Med. J.* (Suppl) 1:62–65, 1877.

Danilevsky, V. Y. Electrical phenomena of the brain. *Fiziol. Sb.* 2:77–88, 1891 (in Russian).

Durup, G., and Fessard, A. Observations psychophysiologiques relatives a l'action des stimuli visuals et auditifs. *Annee. Psychol.* 36:1–32, 1936.

Fischer, M. H. Elektrobiologische Erscheinungen an der Hirnrinde. *Pflügers Arch. Ges. Physiol.* 230:161–178, 1932.

Fischer, M. H., and Lowenbach, H. Aktionsströme des Zentralnervensystems unter der Einwirkung von Krampfgiften: I Mitteilung: Strychnin und Pikrotoxin. *Arch. Exp. Pathol. Pharmacol.* 174: 357–382, 1934.

Fleischl von Marxow, E. Mitteilung betreffend die Physiologie der Hirnrinde. *Zentral. Physiol.* 4:538–539, 1890.

Gibbs, F. A., and Gibbs, E. L. *Atlas of Electroencephalography,* Vol. I. Cambridge, Mass.: Lew A. Cummings Co., 1941. 221 pp.

Gloor, P. Hans Berger on the electroencephalogram of man. *Electroencephalogr. Clin. Neurophysiol.* (Suppl. 28):1–350, 1969.

Jung, R. Ein Apparat zur mehrfachen Registrierung von Tatigkeit und Funktionen des animalen und vegetativen Nervensystems. Elektrencephalogramm, Elektrokardiogramm, Muskelaktionsströme, Augenbewegungen, galvanischer Hautreflex, Plethysmogramm, Liquordruck und Atmung. *Z. Ges. Neurol. Psychiatr.* 165:374–398, 1939.

Jung, R. Neurophysiologische Untersuchungs—methoden, pp. 1206–1420. In L. Mohr and R. Stoehelin, eds. *Handbuch der innern Medizin,* Vol. 5, Pt. 1. Berlin: Springer, 1968.

Jung, R. Some European neuroscientists: A personal tribute, pp. 475–509. In F. G. Worden, J. P. Swazey, and G. Adelman, eds. *The Neurosciences: Paths of Discovery.* Cambridge: MIT Press, 1975.

Jung, R., and Tönnies, J. F. Hirnelektrische Untersuchungen über Entstehung und Erhaltung von Krampfentladungen: Die Vorgänge am Reizort und die Bremsfähigkeit des Gehirns. *Arch. Psychiatr. Nervenkr.* 185:701–735, 1950.

Kornmüller, A. E. Der Mechanismus des epileptischen Anfalles auf Grund bioelektrischer Untersuchungen am Zentralnervensystem. *Fortschr. Neurol. Psychiatr.* 7:414–432, 1935.

Kornmüller, A. E., and Tönnies, J. F. Registrierung der spezifischen Aktionsstrome eines architektonischen Feldes der Grosshirnrinde vom uneröffneten Schädel. *Psychiatr. Neurol. Wschr.* 34:124, 1932.

Práwdicz-Neminski, V. V. Zur Kenntnis der elektrischen und der Innervationsvorgänge in den funktionellen Elementen und Geweben des tierischen Organismus. Elektrocerebrogramm der Säugetiere. *Pflügers Arch. Ges. Physiol.* 209:362–382, 1925.

Rempel, B., and Gibbs, E. L. The Berger rhythm in cats. *Science* 84:334–335, 1936.

Tönnies, J. F. Der Neurograph, ein Apparat zur Aufzeichnung bioelektrischer Vorgänge unter Ausschaltung der photographischen Kurvendarstellung. *Naturwissenschaften* 22:382–384, 1932.

Tönnies, J. F. Die unipolare Ableitung elektrischer Spannungen vom menschlichen Gehirn. *Naturwissenschaften* 22:411–414, 1934.

Walter, W. G. The location of cerebral tumours by electroencephalography. *Lancet* 2:305–308, 1936.

Walter, W. G. An improved low frequency analyser. *Electron. Eng.* 16:236–240, 1943.

Walter, W. G., Dovey, V. J., and Shipton, H. Analysis of the electrical response of human cortex to photic stimulation. *Nature* 158:540–541, 1946.

Chapter IX

AMERICAN DEVELOPMENTS IN ELECTROENCEPHALOGRAPHY

When Berger published his original study in 1929, only a few American laboratories had the equipment and know-how to verify his results. The number grew over the next decade, as suitable amplifiers, cathode ray tubes, and ink-writing recorders became available. Several laboratories had developed amplifying-recording equipment. Those improvising such equipment became skilled at separating the components of the conducted action potential in somatic and autonomic nerves and sought such potentials in the entry zones of the spinal and cranial nerve roots as well. They determined the properties of the several axon groups, as distinguished by their different conduction rates, thresholds, and refractory periods.

At first these American workers, numbering not over a dozen, called themselves *axonologists.*[1] They met yearly in conjunction with the American Physiological Society. By academic recruiting for graduate training, the original group grew to 100 or more and thereafter named itself The Needlework Society, because sewing needles were used for recording within the central nervous system.

By this time, the technology had ripened significantly, and some axonologists thought themselves prepared for the invasion of the brain and spinal cord along incoming paths. Few, however, had any notion of the complexities to be encountered during brain recording. These included alterations in potential form resulting from central tracts being embedded in a volume conductor instead of being isolated, as was a peripheral nerve laid across electrodes in an incubator. Such isolated nerves did not generate spontaneous activity, as did the living nervous system. Thus, there was no interference from brain waves. Nerve potentials, too, were simply explained—in the stimulus-response preparations used for study outside the body—as produced entirely by summations of well-synchronized, rapidly conducting impulses into all-or-none nerve spikes. Such spikes also were recognizable in the central nervous system, but complicated there by the existence of potentials shown to arise from somata and dendrites of neurons and by synaptic delays encountered in the nerve centers.

Some of the Americans who must be mentioned here—because they either paved the way for verification of Berger's results or participated in later developments—are Alexander Forbes and Hallowell Davis of the Department of Physiology at Harvard Medical School; George H. Bishop of the Oscar Johnson Institute, Washington University School of Medicine, St. Louis; Ralph W. Gerard of the Department of Physiology, the University of Chicago; and Lee E. Travis, Professor of Psychology and Speech Pathology at the University of Iowa,

Iowa City. Alexander Forbes introduced electronic amplification of the feeble brain signals. Hallowell Davis led Americans in verifying Berger's results. With Howard Bartley, Bishop published the first evoked potential studies of animal brain. Gerard's forte at the time also was the recording of brain potentials in the experimental situation. He stressed their intrinsic origin and a makeup deriving from the summations of the beats of individual neurons. Travis' laboratory, too, engaged in recording from animals.

One of the most notable accomplishments of the University of Iowa laboratory was the early graduate training of four of the original American electroencephalographers, all destined for distinguished research careers. These were Herbert H. Jasper, who later joined Wilder Penfield in developing a world-renowned center for clinical and basic research in epilepsy at the Montreal Neurological Institute; Donald B. Lindsley, a noted behavioral psychologist, now at the Brain Research Institute, University of California, Los Angeles; Charles Henry, presently of the Cleveland Clinic; and John Knott, who continued his life's work at the University of Iowa.

In the graduate-student days of these men, there was no government support of research training, and stipends came from university funds. One definition of a stipend—a donation given in small coin—describes exactly the graduate-student salaries of those years. One of these Iowans has stated that he received less than 100 dollars a month in his first postgraduate year. Thanks to outstanding work, he was able to double that figure in his second year. Judged by national standards, Iowa was generous. Assistant professors with families were known to work for as little as $1,800 a year. Despite this inadequate support, some remarkable work was done in American institutions.

BEGINNINGS IN EEG AND OTHER ELECTROCORTICAL RECORDINGS

The Harvard Effort

The breakthrough in 1920 by Alexander Forbes (1882–1965) and Catharine Thacher, who adapted electronic amplification to neurophysiological purposes, was noted in Chapter V. A difficulty with the Hindle galvanometer (an American adaptation of the Einthoven galvanometer), used by Forbes as his recorder for amplified signals, lay in the ease with which signal force broke the silver-coated quartz threads of the instrument. Replacement was both irritating and time-consuming. Thus, where possible, the galvanometer was replaced by a cathode ray tube utilizing a beam of electrons that swept across the tube face on the horizontal axis and could be used for on-line recording of a signal on the vertical axis. Hallowell Davis had such equipment available for audiological research. With L. J. Saul, he had used it to follow the central auditory paths of the cat (Davis and Saul, 1931). Soon thereafter, Saul joined Gerard at the University of Chicago for related studies.

In 1933 A. J. Derbyshire, one of the Davis graduate students in audiology, uncovered Berger's first paper (1929) in a routine check of the literature. He promptly brought it to Davis' attention. With his knowledge of the recordings of the potentials of the auditory path, Davis thought it inconceivable that potentials as slow as Berger's alpha rhythm could arise from the brain. He agreed, however, that the recording equipment available was suitable for confirmation and that repetition of Berger's results was necessary. Accordingly, in 1934 A. J. Derbyshire, with Pauline Davis and H. N. Simpson, another audiology student, undertook to record Berger's wave patterns from one another (Fig. 47). After 3 weeks of sterile effort, they asked Davis to help them check their procedure before writing a negative report. He observed their method and agreed that the results were indeed negative, but he suggested, as an added precaution, that they carry out the same procedure on him. With the electrodes in place on his head in the usual paracentral recording positions of Berger, Davis entered the shielded room. The electrodes were attached to the input of the equipment, the door was shut, and Davis closed his eyes.

Almost immediately, he heard shouts from without. Derbyshire and Simpson were looking at his alpha rhythm, presumably the first to be recorded from a human head on this side of the Atlantic. A letter from Joseph Hughes of Philadelphia, however, indicates that in October 1933 or 1934, while working with Herbert Gasser (later a Nobel Prize winner in physiology) at the Rockefeller

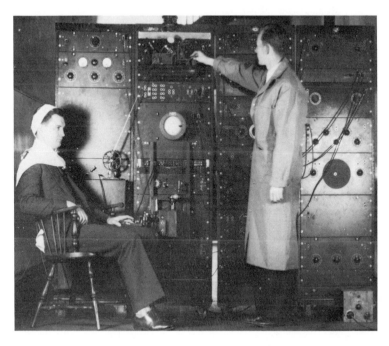

Fɪɢ. 47. Derbyshire (standing) and Lindsley (sitting). Early picture (December 12, 1934) of equipment and American scientists who engaged in confirmation of Berger's ideas.

Institute, they sought to confirm Adrian's reports on the abolition of alpha waves by opening the eyes. Gasser was the subject. Adrian's result was confirmed, but, because of the pressure of other experiments, the matter was dropped. Davis, on the other hand, did continue his interest and was to conduct many important EEG studies. The early American developments in electroencephalography owe much to Davis' efforts (Fig. 48).

Using the available equipment (Fig. 47), it was soon shown that Hallowell Davis, Donald B. Lindsley (a former student of Travis from Iowa City), and Walter B. Cannon, head of physiology at Harvard, had good alpha rhythms. For the remainder of the group, the available amplification was insufficient to record rhythmical brain activity. Davis then decided that further progress would require more subjects and an on-line (i.e., tape) recording system. E. L. Garceau, the department's electronic engineer, obtained an undulator, a recorder developed by Western Union for writing in Morse code on a ticker tape with an ink stylus.

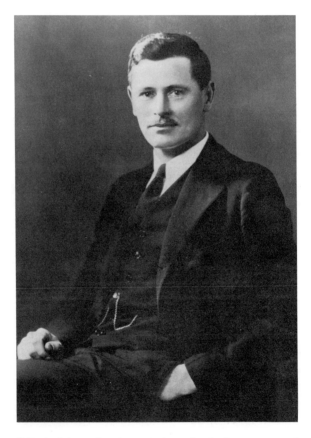

FIG. 48. Hallowell Davis, taken when he was pioneering brain wave recording in the United States.

By replacing its magnets with more powerful ones of nickel, aluminum, and cobalt alloy, and by providing stiffer springs, it became possible to record electronically the amplified alpha rhythm and other frequencies between 1 and 20 per second on-line at a paper speed of three-eighths of an inch per second. After further study of normal subjects, Davis and his associates were ready for a demonstration before a medical group at Harvard. By reflecting their ink-written record on a screen, using an epidiascope (which calls to mind Caton's galvanometric projections from nerve-muscle preparations more than half a century before), they were able to demonstrate brain waves to an audience that was deeply impressed.

Frederic Gibbs saw the demonstration, and shortly thereafter he and his wife, Erna, joined the physiology group expressly to test the utility of the electronic approach in developing a clinical test for epilepsy. Their first subject was a 21-year-old woman, a patient of Professor William G. Lennox, who suffered from frequent petit mal attacks. The repetitive spike-wave discharge appeared as a recognizable pattern after they reduced the sensitivity of the apparatus significantly below that required for recording the relatively feeble normal alpha rhythm through skull and scalp. This recording, so important in the history of epilepsy, and others like it were first reported by Gibbs and his collaborators in 1935. A modern replica is shown in Fig. 49.

Perhaps Berger did not study more epileptic subjects in his early researches because he may well have attributed the epileptic wave-forms either to artifact or to spread of potentials arising from muscle contractions accompanying a seizure. Yet, as indicated in the last chapter, the German reports by Fischer and Löwenbach and of Kornmüller and Tönnies on strychnine convulsions in animals could have caused Berger to reassess his early records taken from epileptics.

By spring 1935, Albert M. Grass, an electrical engineer who had entered this new field in cooperation with the Gibbses, had developed the concept of a three-channel instrument, which he undertook to build for $1,000. This was financed

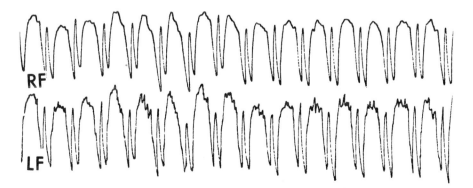

Fig. 49. Scalp traces of a three-per-second spike-wave pattern, such as is recorded during petit mal attacks. RF and LF (right and left frontal).

by a grant Lennox obtained from the Macy Foundation. A year later the equipment, including an ink-writer also devised by Grass, was completed. A Boston group, including Davis, Gibbs, Grass, and Lennox, demonstrated it at an American Medical Association meeting in Kansas City. It had been carried across country in the trunk of an automobile, evidence of the sturdiness of the amplifiers.

Grass and his wife, Ellen, in 1937 provided a four-channel machine for Robert Schwab of Massachusetts General Hospital, another for the Lee Travis group in Iowa City, and two for the Yale University Medical School. One of the latter was placed in the laboratory of Dusser de Barenne, who played an important role in the early investigation of strychnine effects on cerebral cortex, and the other was assigned to Margaret Lennox, an epileptologist, the daughter of William Lennox. The four-channel Grass Model II instrument was brought out in 1938. It was in widespread military use during World War II.

The University of Iowa Laboratory

Lee E. Travis came to the field of brain wave activity because of his theory relating stuttering to cerebral dominance. He first relied on laryngeal electromyography, but came to the conclusion that his theory required the comparative study of brain waves of normal subjects and those of stutterers. About 1932 Travis, with the aid of Theodore Hunter, an electrical engineer, developed a two-channel device for recording the electrical activity of an animal brain. Basically, it was a transformer-coupled amplifier that used a mirror galvanometer as the recording instrument (Travis and Dorsey, 1932). Unfortunately, it did not register the lower frequencies.

Early in the Iowa developments, in 1931, Howard Bartley and E. B. Newman, graduate students at the University of Kansas, visited Travis for advice. These collaborators had developed an amplifier that could register the slow frequencies. Using it, they published two studies on the brain waves of dogs. Incidentally, Travis recognized the priorities of both Caton and Berger. Indeed, he was the first American worker to mention the precedence of Caton in animal recording.

In 1934–1935 Travis obtained drawings of the circuitry used by Howard Andrews to develop the amplifying and recording equipment of Herbert Jasper at Brown University. Working with his electrical engineer Paul Griffith, Travis built a two-channel amplifying system with a Westinghouse galvanometer as the recorder. This equipment followed the frequency band faithfully, and it was used for the first human scalp recordings made by the Iowa City group. Travis also became aware of the Garceau modification of the undulator and was able to obtain two undulators from a local Western Union office. Using one of them, he carried out his classical study of the temporal course of consciousness. In 1937 the group purchased its initial Grass Model I, three-channel instrument. One of the earliest papers published by the Iowans on human electroencephalography compared brain waves in normals and stutterers (Travis and Knott, 1936).

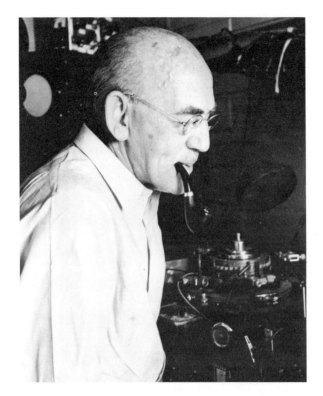

FIG. 50. G. H. Bishop, an associate of Erlanger and Gasser during the formative days of electrophysiology at Washington University Medical School. (Courtesy of Martin Schweig, St. Louis.)

Bartley and Bishop

After publishing with Newman on the brain waves of the dog in 1930–1931, Howard Bartley moved to St. Louis on a Rockefeller Foundation fellowship to work with George H. Bishop (1889–1973). There, the equipment was beyond the exploratory stage. The St. Louis apparatus was an adaptation of that used since the original Gasser-Erlanger-Bishop axonology studies of the early 1920s. The Bartley and Bishop (1932) preliminary studies concerned the interaction of evoked potentials and the phases of the intrinsic cortical rhythm of the rabbit. The camera used for oscillographic recording was locally made. Using bromide paper rolls, it sufficed for direct photographic traces of either a few waves or continuous activity. Potentials were evoked (see EVOKED POTENTIAL in the Glossary) by electric shocks delivered by a rotary wheel that provided movable contacts that could be used to regulate the timing position of the shock with respect to the waxing and waning of the intrinsic rhythm of the animal under study.

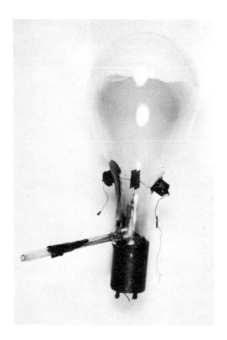

FIG. 51. Original cathode ray tube used by Gasser and Erlanger.

In later studies, Bishop and his co-workers turned to the cat for identical experiments. These provided much additional information about the wave pattern of the evoked response. By varying the depths of the recording electrode tips in the cortex, the components of evoked response excitation could be related to cortical levels of the architectonic six-layer plan (see Chapter VII).

The best recounting of the problems of early American electrophysiology was given by George Bishop (Fig. 50) at the memorial service for Joseph Erlanger on January 14, 1966. It covers the early use of the Braun tube (Fig. 51) as a recording instrument.[2]

Ralph W. Gerard (1900–1974) and His Associates[3]

In late 1930 Wade H. Marshall (1907–1972), recruited from the Physics Department, was developing a cathode ray oscillograph for Gerard. This was in operation when Leon J. Saul joined the project from the Harvard laboratory, where he had been engaged in animal audiological and human EEG studies with Hallowell and Pauline Davis. Together, in 1933, Gerard, Marshall, and Saul undertook some of the earliest American exposed brain studies on animals, using a concentric needle electrode manipulated by a Clarke-Horsley stereotaxic electrode carrier. They explored the entire cranial contents, distinguishing *spontaneous* from *evoked* potentials, terms that they introduced to neuroscience. In a recent letter, Gerard remarks that they ". . . followed afferent visual, auditory, and tactile messages to parts of the brain where they were never believed to go—for example, the cerebellum and hippocampus."

Gerard (Fig. 52) also was to collaborate in 1946 with Judith Graham and later with Gilbert Ling on the early development of the microelectrode for unit recording from the exterior and the interior of the single cell. Especially after others improved the original technique, using such innovations as electrophoresis for injecting transmitters and other agents into neurons through multibarrel electrodes, this development certainly was one of the most important technological breakthroughs in the whole of electrophysiology. Like the cathode ray tube and Clarke's stereotaxic design (see Chapter VII), and unlike the current and voltage measuring devices of earlier times, it dictated a permanent change in the concept of how the nervous system should be studied. Replacement by any radically different design seems inconceivable at this writing. It has since provided important insights into the explosive behavior of the "epileptic neuron" (see Chapter XIII).

Franklin Offner joined Gerard's group in 1934 in an engineering capacity.

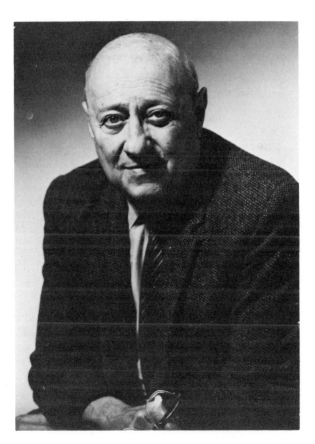

FIG. 52. Ralph W. Gerard (1900–1974).

Among other accomplishments, in 1936 he developed a high-speed, piezoelectric crystal ink-writer with Gerard.

Herbert H. Jasper, Providence, Montreal

In 1933 Herbert Jasper, a former Travis associate, returned from European research with L. Lapique in Paris to work with Leonard Carmichael at Brown University, supported by the Rockefeller Foundation (Fig. 53). Jasper held appointments at Brown University and Butler Hospital. At that time there were rumors that Lord Adrian was taking Berger's work seriously; and, during the summer of 1934, Carmichael and Jasper set out to check some of Berger's findings. Two of their subjects, Carl Pfaffman (now at Rockefeller University) and Jasper himself, had good alpha rhythms; Carmichael and Howard Andrews did not. The studies of normal brain rhythms were published in 1935 in *Science*

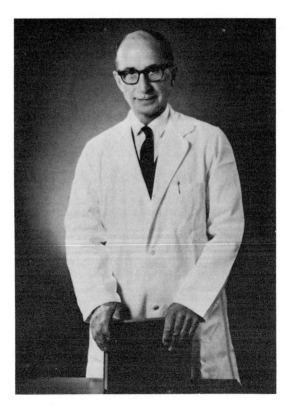

FIG. 53. Herbert H. Jasper, Montreal.

TABLE 1. *Early American clinical electroencephalography after Hans Berger (1930s)*[a]

Normal	Sleep EEGs	Children	Epilepsy	Early records from exposed human brain	Localization of brain tumor
Jasper & Carmichael (1935)	Loomis, Harvey, & Hobart (1935)	Kreezer (1936)	Gibbs, Davis, & Lennox (1935)	Sachs, Schwartz, & Kerr (1939)	Case & Bucy (1938)
Bagchi (1936)	Davis et al. (1937)	Lindsley (1936)	Gibbs, Lennox, & Gibbs (1936)	Scharff & Rahm (1941)	Williams & Gibbs (1938)
H. & P. Davis (1936)			Gibbs & Lennox (1937)		Yeager (1938)
			Jasper & Hawke (1938)		
			Jasper & Nichols (1938)		

[a] Other references to early U.S. literature are provided by D. B. Lindsley (1944).

and were Jasper's first contribution in the EEG field. A summary of these early studies was also published by Jasper in the same year as a second doctoral thesis at the University of Paris.

The equipment Jasper used in Providence was devised by Howard Andrews, a physicist and electronic engineer of Brown University, mentioned previously. Jasper believes that its excellence was due to the use of low-noise-level vacuum tubes in the input of the amplifier (personal communication, 1973). This was also true of the Bishop-Bartley equipment.

For transcription, a Western Electric mirror oscillograph and photographic recording were used. The bromide paper came in rolls; by using a drum, seemingly endless quantities were developed each day, also in line with Bishop's experience. The ensemble provided very accurate traces. Jasper says, for example, that he was able to identify the fast *beta rhythm* of Berger recorded from closely spaced electrodes applied to the scalp, an observation confirmed later in open brain studies conducted with Wilder Penfield as a prelude to surgical removal of epileptogenic foci at the Montreal Neurological Institute.

The first ink-writers used by Jasper were crystographs (made of piezoelectric crystals) as developed by Offner and Gerard. During the year preceding Jasper's move to Montreal, he used a portable version of the Andrews amplifiers, which could be transported between Providence and Montreal in the trunk of a car. The equipment Jasper used in Montreal was built by Andrew Cipriani, who also developed the recording pens used with it.

The first EEG recording done in Montreal was in the winter of 1937. Thereafter, Wilder Penfield and Jasper were frequent collaborators in the operating room, taking volumes of records during craniotomies in which accurate localization of an epileptogenic focus was the prelude to its eradication. The patients came from all over the world.

Table 1 presents the major developments in early American clinical electroencephalography.

EXPANSION OF BRAIN WAVE RECORDING DURING WORLD WAR II

The EEG was uniquely suited to the diagnostic needs of neuropsychiatric and neurosurgical services in World War II. Aside from its use in epilepsy, it became a valuable asset in encephalopathy, penetrating wounds of the head, and in a variety of other wartime neurological conditions. The Grass Instrument Company provided most of the instruments from its Model II, four-channel equipment, Grass and his wife wiring and assembling the parts in the basement of their home. They estimate that 100 intruments were delivered to the armed services between 1942 and 1946 (personal communication). Some of these were used exclusively for research or diagnosis in what the military called the Zone of the Interior. Others were packed in waterproof crates for overseas shipment; one actually was rescued from the sea off a landing area and set up in a combat zone.[4]

U.S. Army

Thirty-five four-channel instruments were installed in the general hospitals of the Zone of the Interior and in six Air Force installations. Five others were sent to the European-Mediterranean theater and six to the Pacific.

By 1944, the widespread need for diagnostic EEGs had become quite evident. Technicians for recording and maintenance, and medical officers capable of supervision and interpretation of tracings, were not available in the numbers needed. Major William H. Evarts of the Office of the Surgeon General, Neuropsychiatry Division, began a systematic attack on the problem. Since that time, electroencephalography has been linked to neurology as an important subspecialty.

Frederic A. Gibbs, whose work had figured prominently in the American development of electroencephalography, was retained as consultant. He furnished the salient information on the uses and limitations of the EEG, providing standard electrode positions, combinations to be used in each recording sequence, and a uniform calibration in microvolts, so that tracings could be compared in a center of definitive care with those taken earlier in one of a succession of hospitals along a chain of evacuation. This information was succinctly developed in TB Med 74 (July 27, 1944), written by Gibbs and Evarts for the Surgeon General's Office.

A School of Electroencephalography was developed as a subsidiary to the School of Military Neuropsychiatry, Mason General Hospital, Brentwood, Long Island, of which Col. W. C. Porter was director. Gibbs visited the school to start its program of instruction. He provided more than 100 record strips as examples of tracings seen in epilepsy and organic conditions of the nervous system. Their use as teaching aids was supplemented by the Gibbses' *Atlas of Electroencephalography* (1941) and on-the-job interpretations of tracings as they were being recorded. Medical officers also were trained for laboratory supervision, Women's Army Corps (WAC) enlistees to run tracings, and graduates of army radar schools as maintenance technicians. By the war's end, the school had graduated 56 medical officers and 23 enlisted men and women who had been trained for these several purposes. By October 1945, 21,217 EEGs had been recorded in Zone of Interior hospitals, of which approximately 6,000 were from cases of post-traumatic encephalopathy, 2,697 of epilepsies, and 165 of expanding lesions, such as brain tumors.

The only American EEG laboratory in the European Theater was at the 96th General Hospital in England. It was under the supervision of Maj. Alexander Ross. In the Mediterranean Theater, Col. Theodore von Storch of the 33d General Hospital had Grass equipment mounted on an ordnance truck for field use in the Italian campaign. His team studied blast concussion cases shortly after injuries occurred. Colonel Benjamin Boshes operated a laboratory at the 12th General Hospital, where EEGs were taken on head injuries and in a variety of seizure situations.

Information on the use of brain wave recording in the Air Corps is scanty. Melvin Thorner was active in experimental studies and in pilot screening. Several thousand pilot candidates were examined during World War II by electroencephalography.

U.S. Navy

The EEG was first used in Navy medicine for research purposes. In collaboration with Dr. Robert Cohn, tests were conducted under hyperbaric (excessive oxygen pressure) conditions by the experimental Diving Unit at the Washington Navy Yard. EEGs were used in studying concomitants of nitrogen intoxication. Recordings were made during simulated dives to investigate the effect of air at depth equivalents of 275 feet (83.8 meters). The first recordings of EEGs during breathing of 100% oxygen under pressure and a study of helium-oxygen mixtures under simulated, high-pressure conditions were done there. Some of this work was published in the *Naval Medical Journal,* but because of military security regulations, most of it remained unpublished elsewhere.

For clinical recording purposes, the EEG was first used by the Navy at St. Elizabeths Hospital in Washington, D.C., where the service referred patients for diagnostic evaluation of epilepsy by Robert Cohn, the electroencephalographer. When Cohn entered active Naval duty, early in 1943, an instrument was installed at the U.S. Naval Hospital at Bethesda, Md. It was used primarily for differential diagnosis of epilepsies and for localization of brain tumors.

Experimental studies also were conducted by R. H. Pudenz and C. H. Sheldon, who had developed a plastic clavarium. An experimental study on cats of the effect of 100% oxygen under hyperbaric conditions was also undertaken with Dr. Isidore Gersh at the Naval Medical Research Institute. The work showed the rather precise sequence of seizure events that ensued under those conditions. The convulsive side-effects of newly developed antimalarial drugs were screened by electroencephalography, and EEG abnormalities that developed in experimentally induced subdural hematomata of the cat also were analyzed.

In 1944 an EEG facility was established at the Naval Hospital at Portsmouth, Va., and used by G. N. Raines and Ralph Rossen for clinical purposes. Shortly thereafter, EEG instrumentation became available at St. Albans, New York, and at Chelsea Naval Hospital at Chelsea, Mass., under Robert Schwab. By the end of World War II, a large number of EEG units had been installed for clinical purposes. It was not until the Korean War, however, that electroencephalography became an integral activity of Navy medicine under combat conditions.

POSTWAR DEVELOPMENTS

After the war came a considerable expansion in the number of hospitals and other laboratories available for electroencephalography, rapid growth in the number of competent electroencephalographers and technicians, the establishment of examining boards to certify the competence of both electroencephalographers and technicians, and the founding of national societies by them.

With Penfield and Jasper (1954) leading the way, direct electrical recording from the surface of the brain in search of epileptogenic foci had become a very useful routine. Grids of electrodes distributed over the cortical surface made it possible to recognize sites of focal epileptogenic disturbance in selected cases, and to use the data to determine the limits of the cortical area required to eradicate a focus. In other hands, arrangements of electrodes have since been implanted for several days at a time and records have been taken by telemetry with the patients walking about under observation. Electrodes implanted in the depths of the brain also have been used to establish the sites of deep-lying disturbances in brain activity. In this way, temporal lobectomy for psychomotor seizures in selected patients has become a quite precise procedure.

Electroencephalography equipment developed concurrently. For example, the Grass instrument, frequently mentioned in these pages, was built in successive models III (1946), IV (1955), VI (1960), and VIII (1972). Late instrumentation is housed in aluminum modules and includes much solid-state circuitry. It is light enough to be shipped by air.

A standard distribution of scalp electrodes was adopted by the International Federation of EEG Societies (1958) and is now widely used for recording purposes. The sites of application and the method of positioning are too detailed for description here. Substantial agreement has been reached on the significance of various abnormal wave-forms that indicate the existence of an epileptic process. Electroencephalography also has entered into the criteria used for establishing cerebral survival through monitoring in intensive care units. The principles laid down during the pre-World War II period are still followed. The tracings, although now recorded effortlessly and cleanly, are no different, save for the electrode combinations, than those seen and interpreted by pioneers.

COMMENT

The value of the EEG lies in its use as a tool for physical diagnosis. It has applications as broad in the field of epilepsy as the electrocardiogram has in heart disease. To an extent, the technological developments that led to electrocardiography and electroencephalography ran parallel, the former having lesser obstacles to surmount because the source of signals is not largely encased in bone and the obstacles to amplification are easier to overcome.

The field of usefulness of the EEG is not restricted to the estimated two million or more Americans who have epilepsy. There are several other common causes of syncope (fainting attacks) in which some aspects of symptomatology may be similar. Upon repeated testing, many individuals prove negative for epilepsy who might otherwise remain under suspicion. The EEG also has been used for other purposes, for example, establishing the sites of brain tumors and cerebrovascular softenings and contributing to proof of other neurological diseases that affect the cerebrum. It also has shown itself to be a useful monitor of brain activity in intensive care units and for establishing cerebral survival in the near moribund patient.

Berger's desire in his momentous studies was to relate the EEG to the psychic manifestations of brain activity, thus increasing knowledge of mental processes and also of their aberrations. His outstanding success was a spin-off of immense value to the neurologist and neurological surgeon. That Berger's original goal was not reached does not mean that this approach to mental disorders is inefficacious. We need only look back over the last two centuries to see in perspective the knowledge of diagnosis and treatment that has developed and to recognize that as knowledge continues to accumulate, Berger's goal may yet be reached unexpectedly. We must maintain the momentum of research and training.

NOTES

[1] In 1972 a short history of the axonologists was published in the quarterly publication of the Society for Neuroscience. (*Neuroscience Newsletter,* Vol. 3, No. 2, p. 6, June, 1972.) The following quotation is from that article:

> There are no records, but general agreement is that about a dozen axonologists met at the home of Ralph Gerard when the APS met in Chicago in 1930. Among those who took part were George Bishop, Detlev Bronk, Hallowell Davis, Joseph Erlanger, Wallace Fenn, Alexander Forbes, Herbert Gasser, H. K. Hartline, Lorente de Nó, Grayson McCouch, F. O. Schmitt, and perhaps others. Fenn in his history, "The Third Quarter Century of the American Physiological Society," credits Forbes as having originated the terms "axonology" and "soup at the synapse" at one of the early meetings, which were unstructured and larded with good fun and hot arguments. The group agreed early in its discussions to jettison the term "sigma" in favor of millisecond. It continued to meet informally in private homes until it became too large and unwieldy due to the popularity of the skits and discussions, and finally disbanded by common consent.

[2] From a tape recording of George H. Bishop's remarks at a memorial exercise for J. E. Erlanger, January 14, 1966. The tape is used through the courtesy of the Grass Instrument Company.

> At this stage a cathode ray oscillograph, the Braun tube, requiring the extremely high driving potential of 10,000 volts but of low sensitivity, was supplied with a hot cathode permitting operation at only 300 volts. Gasser and Erlanger saw in this instrument a final answer to their problem. The new tube was still in the experimental stage and not available to them. They attempted to make one, which blew out on its first trial. Meanwhile negotiations with the manufacturer resulted in the release of this early model for strictly experimental use and their project was on its way. These two men were not particularly sophisticated in either electronics or physics, and their troubles were varied and cumulative. Noise in the amplifier, noise in the environment, vibration from trucks and sparks from the trolley line, called for shielding and insulation. Switches had to be devised which would operate in fractions of a thousandth of a second, without chatter, etc. Finally, no camera would photograph the dim trace obtainable at the speed required to record the nerve impulse. The first records were obtained by holding a photographic film against the end of the tube and repeating the stimuli until an accumulation of superimposed traces induced a bleary line on a somewhat fogged background. I can only compare their progress to the trek of the pioneers in oxcarts across the plains and mountains of the West. They were pioneers of electrophysiology and they encountered every conceivable obstacle but the Indians. Far more time was spent on reconstruction than on recording of nerve, when one good record occasionally made a successful day.
>
> I have gone back and read again those early papers. The problems now look so simple, the results so elementary, the difficulties met so trivial, that one has to think in terms of an era

when electronics was at as elementary a stage as was the sophistication of the workers learning how to deal with both. This was the first application of the cathode ray device to biology and one of the first, at least, to any specific problem.

[3] Robert A. Cohen of the National Institute of Mental Health is the source of information about Gerard's laboratory at the University of Chicago.

[4] One source for information given here regarding its use of the equipment comes from official Army records (Anderson et al., 1966). Navy and Air Corps information was given by former officers who engaged in electroencephalography as a wartime activity.

REFERENCES AND BIBLIOGRAPHY

Adrian, E. D., and Matthews, B. H. C. The Berger rhythm: Potential changes from the occipital lobes in man. *Brain* 57:355–385, 1934.

Anderson, R. S., Glass, A. J., and Berucci, R., eds. *Neuropsychiatry in World War II. Vol. I. Zone of Interior.* (Dept. of the Army, Office of the Surgeon General.) Washington, D.C.: U.S. Government Printing Office, 1966. 898 pp.

Bagchi, B. K. The adaptation and variability of response of the human brain rhythm. *J. Psychol.* 3:463–485, 1937.

Bartley, S. H., and Bishop, G. H. Cortical response to stimulation of the optic nerve. *Proc. Soc. Exp. Biol. Med.* 29:775–777, 1932.

Bartley, S. H., and Newman, E. B. Studies on the dog's cortex. I. The sensori-motor areas. *Am. J. Physiol.* 99:1–8, 1931.

Berger, H. Über das Elektrencephalogramm des Menschen. *Arch. Psychiatr. Nervenkr.* 87:527–570, 1929.

Case, T. J., and Bucy, P. C. Localization of cerebral lesions by electroencephalography. *J. Neurophysiol.* 1:245–261, 1938.

Davis, H., and Davis, P. A. Action potentials of the brain in normal persons and in normal states of cerebral activity. *Arch. Neurol. Psychiatry* 36:1214–1224, 1936.

Davis, H., Davis, P. A., Loomis, A. L., Harvey, E. N., and Hobart, G. Changes in human brain potentials during the onset of sleep. *Science* 86:448–450, 1937.

Davis, H., and Saul, L. J. Action currents in the auditory tracts of the midbrain of the cat. *Science* 74:205–206, 1931.

Forbes, A., and Thacher, C. Amplification of action currents with the electron tube in recording with the string galvanometer. *Am. J. Physiol.* 52:409–471, 1920.

Gerard, R. W., Marshall, W. H., Saul, L. J. Cerebral action potentials. *Proc. Soc. Exp. Biol. Med.* 30:1123–1125, 1933.

Gibbs, F. A., and Gibbs, E. L. *Atlas of Electroencephalography,* Vol. I. Cambridge, Mass.: Lew A. Cummings Co., 1941. 221 pp.; Vol. II, *Epilepsy.* Cambridge, Mass.: Addison-Wesley Press, Inc., 1952. 422 pp.

Gibbs, F. A., and Lennox, W. G. The electrical activity of the brain in epilepsy. *N. Engl. J. Med.* 216:98–99, 1937.

Gibbs, F. A., Davis, H., and Lennox, W. G. The electroencephalogram in epilepsy and in conditions of impaired consciousness. *Arch. Neurol. Psychiatry* 34:1133–1148, 1935.

Gibbs, F. A., Lennox, W. G., and Gibbs, E. L. The electroencephalogram in diagnosis and in localization of epileptic seizures. *Arch. Neurol. Psychiatry* 36:1225–1235, 1936.

Graham, J., and Gerard, R. W. Membrane potentials and excitation of impaled single muscle fibers. *J. Cell. Comp. Physiol.* 28:99–117, 1946.

Jasper, H. H., and Carmichael, L. Electrical potentials from the intact human brain. *Science* 81:51–53, 1935.

Jasper, H. H., and Hawke, W. A. Electroencephalography. IV. Localization of seizure waves in epilepsy. *Arch. Neurol. Psychiatry* 39:885–901, 1938.

Jasper, H. H. Report of the Committee on Methods of Clinical Examination in Electroencephalography, 1957. Appendix. The ten twenty electrode system of the International Federation. *Electroencephalogr. Clin. Neurophysiol.* 10:371–375, 1958.

Jasper, H. H., and Nichols, I. C. Electrical signs of cortical function in epilepsy and allied disorders. *Am. J. Psychiatry* 94:835–850, 1938.

Kreezer, G. Electric potentials of the brain in certain types of mental deficiency. *Arch. Neurol. Psychiatry* 36:1206–1213, 1936.

Lindsley, D. B. Brain potentials in children and adults. *Science* 84:354, 1936.

Lindsley, D. B. Electroencephalography, pp. 1033–1103. In J. McV. Hunt, ed. *Personality and the Behavior Disorders,* Vol. II. New York: The Ronald Press, 1944.

Loomis, A. L., Harvey, E. N., and Hobart, G. Potential rhythms of the cerebral cortex during sleep. *Science* 81:597–598, 1935.

Offner, F., and Gerard, R. W. Scientific apparatus and laboratory methods. A high speed crystal ink writer. *Science* 84:209–210, 1936.

Penfield, W. G., and Jasper, H. H. *Epilepsy and the Functional Anatomy of the Human Brain.* Boston: Little, Brown and Co., 1954. 896 pp.

Sachs, E., Schwartz, H. G., and Kerr, A. S. Electrical activity of the exposed human brain. *Trans. Am. Neurol. Assoc.* 65:14–17, 1939.

Scarff, J. E., and Rahm, W. E., Jr. The human electro-corticogram. A report of spontaneous electrical potentials obtained from the exposed human brain. *J. Neurophysiol.* 4:418–426, 1941.

TB MED 74. War Department Technical Bulletin. Electroencephalography: Operative technique and interpretation. Washington, D.C.: U.S. Government Printing Office, 27 July 1944. 6 pp.

Travis, L. E., and Dorsey, J. M. Action current studies of simultaneously active disparate fields of the central nervous system of the rat. *Arch. Neurol. Psychiatry* 28:331–338, 1932.

Travis, L. E., and Knott, J. R. Brain potentials from normal speakers and stutterers. *J. Psychol.* 2:137–150, 1936.

Williams, D., and Gibbs, F. A. The localization of intracranial lesions by electroencephalography. *N. Engl. J. Med.* 218:998–1002, 1938.

Yeager, C. L. Electro-encephalography as an aid in localizing organic lesions of the brain: Report of a case. *Mayo Clin.* 13:422–426, 1938.

Chapter X

RETICULAR CORE

Localization of function remained subordinate to the diffuse mentalistic view of cerebral activity through much of the nineteenth century. Yet localization won out in the end, prospering anatomically from the general acceptance of the neuron doctrine and physiologically from the evidence for cerebral excitability developed by Fritsch and Hitzig and by Ferrier. It soon became evident, however, that important generalizing functions such as sleep and consciousness had been largely neglected by the localizers.

The reticular substance of the brainstem was known to the classical neuroanatomists of the late nineteenth century as a separate part of the brain in which the nuclei of the cranial nerves were embedded. It was considered a composite of centers for respiration, cardiovascular control, and other generalized bodily functions. Its importance to the maintenance of consciousness and the control of the sleep-waking cycle was unforeseen.

In the 1940s E. W. Dempsey and R. S. Morison, using electrophysiological methods, showed the significance of cellular aggregates of the midline thalamus in exercising diffuse control over the electrical activity of the cortex, and in 1949 G. Moruzzi and H. W. Magoun (1949) published their now classic work concerning activation of the electrocorticogram by repetitive electrical stimulation of the reticular substance. This rapidly led to a series of studies enunciating the roles of reticular substance and midline thalamus as channels that funnel off a part of the information coming from spinal and cranial nerves, including special sense nerves, and disperse it widely over the cerebral cortex. This spino-reticulo-thalamo-cortical system should not be confused with the more direct and localized paths, which early neuroanatomists referred to as *sensory*. After relay in circumscribed loci of the thalamus—sensory relay neuron aggregates—those direct paths project to the cerebral cortex in localized fashion. The contrast between the generalized reticular core routing and that over the localized paths to the confined sense areas of cerebral cortex (tactile, auditory, visual) will become clear as the chapter proceeds.

RETICULAR CORE OR RETICULAR SUBSTANCE

Reticular substance occupies an expanse of the hind- and midbrain underlying both the floor of the posterior ventricle and the aqueduct leading from the anterior parts of the ventricular system (Fig. 1). The reticular core is made up of neuronal clusters with diffusely drawn borders that separate them into aggregates. A wealth of axons, which pass in all directions but chiefly longitudinally, make up the core remainder. In the forward direction, its makeup blends with the more structured neuron groups of the thalamus; backwards, with the central gray matter of the spinal cord. The left side of Fig. 54 illustrates seven cross-sections of the brainstem (Olszewski and Baxter, 1954). (A) through (G) indicate by diagonal shading the position of the reticular substance in transverse sections drawn at equal intervals between the lower brainstem terminus (A) and the upper midbrain (G). The right side shows dorsal (upper) and lengthwise (lower) perspectives of the brainstem, with the extent of the reticular aggregate of each indicated by dots. Figure 55, comparable with the lower right sketch of the

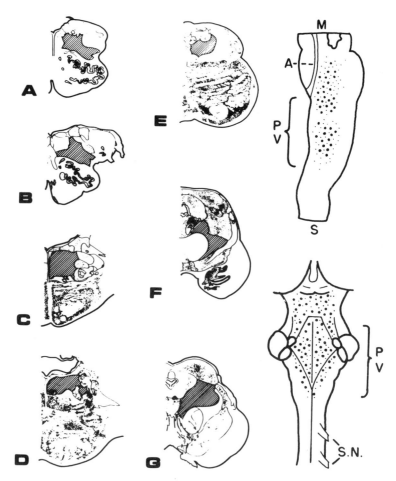

Fig. 54. Redrawn and modified from the Olszewski and Baxter (1954) atlas of the human brainstem. A: Lower medulla. B-G: Successively higher transverse sections of the stem to G, upper midbrain. Reticular core indicated in diagonal lines. Sketch, upper right, longitudinal view, brainstem, reticular core in dots. (M) Midbrain; (A) aqueduct; (PV) posterior ventricle; (S) spinal cord. Sketch, lower right, brainstem viewed from above. Dots identify position of reticular core. (PV) Lozenge-shaped posterior ventricle; (SN) spinal nerve roots.

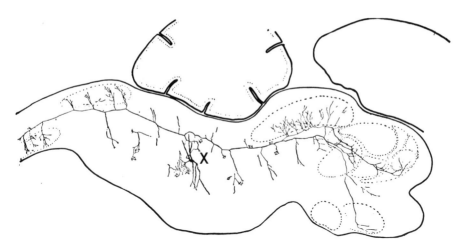

Fig. 55. Longitudinal sketch, brainstem of 2-day-old rat, showing a single reticular neuron *(X)* and an axon that arborizes forward and backward through the reticular core. (From Scheibel and Scheibel, 1958.)

preceding figure, is a lengthwise outline of an animal brainstem showing a single reticular neuron with the entirety of its longitudinally coursing axon—including terminal collaterals—as drawn by Scheibel and Scheibel (1958). Figure 56, also courtesy of the Scheibels, is a horizontal Golgi-stained section of upper brainstem showing the terminus of the reticular substance and the commencing dispersion through the thalamus of those reticular axons that scatter before reaching their endings in the cerebral cortex.

Historically, the earliest insight into the structure of the human brainstem was provided in 1846 by B. Stilling, who cut it freehand with a razor into a succession of either transverse or longitudinal planes, after hardening in spirits of wine (impure alcohol). Even in those early days, a microscope could reveal the sharp contours of the cranial nerve nuclei embedded within the reticular substance. At that time, the reticular core was also identifiable from longitudinal axon bundles and the routes of ingress and egress of cranial nerves passing to the exterior of the brain. Later, in thinner sections—cut on a microtome and stained by Weigert for the axon sheaths and by carmine for the cell bodies—the meshwork appearance of the reticular substance became clearly evident.

Reticular neurons and their neighboring neuropil fill in the spaces that lie between the bundles of axons. Near the midline of the brainstem, reticular neurons are larger and fewer. Farther outward they become smaller and more numerous, the neuropil increases in amount, and the axons become more scattered. W. Nauta and H. G. J. M. Kuypers (1957) undertook an experimental study in which spinoreticular collaterals arising from the localized ascending sensory systems were shown to have a wide distribution within the reticular core.

Many efforts have been made to subdivide reticular neurons into identifiable aggregates, but the cell assemblies have ill-defined margins, and no two

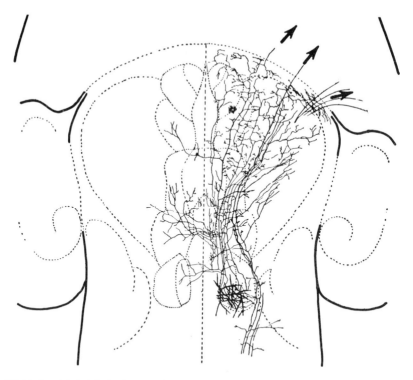

Fig. 56. Horizontal sketch, brainstem of 12-day-old mouse, showing the reticulocortical radiation fanning out toward the cortex (*arrows*). (From Scheibel and Scheibel, 1957.)

neuroanatomists agree exactly upon the subdivisions. Their appearance resembles a suburban area built up without a plan relating units of different sizes and separations. But such appearances are deceiving. There is a well-formed organization that is in the process of being uncovered by the arduous work of A. B. and M. E. Scheibel (1957). Using Golgi thick sections (Fig. 55), they have studied reticular neurons as they appear in lengthwise and transverse planes of the brainstem of the immature animal. The dendritic arbors of individual neurons occur in overlapping series throughout the longitudinal extent of the reticular core. The maximal dendritic arborizations always develop in a plane perpendicular to the long axis of the brainstem. Each axon provides a variety of neighboring terminals at different levels of the brainstem and those form synapses with other reticular elements. In the forepart of the reticular substance, the axons of many neurons project to the cerebral cortex. Figure 57 shows a drawing from D. B. Lindsley (1957) that illustrates by thick diverging arrows how the reticular projection spreads upward to disperse to different cortical regions. Upon arrival in the cortex, these axons arborize widely across all cell layers, whereas, by contrast, the thalamocortical axons reaching upward to each of the circumscribed sensory cortical areas (tactile, visual, auditory) terminate only in the middle level of cortical thickness.

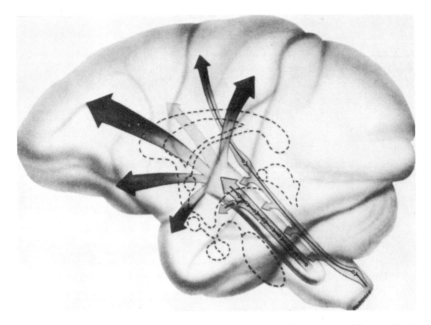

Fig. 57. Ascending reticular activating system projected onto a lateral view of the monkey brain. (From Lindsley, 1957.)

Many studies have indicated that the reticular neurons are capable of intrinsic activity. They are driven also by impulses pumped into the reticular substance over axon collaterals, reaching them from the specific sensory systems. Such afferents bring information from the general and special sense organs at the periphery of the body. Reticular neurons are also driven by impulses from cerebral cortex, subcortical gray matter, and cerebellum. Thus, each reticular neuron is of itself a minute integrative center capable of moment-to-moment compromises in its responses to several inputs.

The essential morphological concept of the reticular core has been touched on in René Dubos' column, *The Despairing Optimist* (1971–1972). Dubos thinks of a solitary ant as a ganglion on legs, and perhaps that is also a satisfactory simile for each of the many neurons that comprise the reticular substance. Thousands of ants crowded together and working on an anthill behave collectively as reticular substance (or as an organism) does. The workers of a given anthill are linked in a complex system for collection, storage, processing, and retrieval of an immense variety of information that is the collective property of the hill. But, instead of speaking further of the anthill, we will revert to the term that describes it, *reticular core.*

CHANGES IN CORTICAL RHYTHMS AND BEHAVIORAL CORRELATES

It is necessary, first, to explain how activity carried to the cerebral cortex via the reticular route is registered on the electrocorticogram of an experimental animal or the electroencephalogram (EEG) of man. The specific localizing systems for touch, hearing, and vision convey signals rapidly over the well-trodden, direct paths to the respective circumscribed cortical receiving areas allotted to these sensations. Each such path is a closely confined one along which routed signals pass no more than two synapses in reaching cortex. A genetic pattern dictates that the left cerebral cortex is related to the right side of the body and vice versa, and the decussation and course of the paths correspond. At their cortical terminus, the signals activate a rapidly consummated, specific response, the *evoked potential.*

By contrast, identical signals, which pass from the mother axon along collaterals, enter the labyrinthine connections of the reticular net, thereafter to synapse with other reticular neurons, the axons of which fan widely to enter cerebral cortex. There the signals arriving over reticular axons block the intrinsic alpha rhythm in man or the corresponding spontaneous rhythm in the experimental animal. Such blocking had been suspected long ago—by A. Beck in 1890 and his successors—during the early development of electrocorticography. In the visual system, the blocking can last as long as 10 seconds following a single flash of light. It is the equivalent of the disappearance of alpha rhythm in a human subject as he opens his eyes, and results from a diffuse desynchronization of neuronal activity. In the terminology of behaviorists, the desynchronized pattern is called an *activation trace.*

Rapid electrical stimulation (i.e., tetanization) of the reticular core in an anesthetized animal, using stimulating electrodes, can produce an identical result, which likewise is a nonspecific response to the stimulus. If anesthesia is lightened somewhat, a simultaneous pricking up of the animal's ears may occur upon stimulation. This is called *arousal,* another behavioristic term. A lesion made in the reticulocortical path of one cerebral hemisphere of an anesthetized animal abolishes the activation effect on the side of the lesion, converting the brain rhythms of that side to a slow frequency pattern identical with that seen in man in deep sleep. F. Bremer (1938), the Belgian neurophysiologist, who first saw this abolition of pattern following a bilateral lesion, called it "permanent sleep," and designated the animal with the bilateral lesion that produces it a *cerveau isolé* preparation. Such a preparation is a useful experimental model for studying the spread of the epileptic attack.

EVOKED AND UNIT RECORDING FROM NEURONS OF THE RETICULAR CORE

Potentials can be evoked in the reticular core by local stimulation of outlying nerves deriving from the skin, the viscera, or the special sense organs. The first convey tactile sensibility; the second, visceral; and the last, taste, olfactory, visual, and auditory sense data. Potentials from each source can be evoked widely in the reticular substance. In other words, their endings are not localized.

G. Moruzzi and H. W. Magoun (1949) recorded randomly through fine wire recording electrodes inserted into various parts of the reticular core and were successful in recording the same potential at several sites. Regional stimulation of cerebral cortex by single shocks also evokes such potentials, and the same cellular region can be activated from cerebral cortex and from stimuli given one or another spinal or cranial nerve.

Such data indicate wide overlaps in the effects of cortical and of outlying nerve activation on the reticular substance. When two shocks are given in widely different cortical areas, the one leading the other by a few thousandths of a second, the reticular potential evoked by the first shock may occlude that produced by the second. This is added proof that physiological effects of disparate origins converge on *one and the same neuron* in contrast to reticular activation effects, where such occlusions or convergences do not happen. In the specific localizing systems described here, close identification of the source of a stimulus may be expected.

Reticular neurons, as well as neuron clusters, can be recorded by still finer electrodes. This also strongly suggests the convergence of different modalities of sensation (as visual and tactile) on the same reticular neuron. Using microelectrodes, P. R. Huttenlocher (Evarts, 1961) showed by unit-discharge studies that reduction in auditory-click-evoked cell spikes occurs during both slow-wave and REM (rapid eye movement) sleep. He did not observe a corresponding reduction in spontaneously discharging unit activity, however. In fact, during REM sleep, spontaneous discharges were much more frequent than in either the waking state or in slow-wave sleep.

INHIBITION AND FACILITATION ARISING FROM THE RETICULAR CORE

The reticular core produces downstream as well as upstream effects. This is evident in studies of the spinal reflexes. An inhibitory center is reported to exist in the reticular substance of the hindbrain (Magoun and Rhines, 1946). Tetanic stimulation in anesthetized animals yields decrease or abolition of eye blink, knee jerk, and other phasic reflexes; decrease of fore- and hind-limb flexion; and tonic stretching of extensor muscles. These reflexes were concurrently activated, with and without inhibitory stimulation.

Facilitation (enhancement of reflexes) is affected by activation within a length of the lateral reticular core extending from midline thalamus downward to a facilitatory center in the hindbrain (Magoun, 1950). From there, activity directed toward the spine facilitates spinal reflexes. This system operates through short relays, as do the ascending reticular paths. Cerebellar inhibitory influences can be propagated spinally from the anterior area of the cerebellum. On the other hand, high-frequency stimulation in the region of the central cerebellar nuclei evokes spinal facilitation.

RETICULAR ACTIVATION RESULTING FROM HUMORALLY MEDIATED AGENTS

Experimental observations indicate that activation of the cortical brain wave pattern can also be mediated humorally. A. Hugelin, M. Bonvallet, and P. Dell (1959) showed that activation of the electrocorticogram occurs in a tripartite sequence, e.g., after sciatic stimulation, an initial activation, followed by return to slow waves, and those, in turn, succeeded by a much longer activation sequence. A rise in blood pressure separates the two activation sequences. The late, but not the early, phase of activation can be reproduced by either the injection of epinephrine into a vein or the stimulation of the splanchnic nerve; the latter is a procedure that liberates epinephrine from the adrenal gland. The epinephrine effect does not act directly on the cortex, but rather through the ascending reticular activating system. This is proved abundantly by division of one-half the brainstem just above the midbrain. In that case, humoral activation through systemic injection of epinephrine continues to occur on the side still connected through its reticular links, but is missing on the separated side. Thus, epinephrine must affect the reticular neurons at their source and not at the endings of the system in the cortex.

Such observations show the existence of a diffusely distributed ascending reticular activating system that extends through all levels of the cerebrospinal axis. It responds to and works with the specific systems in their functioning. The chief result of the operations of the upgoing system is coterminous *activation of the cerebral cortex* (a diffuse change in the electrocorticogram) and *arousal* (a behavioral change). The chief downstream effects of the system are facilitation or inhibition of spinal and brainstem reflexes, regulating the balance between these opposing influences on intercalary neurons and motoneurons. Optimal balances may and do vary between waking, REM, and slow-wave sleep states. They also must meet the neuromuscular requirements of postural control as mediated through brainstem mechanisms. Humoral agents carried in the blood stream act on reticular neurons directly and can modify activating, facilitatory, and inhibitory effects.

INTEGRATIVE ACTION OF THE DIFFUSE THALAMIC PROJECTION SYSTEM

In a series of provocative researches leading toward proof of the existence of a diffuse thalamic integrating system, which is paralleled by and articulated with the specific sensory systems at thalamic and cortical levels, E. W. Dempsey and R. S. Morison (1941) showed that low-frequency stimulation (8 to 13 per second) of midline thalamic neuron aggregates exercises a widespread influence over cerebral cortical rhythms. Described elsewhere, these are called *recruiting responses.*

R. W. Doty (1969) reviewed current neurophysiological thought concerning the effect of electrical stimulation on the brain. He concluded that the neural organization responsible for any complex outcome of a localized artificial stimulus lies remote to the neurons stimulated. In the instances compared in the Morison-Dempsey experiments, the thalamic source lay within either a midline or a relay neuron aggregate. The first gave rise to a widespread cortical "recruiting" (incrementing) response that follows repetitive stimulation. The second produced a cortical-evoked response that drops in amplitude when activated repetitively. In each instance, the site of activation was provable by a survey of histological sections through the thalamus.

The evoked potential activated from a sensory relay nucleus is invariably localized to its corresponding cortical site. It is a rapid diphasic signal, initially surface-positive in polarity and secondarily, surface-negative. It *declines in amplitude on repetitive stimulation.* S. Sharpless and H. H. Jasper (1948) aptly illustrate the meaning of decrement in this instance by reference to a sea anemone (a whole organism instead of a neuron) afloat upon the water. It contracts vigorously when a drop of water falls upon it. A second drop falling minutes later evokes a less vigorous contraction, and, with a third and fourth drop, the contraction disappears altogether. That is the equivalent of the decremental response of the specific systems mentioned above, with the exception that repetitive neural stimuli fall at intervals of milliseconds, not minutes.

To the contrary, the widespread recruiting (incrementing) response to midline thalamic stimulation gives only a slight blip after the initial stimulus of a series and *grows in amplitude over a stimulus succession* (Fig. 58). Growth reaches a limit, of course, after which the response wanes again. The optimum growth rate is achieved at 8 to 12 stimuli per second. That, incidentally, is the frequency of the animal cortical rhythm, which is the presumed equivalent of the human alpha rhythm.

Recruiting is characteristic of the graded cortical responses attributed by G. H. Bishop (1956) to cortical dendrites. Decrementing-evoked responses, to the contrary, are presumed due to neuron soma activities. A. Arduini and C. Terzuolo (1951, 1957) believe that the organization of the recruiting effect occurs at the stimulus site in the circuitry of the midline thalamus. An alternative explanation attributes recruiting to a cortical recording site overlying the surface dendritic arbors of the cortical pyramids.

The latency of the recruiting response at corresponding sites in the cortices of the two hemispheres is the same only when the stimulating electrode tip lies exactly in the midline (Kerr and O'Leary, 1957). Moving the tip toward right or left diminishes latency to cortex in the direction in which the tip is moved and lengthens it for recruiting responses of the other hemisphere. This indicates that the midline circuitry in the environs of the stimulus tip does play an important role in organizing the cortical recruiting response.

Herbert Jasper (1949) extended the observations of Morison and Dempsey, mapping the cortical sites that showed maximal recruiting. Jasper and J. Droogleever-Fortuyn (1947) also related the results to epilepsy research by showing

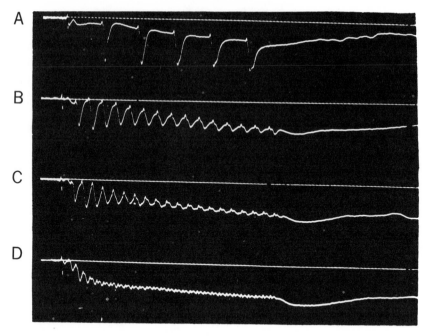

FIG. 58. A: Cortical-recruiting response stimulus to midline thalamus, recorded with direct-coupled amplifier and showing underlying slow potential shift. **B-D:** Same stimulus strength and increasing stimulus frequency, showing transition from recruiting to activation type of tracing. Straight white lines, zero of the amplifier, from which slow potential shift develops during stimulation.

that stimuli at three to four per second in the midline of the animal thalamus activated an approximation of the spike-wave sequence of petit mal epilepsy in widespread cortical areas of the two hemispheres. This is only one of the important dividends for epilepsy paid by experimental studies, which indicate in this instance the existence of a diffuse thalamic system exercising control over both sides of the brain. The cerebral commissure called corpus callosum does not serve that purpose. Experimentally, it can be sectioned entirely, yet bilateral recruiting still develops on midline stimulation.

Using a chopper-stabilized, capacity-coupled amplifier and nonpolarizing electrodes (which also minimize baseline drift) to record the slower components of cortical potential, the recruiting sequence in animals can be shown to be underlaid by an enduring negative shift reaching 1 to 2 millivolts in amplitude. The shift develops during stimulation, together with the series of recruiting waves, and persists into the poststimulus period (Goldring and O'Leary, 1957) (Fig. 58). This is another instance of midline activation suggestive of a dendritic origin of the recruiting response. A slow shift of similarly negative polarity also occurs in cortical activation due to tetanizing stimulation of either forward reticular core or midline thalamus. It is evidence of interlocking between reticular and midline thalamic routes to cerebral cortex.

Slow-potential shifts of long duration also underlie all seizure discharges of animals and man that have been studied by such electrocorticographic recording. In human scalp EEGs, such shifts also have been shown to accompany the bursts of spike-wave discharge of petit mal epilepsy (Cohn, 1954).

NEURAL MECHANISMS RELATED TO SLEEP

Sleep is of special importance to the epileptologist. Epileptic attacks occur in some subjects during both sleeping and waking states, in others during sleep alone. In still others, attacks are related to a particular phase of sleep, or occur on awakening. Significantly, what is called "slow-wave sleep" in man is replaced periodically by an activation-like trace sometimes designated as paradoxical sleep (Fig. 59). Dreams occur during the latter. The equivalent phase of sleep in animals is also accompanied by rapid eye movements (REM) and a loss of tone in the neck muscles. In animal experiments, this sleep occurrence is designated as *activated* sleep.

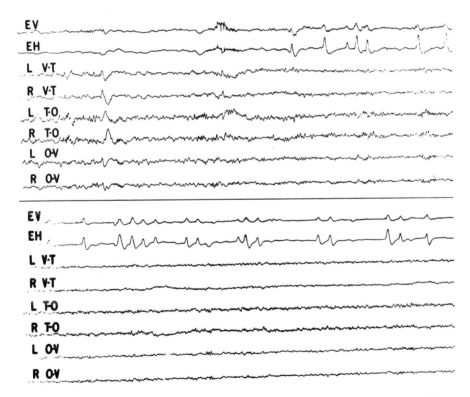

FIG. 59. Human EEG showing "activated" sleep. Upper two traces of each strip show rapid eye movement (REM) recorded electrically from vertically and horizontally placed ocular electrodes. Other traces are of brain activity. (From O'Leary Landau, and Brooks, 1971.)

In experimental studies, H. Jasper and J. Tessier (1971) examined the rate of liberation of free acetylcholine (the excitatory neurotransmitter) at the surface of the cerebral cortex during slow-wave sleep, activated or REM sleep, and waking states. They found the acetylcholine release to increase in relation to the activation pattern rather than to the behavioral alertness of the animal.

THEORIES OF SLEEP

The nature of sleep seems to have been among the more puzzling questions of mankind. In a historical review, Moruzzi (1964) followed the development of theories of sleep causation from Lucretius, who died in 55 B.C., to modern times. Within the limits of an obsolete teminology and hampered by ancient physiological misconceptions, Lucretius had ideas germane to a widely held modern theory that ascribes sleep to a temporary loss in sensory inflow to the cerebral mechanism (deafferentation).

As used in discussing theories of sleep, "deafferentation" should not be confused with the pathological state of neurons adjoining an epileptic lesion. In this context, it denotes a temporary interruption in the flow of afferent impulses that maintains a state of waking tone at the higher brain levels. This awareness is assured by the ascending reticular activating system. Lucretius, of course, held no such modern ideas, nor did Burdach[1] 2,000 years later, although the latter's views also were couched in a scientifically primitive terminology.

L. Rolando and P. Flourens, whose studies are reviewed in Chapter VI, were the first to engage in ablative experiments, including assessment of the deficit incurred in animals after removal of the cerebrum. In 1809 Rolando reported that birds behaved as if asleep after such removals. So did Flourens' report in 1822, after making bilateral extirpations of the cerebral hemispheres. The universally admired Purkinje[2] (1846) theorized on the basis of those results that sleep resulted from functional interruption of the relation between cerebrum and brainstem occurring at the site where the localizing systems traverse the capsular white matter between brainstem and cortex. Naturally, his assumptions were couched in mechanistic terms foreign to later electrophysiological observations.

Anatomicoclinical studies of sleeping sickness, a lethargic encephalitis epidemic that occurred during World War I, by C. von Economo (1926) led him to hypothesize an elongate wakefulness center on either side of the cerebral aqueduct and third ventricle. His sleep center was postulated to exert an active inhibition over other parts of the brain, thus producing sleep.

F. Bremer (1938), observing the electrocorticogram of the experimental animal before and after a complete midbrain transection, showed that the aftermath was a replica of normal sleep, including transition to high-voltage slow waves in the electrocorticogram, divergence of the eyes, and constriction of the pupils. Thus, he offered the earliest tangible support of the "deafferentation" hypothesis.

Passing over theories unrelated to the scientific base of epilepsy, one looks to the reticular core hypothesis of sleep. This stems from the work of H. W. Magoun,

G. Moruzzi, and associates beginning in 1949. It involved projection of the ascending reticular activating system to the cerebral hemispheres. They found indications of activation of cortex by rapid repetitive stimulation of the reticular core at the midbrain level. Conversely, destruction of the reticular core by lesions made the cortex unresponsive to activation by electrical stimuli applied at lower brainstem levels. Moruzzi (1964) concluded that under normal circumstances in the alert animal, the cortex is maintained in a state of tonic activation by a steady ascent of impulses along the spino-reticulo-cerebral activating system. This exerts the diffuse facilitating influence on the cerebrum necessary to maintain wakefulness. When the cortical tone derived from the ascending system falls below a critical level, the maintenance of a waking state is no longer possible. That is the equivalent of falling asleep.

TEMPORAL LOBE SEIZURES AND EEG RECORDING DURING SLEEP

Some epileptics afflicted by temporal lobe seizures (Chapter II) show low-voltage spikes that rise from one or another (or both) of the temporal scalp regions during sleep. Their waking trace can be quite normal (Gibbs, Gibbs, and Fuster, 1947). The average adult spends one-third of his life asleep, so the occurrence of grand mal or other seizures during sleep should not be surprising. This is one more reason why the physiology of sleep is of interest to the scientific investigation of epilepsy.

COMMENT

The operations of the reticular core as a generalized integrative mechanism that regulates transitions between waking and sleep, and in the waking state participate importantly in the maintenance of consciousness, exemplify the holistic concept of cerebral functioning. If the need for a working relationship between brainstem and cerebral hemispheres is recognized as basic to higher brain activity, this chapter has made its major point.

At the psychological level, there is a more erudite instance of whole brain integration that also requires the cortices of the cerebral hemispheres. The corpus callosum and other lesser connections between the cerebral hemispheres integrate effectively the mental activities unique to the half-brains. R. W. Sperry has used advanced perceptual analysis to study the deficit incurred in several individuals whose commissures had been divided surgically at an earlier date to aid the control of advanced, intractable epilepsy. Remarkably, the absence of the cerebral commissures does not prevent the spread of bursts of spike-wave activity of petit mal type to both hemispheres (Hursh, 1945). This shows that the deficit incurred by commissurectomy need not include functions mediated by the reticular activating system.

In analyzing the mental aspects of the deficit incurred by commissural lesions, Sperry (1970) speculated that like electrical, chemical, and physical properties of brain excitation, the conscious properties are embedded within the brain process as an essential constituent of the action. He views conscious forces as encompassing and transcending the details of neural processes in somewhat the same way that others have viewed the relations of atom, molecule, cell, and so on, each a higher stage of hierarchical system, the topmost of which adds an intangible something to the whole of what lies below it. The reader need only reflect upon the developments that arose from the pursuit over preceding centuries of what our progenitors called a *mysterious force,* and thereafter harnessed as a new source of energy, *electricity.* Is it too much to expect that someday mental "energy" will become comprehensible in the same way?

Both experimentally and clinically, seizure-discharges have been shown to spread across the corpus callosum, but that spread is more topically organized than is that of the reticular activating system. Wilder Penfield and Herbert Jasper (1954) designated the latter as the *centrencephalic system.* It is presumed to be the route of spread of all generalized seizures, and particularly of those designated as petit and grand mal. These are sometimes called *centrencephalic seizures,* and it has been recognized of late that such epilepsy may have a hereditary significance.

NOTES

[1] K. F. Burdach's work, *Vom Baue und Leben des Gehirns* (1826), was not available to the writer.

[2] V. Kruta (1967, p. 284) considers Purkinje's notion of a mechanical interruption as involving "strangling and compressing" of the nervous connections between the cerebrum and the more caudal parts of the central nervous system. "It reflects a time," in Kruta's words, "in which knowledge of the nature of nervous processes was just elementary." On the other hand, Purkinje was sophisticated enough to view nerve cells as generators and nerve fibers as distributors.

REFERENCES AND BIBLIOGRAPHY

Arduini, A. Enduring potential changes evoked in the cerebral cortex by stimulation of brain stem reticular formation and thalamus, pp. 333–351. In H. H. Jasper, L. D. Proctor, R. S. Knighton, W. C. Noshay, and R. T. Costello, eds. *Reticular Formation of the Brain.* Boston: Little, Brown and Co., 1957. 766 pp.

Arduini, A., and Terzuolo, C. Cortical and subcortical components in the recruiting responses. *Electroencephalogr. Clin. Neurophysiol.* 3:189–196, 1951.

Bishop, G. H. Natural history of the nerve impulse. *Physiol. Rev.* 36:376–399, 1956.

Bremer, F. Effets de la deafferentation complète d'une région de l'écorce cérébrale sur son activité électrique spontanée. *C. R. Soc. Biol. (Paris)* 127:355–359, 1938.

Cohn, R. Spike-dome complex in the human electroencephalogram. *Arch. Neurol. Psychiatry* 71: 699–706, 1954.

Dempsey, E. W., and Morison, R. S. The production of rhythmically recurrent cortical potentials after localized thalamic stimulation. *Am. J. Physiol.* 135:293–300, 1941.

Doty, R. W. Electrical stimulation of the brain in behavioral context. *Annu. Rev. Psychol.* 20:289–320, 1969.

Dubos, R. The despairing optimist. *American Scholar* 41(1):17, 1971–1972.

von Economo, C. Die Pathologie des Schlafes, pp. 591–610. In A. Bethe, G. v. Bergmann, G. Embden, and A. Ellinger, eds. *Handbuch der normalen und pathologischen Physiologie,* Vol. 17. Berlin: Julius Springer, 1926.

Evarts, E. V. Effects of sleep and waking on activity of single units in the unrestrained cat, p. 171–182.

In G. E. W. Wolstenholme and M. O'Connor, eds. *Ciba Foundation Symposium on The Nature of Sleep.* Boston: Little, Brown and Co., 1961.

Gibbs, F. A., Gibbs, E. L., and Fuster, B. Anterior temporal localization of sleep-induced seizure discharges of psychomotor type. *Trans. Am. Neurol. Assoc.* 72:180–182, 1947.

Goldring, S., and O'Leary, J. L. Cortical DC changes incident to midline thalamic stimulation. *Electroencephalogr. Clin. Neurophysiol.* 9:577–584, 1957.

Hugelin, A., Bonvallet, M., and Dell, P. Activation réticulaire et corticale d'origine chémoceptive au cours de l'hypoxie. *Electroencephalogr. Clin. Neurophysiol.* 11:325–340, 1959.

Hursh, J. B. Origin of the spike wave pattern of petit mal epilepsy. *Arch. Neurol. Psychiatry* 53: 274–282, 1945.

Jasper, H. H. Diffuse projection systems: The integrative action of the thalamic reticular system. *Electroencephalogr. Clin. Neurophysiol.* 1:405–419, 1949.

Jasper, H. H., and Droogleever-Fortuyn, J. Experimental Studies on the functional anatomy of petit mal epilepsy. *Res. Publ. Assoc. Res. Nerv. Ment. Dis.* 26:272–298, 1947.

Jasper, H. H., and Tessier, J. Acetylcholine liberation from cerebral cortex during paradoxical (REM) sleep. *Science* 172:601–602, 1971.

Kerr, F. W. L., and O'Leary, J. L. The thalamic source of cortical recruiting in the rodent. *Electroencephalogr. Clin. Neurophysiol.* 9:461–476, 1957.

Kruta, V. J. E. Purkyně's conception of the physiological basis of wakefulness and sleep. *Scripta Med.* 40:281–290, 1967.

Lindsley, D. B. The reticular system and perceptual discrimination, pp. 513–534. In H. H. Jasper, L. D. Proctor, R. S. Knighton, W. C. Noshay, and R. T. Costello, eds. *Reticular Formation of the Brain* (Henry Ford Hospital International Symposium.) Boston: Little, Brown and Co., 1957.

Magoun, H. W. Caudal and cephalic influences of the brainstem reticular formation. *Physiol. Rev.* 30:459–474, 1950.

Magoun, H. W., and Rhines, R. An inhibitory mechanism in the bulbar reticular formation. *J. Neurophysiol.* 9:165–171, 1946.

Moruzzi, G. The historical development of the deafferentation hypothesis of sleep. *Proc. Am. Philos. Soc.* 108:19–28, 1964.

Moruzzi, G., and Magoun, H. W. Brain stem reticular formation and activation of the EEG. *Electroencephalogr. Clin. Neurophysiol.* 1:455–473, 1949.

Nauta, W. J. H., and Kuypers, H. G. J. M. Some ascending pathways in the brainstem reticular formation, pp. 3–30. In H. H. Jasper, L. D. Proctor, R. S. Knighton, W. C. Noshay, and R. T. Costello, eds. *Reticular Formation of the Brain.* (Henry Ford Hospital International Symposium.) Boston: Little, Brown and Co., 1957.

O'Leary, J. L., and Coben, L. The reticular core—1957. *Physiol. Rev.* 38:243–276, 1958.

O'Leary, J. L., Landau, W. M., and Brooks, J. E. Electroencephalography and electromyography, pp. 1–64. In A. B. Baker and L. H. Baker, eds. *Clinical Neurology,* Vol. I. New York: Harper & Row, 1971.

Olszewski, J., and Baxter, D. *Cytoarchitecture of the Human Brain Stem.* Philadelphia: J. B. Lippincott Co., 1954. 199 pp.

Penfield, W. G., and Jasper, H. H. *Epilepsy and the Functional Anatomy of the Human Brain.* Boston: Little, Brown and Co., 1954. 896 pp.

Purkinje, J. E. Wachen, Schlaf, Traum und verwandte Zustände, pp. 412–480. In R. von Wagner, ed. *Handworterbuch der Physiologie, mit Rücksicht auf physiologische Pathologie.* Abth. 2. Braunschweig: F. Vieweg und Sohn, 1846.

Rasmussen, A. T. *Some Trends in Neuroanatomy.* Dubuque, Ia.: W. C. Brown Co., 1947. 93 pp.

Scheibel, M. E., and Scheibel, A. B. Structural substrates for integrative patterns in the brain stem reticular core, pp. 31–55. In H. H. Jasper, L. D. Proctor, R. S. Knighton, W. C. Noshay, and R. T. Costello, eds. *Reticular Formation of the Brain.* (Henry Ford Hospital International Symposium.) Boston: Little, Brown and Co., 1957.

Sharpless, S., and Jasper, H. H. Habituation of the arousal reaction. *Brain* 69:655–680, 1948.

Sperry, R. W. Perception in the absence of the neocortical commissures, pp. 123–138. In D. A. Hamburg, K. H. Pribram, and A. J. Stunkard, eds. *Perception and its Disorders. Proceedings of the Association for Research in Nervous and Mental Disease,* Vol. 48. Baltimore: Williams and Wilkins Co., 1970.

Starzl, T. E., Taylor, C. W., and Mahoun, H. W. Ascending conduction in reticular activating system, with special reference to the diencephalon. *J. Neurophysiol.* 14:461–477, 1951.

Chapter XI

NEUROPATHOLOGY OF EPILEPSY

Some set the scene to make it unimportant, others very important.

Anon.

Throughout this book epilepsy is called a disorder rather than a disease. That may seem at variance with the opinion of A. Pope (1969), a leading neuropathologist who views most human epilepsy as the result of brain damage. W. Gowers (1885), famed nineteenth-century epileptologist, held that the appearance of affected nerve centers is for the most part the same as that of healthy organs, an appraisal with which this book agrees. Nevertheless, Gowers' opinion, expressed in 1885, was limited largely by naked eye inspection, whereas today's observation has the advantages of the universal use of light microscopy and of a giant step forward to electron microscopy. The latter gives an immense increase over the light microscope in both magnification and resolution of tissue detail.

In considering the relevance of neuropathological findings within the epileptic's brain to attacks during life, it must be kept in mind that epilepsy is very prevalent, that its occurrence is worldwide, and that its manifestations vary from mild to severe. As a result, there are formidable sampling differences between lesser manifestations as seen in the outpatients of an epilepsy clinic and the more severe ones found in inpatients of a hospital for chronic cases. Epilepsy is an umbrella term covering both the cases in which only a few isolated attacks occur over a lifetime and those with severe recurring manifestations. Most cases lie between the two extremes.

If the most advanced microscopic technologies could establish that one epileptic person had an unequivocally normal brain, there would be strong vindication of the proposition that epilepsy is a disorder. There is always the reservation that as yet we know next to nothing of the microscopy of brain organization at the molecular level. It seems improbable that this hurdle will be surmounted in our generation. Moreover, there are several primary diseases of the nervous system in which convulsions are a cardinal symptom; and head injuries, especially at birth, are an important predisposing factor in epileptic attacks.

Thus, it is difficult to draw a clear line between epilepsy, which is a symptom of organic brain disease (including the residual effects of trauma), and those cases in which the condition is due exclusively to the faulty operations of normal brain. With this caution in mind, attention is given first to those pathologic findings that occur in the brains of epileptics but are not found ordinarily in those of nonepileptics.

NEUROPATHOLOGICAL FINDINGS

In idiopathic epilepsy (including cases of generalized seizures not having a focal origin) the following occurrences are reported for the cerebral hemispheres. Gliosis (overgrowth of neuroglial connective tissue) may affect the outer margin of cerebral cortex to a variable extent and also appear at the white matter rim of the brain ventricles. Isolated neurons, scattered throughout the cerebral cortex, present bizarre shapes in some brains of epileptics. In others, many neurons show excessively pale or dark tints compared with the usual intermediate blue or violet of normal nerve cells colored by conventional stains.

In very rare cases, the death of a child epileptic may occur as the conclusion of a series of rapidly recurring severe seizures *(status epilepticus)*. Under that circumstance, laminar deterioration of neurons may involve the intermediate strata of cerebral cortex (Meyer, Beck, and Shepherd, 1955). This condition is called "laminar" necrosis because of the massive cell destruction that takes place within the involved transverse layers. Identical necrosis also develops as a result of any prolonged illness complicated by a severe oxygen deficit, even when there are no accompanying seizures. In status epilepticus, such necrosis is blamed on extreme sensitivity of cortical neurons to a deficiency in oxygen supply.

The pathologist may unexpectedly encounter a cortical scar to which the enveloping membranes of the brain are attached locally. Such occurrences ordinarily relate to an earlier head injury. The cortex near the scar may contain many "deafferented" neurons. In these, as will be discussed in more detail later, the somata and dendrites are almost bare of synapses. This is also seen in experimental epilepsy in animals. In electrophysiological recordings, such deafferented neurons show burst discharges of a type similar to those seen in the epilepsy of experimental animals (see Chapter XIV).

SCLEROSIS OF AMMON'S HORN AS A FINDING IN EPILEPTIC BRAINS

Ammon's horn (technically the hippocampus) and its adnexa, the dentate fascia, are formed by a rolling-in of the margin of the exposed cerebral cortex along a line separating the lower inner surface of the temporal lobe and the inside of the inferior horn of the lateral ventricle (Grünthal, 1968). A dissection of the right hippocampal formation exposed within that part of the lateral ventricle is shown in Fig. 60. Hardening, atrophy, or softening was first detected in Ammon's horn by Bouchet and Cazauvieilh (1825). That was too long ago for the use of light microscopy, and those pioneers had to depend on naked eye appearances and the feel of the parts involved.

The region that lies at the transition between the outside and inside of the turned-in cortex is most susceptible to oxygen lack, due presumably to special vulnerability of its blood supply. It is sometimes called the *Sommer sector* in memory of W. Sommer (1880), who first described the degeneration of neurons in that hippocampal region. Figure 61 is a sketch of a normal human hippocampus; Fig. 62, the corresponding cellular architecture of the horn as seen by Ramón y Cajal in an animal Golgi preparation.

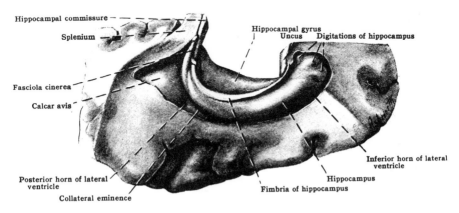

FIG. 60. Hippocampus from the inside of the lateral ventricle. (From Schaeffer, 1942.)

Sclerosis (hardening) of the hippocampal region has been reported as occurring on one or both sides of the brain in up to 50% of a series of epileptic brains examined thoroughly. In the aggregate of all case material so examined, however, it is a far less common occurrence. K. Earle, M. Baldwin, and W. Penfield (1953) wrote of a herniation of one or both hippocampi beneath the edge of tentorium, a fold of the outer tough dural cover of the brain that forms an inner shelf separating the cerebrum from the cerebellum along the curve of the hippocampal formation.

In the newborn, the temporal lobe is not well developed. Due to the pressure built up in the head as the infant passes downwards through the birth canal, herniation of the hippocampal formation may develop. This can cause local damage that may not be immediately evident, yet may relate to seizures in adult life. In fact, birth herniation is a probability in the brains of a significant proportion of adult victims of temporal lobe seizures. Evidence for such herniations can be obtained in adult life from the combined use of pneumoencephalography, arteriography, and electrodes implanted in depth for electrocorticographic recording. All these are neurosurgical procedures.

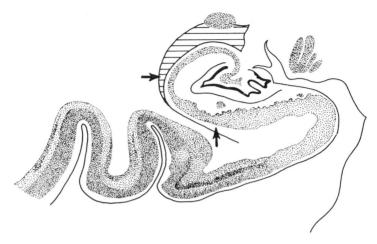

Fig. 61. Sommer sector of the normal human Ammon's horn. (Redrawn from E. Grünthal, Ammon's horn, pp. 707–711 in *Pathology of the Nervous System*, E. Minckler, ed. Copyright 1968. Used with permission of McGraw-Hill Book Co.)

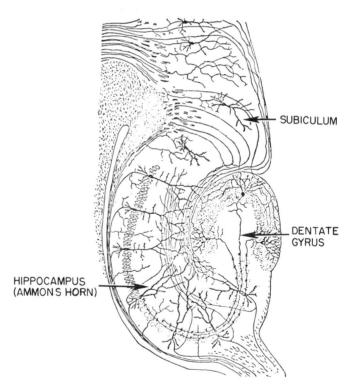

Fig. 62. Sketch of hippocampus, lesser animal, showing nerve cells, dendrites, and axon plexuses. [Fig. 41 reproduced by kind permission from *Studies on the Cerebral Cortex* (1955, p. 78), by S. Ramón y Cajal. London: Lloyd-Luke (Medical Books) Ltd.]

WHOLE NEURON STUDIES OF EPILEPTOGENIC CORTEX IN MAN

Fine structure alterations in epileptogenic cortex also claim attention. The best known example is loss of spines that adhere to the dendrites of the pyramidal neurons. These can be seen in Golgi whole neuron preparations, especially in the neurons of Ammon's horn. They also may occur in the neighborhood of any cortical scar, whether resulting from cortical birth trauma or brain damage occurring in later life. Spines are bits of broken-off synapsing axons seen in Golgi sections of normal animals. When they lose contact with their axons of origin, affected endbulbs degenerate and leave the dendrite surface smooth. This has been shown experimentally, as well as in human brains at autopsy.

J. DeMoor (1898) first utilized Golgi methods to study whole neurons in epileptogenic cortex. He found the widespread loss of spines as well as nodular deformities of the dendritic shafts, both attributable to vascular insufficiency. L. Westrum, L. White, and A. Ward (1964) used similar whole neuron preparations to study the cellular margins of epileptogenic cortical lesions in monkeys, producing them by local application of a substance called *alumina gel.* At the edges of the scar lesion, they observed neuron depopulation, reactive gliosis, and marked changes in the upward arborization of the shaft dendrites of cortical pyramids. This included absence or severe reduction in the number of dendritic spines, each formerly the site of a cerebral synapse. Investigators concluded that damaged neurons were the likely cause of epileptogenesis in human cortical scars, since the same neurons, studied in animal electrophysiological experiments, were prone to burst discharges.

By comparable Golgi methods, M. E. and A. B. Scheibel (1973) studied the human Ammon's horn from surgical patients who had had verified temporal lobe seizures. The tissue was obtained from medically incurable cases in which the existence of a discharging lesion was verified by the introduction of depth electrodes into the Ammon's horn region (see Chapter II, Case Report I). Because neurosurgical removal of the affected tissue had proved efficacious in other cases, P. Crandall of the Division of Neurosurgery, University of California, Los Angeles, removed it in the Scheibel series and had it prepared for pathological study, including the use of the Golgi method.

In addition to the changes mentioned previously, the Scheibels observed leafy excrescences upon the dendrites, bulbous and horn-shaped outgrowths, and "string-of-beads" appearances of the dendritic shafts. There also was a final stage of neuronal disintegration in which swelling and shriveling of neuron bodies could be seen. In areas within the tissue examined, the dendritic arbors showed nonuniformity in shape and size and the loss of their normal vertical look. Thus, the dendritic arbors lay sidewise, having a "windblown" look (Fig. 63). Glial connective tissue scarring is another prominent feature of such epileptogenic lesions, and the distortions of dendritic arbors spoken of above could relate to contraction of the scar.

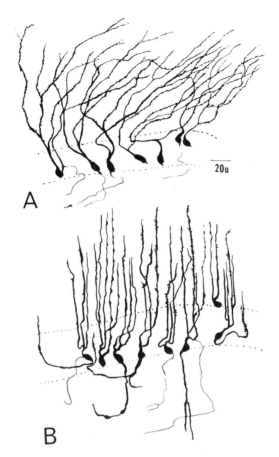

FIG. 63. A: A drawing of cluster of human dentate granules showing the "windblown" appearance found in limited areas of some specimens of human dentate gyrus. The distortion of dendrite patterns may be due to adjacent scar formation. From a subject of temporal lobe epilepsy; tissue removed surgically for control of seizures. Rapid Golgi variant; magnification 250. **B:** Dentate neurons showing loss of dendrite spines, nodulation, and inward collapse of dendrite domains called the "closed parasol effect." Drawn at magnification 250. (Both drawings from Scheibel and Scheibel, 1973.)

ZINC IN TEMPORAL LOBE EPILEPSY

The most recent developments relating the hippocampus to the causation of epilepsy commenced with the discovery in Germany by H. Maske (1955), confirmed by K. Fleischhauer and E. Horstmann (1957), that dithizone, a colorimetric zinc detector, when made up in weak alcoholic, alkaline solution and injected intravenously into small animals, showed in the cell layers of the hippocampus the red coloration characteristic of the islets of Langerhans of the pancreas, where zinc is incorporated into the antidiabetic hormone, insulin. In the pancreas, the color is restricted to granules; in the hippocampus, it is evidently distributed through the neuropil. A. Barbeau and J. Donaldson (1974) proposed that hippocampal zinc is involved in its epileptogenicity and that taurine, a nonessential amino acid, has an anticonvulsant effect plausibly related to the zinc content. This is a field now under active investigation in several American and Canadian laboratories.

COMMENT

The opinions cited here indicate that the brains of many epileptics can be normal, at least in appearance to the naked eye and perhaps after light and electron microscopic study as well, although the latter technology has yet to be used extensively in analysis of human epileptic tissue. The case for focal lesions causing either partial or generalized seizures is indubitable, and either a growing tumor or the effect of cortical trauma can produce an epileptogenic focus anywhere within the cortex of the brain. That is why a first seizure occurring in an adult may presage the growth of a brain tumor (see Chapter II, Case Report V). The evidence for birth trauma as a cause of seizures is best documented in the temporal lobe seizures.

REFERENCES AND BIBLIOGRAPHY

Barbeau, A., and Donaldson, J. Zinc, taurine, and epilepsy. *Arch. Neurol.* 30:52–58, 1974.

Bouchet, and Cazauvieilh. De l'épilepsie considereé dans ses rapports avec l'aliénation mentale. Recherches sur la nature et le siege de ces deux maladies. Memoire qui a remporté le prix au concours établi par M. Esquirol (2 Septembre, 1825). *Arch. Gén. Méd.* 9:510–542, 1825.

Brazier, M. A. B., ed. *Epilepsy: Its Phenomena in Man.* (UCLA Forum in Medical Sciences, No. 17.) New York: Academic Press, 1973. 391 pp.

Colonnier, M. Experimental degeneration in the cerebral cortex. *J. Anat.* 98:47–53, 1964.

Demoor, J. Le mécanisme et la signification de l'état moniliforme des neurones. *Ann. Soc. R. Sci. Med. Nat. Brux.* 7:205–250, 1898.

Earle, K., Baldwin, M., and Penfield, W. Incisural sclerosis and temporal lobe seizures produced by hippocampal herniation at birth. *Arch. Neurol. Psychiatry* 69:27–42, 1953.

Fleischhauer, K., and Horstmann, E. Intravitale Dithizonfärbung homologer Felder der Ammonsformation von Säugern. *Z. Zellforsch.* 46:598–609, 1957.

Gowers, W. R. *Epilepsy and Other Chronic Convulsive Diseases: Their Causes, Symptoms and Treatment.* New York: William Wood and Co., 1885. 255 pp.

Greenwood, J. G., Blackwood, W., McMenemey, W. H., Meyer, A., and Norman, R. M. *Neuropathology,* "Chapter 10," pp. 550–565. London: Edward Arnold, 1968.

Grünthal, E. Ammon's horn, pp. 707–711. In J. Minckler, ed. *Pathology of the Nervous System,* Vol. I. New York: McGraw-Hill Book Co., 1968.

Maske, H. Über den topochemischen Nachweis von Zink in Ammonshorn verschiedener Säugetiere. *Naturwissenschaften* 42:424, 1955.

Meyer, A., Beck, E., and Shepherd, M. Unusually severe lesions in the brain following status epilepticus. *J. Neurol.* 18:24–33, 1955.

Pope, A. Perspectives in neuropathology, pp. 773–781. In H. H. Jasper, A. A. Ward, and A. Pope, eds. *Basic Mechanisms of the Epilepsies.* Boston: Little, Brown and Co., 1969.

Ramón y Cajal, S. *Studies on the Cerebral Cortex, Limbic Structures.* (Trans. from the Spanish by L. M. Kraft.) London: Lloyd-Luke, Ltd., 1955. 179 pp.

Schaeffer, J. P., ed. *Morris' Human Anatomy,* 10th ed. Philadelphia: The Blakiston Co., 1942. 1641 pp.

Scheibel, M. E., and Scheibel, A. B. Hippocampal pathology in temporal lobe epilepsy. A Golgi survey, pp. 311–337. In M. A. B. Brazier, ed. *Epilepsy: Its Phenomena in Man.* (UCLA Forum in Medical Sciences, No. 17.) New York: Academic Press, 1973.

Sommer, W. Erkrankung des Ammonshorns als aetiologisches Moment der Epilepsie. *Arch. Psychiatr. Nervenkr.* 10:631–675, 1880.

Wertham, F., and Wertham, F. E. *The Brain as an Organ.* New York: The Macmillan Co., 1934. 538 pp.

Westrum, L., White, L., and Ward, A. Morphology of the Experimental epileptic focus. *J. Neurosurg.* 21:1033–1046, 1964.

Chapter XII

PERSPECTIVES IN FINE STRUCTURE ANALYSIS

Nothing demonstrates more clearly the growth of neuroscientific knowledge than a comparison of present-day concepts of fine structure with those of the late nineteenth century (see Chapter IV). A productive surge in the 1890s culminated in the establishment of the neuron doctrine. But progress was slow until a few decades ago. Then, in the 1950s there was an explosion of new information.

Technological innovations, well-nigh sensational in their capacity to reveal the hitherto unobservable, were developed almost simultaneously and were promptly utilized in neuroscientific research. The electron microscope made possible a new high order of magnification. Radioactive tracer atoms enabled the researcher to follow the migration of embryonic neuroblasts and the transportation of materials along axons. Modification of reduced silver methods permitted the tracing of axons, severed at their neuron origins, from one level of the nervous system to another. And histochemical methods were developed to identify sites of enzyme action within cells or axons. Furthermore, government grants became available for research and training. Thus, investigators were brought to the verge of meshing the facts of nerve structure with those of nerve functioning. An impressive new advance in knowledge now seems almost inevitable.

THE UNIT MEASURE

A plasma membrane envelops the neuron (and probably all cells). It consists of a biomolecular layer of lipids between monolayers of large molecule assemblies composed primarily of protein. Such a three-layer covering of the cell's exterior and its internal organelles is the basis of the unit-membrane hypothesis of J. D. Robertson (1966). That is the underlying structural concept. What A. L. Lehninger (1968) calls "greater membrane" includes, in addition, an outside zone of "fuzz"—complex but related composition, extending fingerlike from both neuronal and glial membranes to invade the spaces between cells (Fig. 64).

Glial cells—nervous connective tissue—are connected end-to-end and side-to-side by "tight junctions" that provide electronic coupling over significant distances. This is especially important to neuropil, where the glia loosely clothe synaptic endbulbs (see Chapter XIV).

Figure 65 shows G. H. Turner's schema of a cell with its internal organelles, which carry the load of its functioning. In neurons, for example, the organelles utilize the oxygen the cell requires for respiration, provide energy resources, and build structural and other proteins, including enzymes. The proteins are used locally within the soma—metabolic center of the neuron—or are transported to the tips of the axon branches. The soma also manufactures and packages neuro-

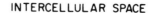

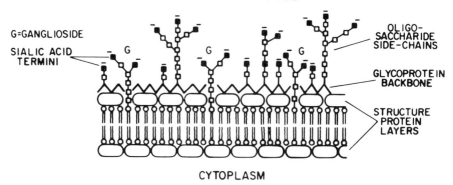

CYTOPLASM

THE GREATER MEMBRANE

FIG. 64. Model of the greater membrane, illustrating the fuzz of carbohydrate-rich material extending upward into the intercellular space. (From Lehninger, 1968.)

transmitters for transport and release at the axon terminals (see Chapter XIII). Those terminals are often a long distance from the neuron soma.

It is the covering membrane of soma, dendrites, and axon that accomplishes most of the specific work of the nervous system. Neuron doctrine is a modification of cell doctrine. Other nonnervous animal cells, such as the columnar epithelial cells that line intestinal glands, are joined sidewise by spot welds between the membranes. Like glial welds, they are called "tight" junctions (Weinstein and McNutt, 1972). They are quintuple-layered plaques. A "gap" junction differs. It shows a slender cleft (20 to 30 Å) at the fusion plane between the opposed trilaminar membranes and contains electron-dense (i.e., dark) material. Such fusion points also tie together parts of adjoining neurons, thus bonding the cellular elements that make up the neuronal web. Unlike synapses, they play no role in the transfer of information from one neuron to another.

In the nervous system there also are innumerable other specialized junctures called *synapses*, of which much already has been said. They participate in the transfer of information from neuron to neuron. This transmission of signals across synapses obeys the *law of dynamic polarization*, impulses passing from the axonal terminals of one neuron to the soma or dendrites of another, not conversely from dendrite to axon. Historically, all synapses of the light microscopy period were axodendritic or axosomatic. Recently, electron microscopists have become certain of the existence of axoaxonic, somasomatic, and dendrodendritic synapses as well (Fig. 66). Any of these should also be capable of providing side-to-side communication between neighboring neuron bodies, just as axosomatic or axodendritic synapses conduct in series in accordance with the orthodoxy of neuron doctrine.

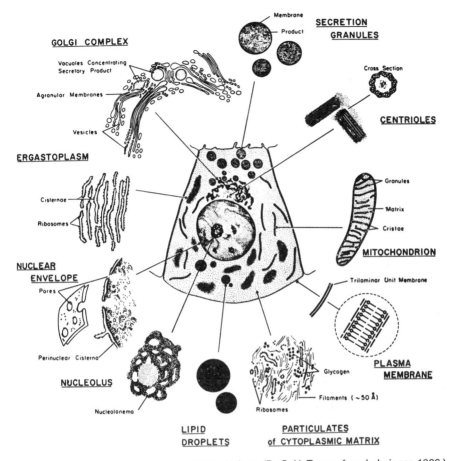

FIG. 65. Ultrastructure of cell organelles and inclusions. (By G. H. Turner, from Lehninger, 1966.)

Recently, F. O. Schmitt and P. F. Davison (1967) have recalled the view of Langmuir (1881–1957), a Nobel Prize-winning chemist of a generation ago whose forte was the study of the molecular monolayers of surface chemistry. Langmuir observed that cell shapes may reflect the shapes and highly specific properties of the protein molecules that compose their plasma membranes. Should that guess prove correct for neurons, it could explain their very numerous assortment of shapes in terms of a widely variable composition of the macromolecules making up their sheathing. Neurons, in fact, occur in greater variety than the cells of all other body tissues taken together. Their adaptive features with respect to size, number, branching of processes, and synaptic connections are countless. The many varieties are a feature of the brain's fine structure that is unique. No other organ can compare with it.

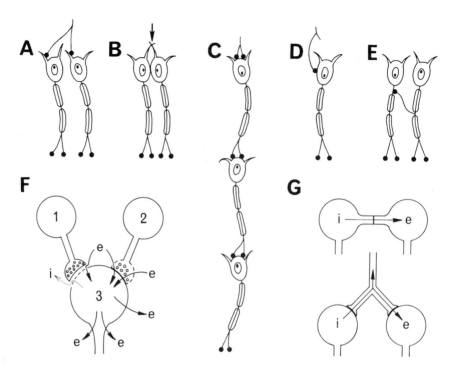

FIG. 66. Diagrams of **A:** axodendritic; **B:** dendodendritic and somasomatic; **C:** axosomatic (in tandem); **D:** axosomatic single neuron; and **E:** axoaxonic synapses, respectively. Redrawn and modified after Bodian (1972b). **F:** Diagram of chemical (left) versus electrical (right) transmission, excitatory synapses (e), inhibitory (i). **G:** dendrodendritic electrical synapse, top; electrically mediated axosomatic synapses relating to two neurons, bottom. (From Bennett, 1972.)

SIZES AND ARRANGEMENTS OF NEURONS AND THEIR SYNAPTIC CONTACTS

The disparity in neuron size is remarkable. The largest are almost visible to the naked eye; the smallest are the size of a red blood corpuscle, of which 4 million occur in a single droplet of blood. Small neurons tend to be closely packed, to show far less intervening neuropil, and to have short axons. In a given location such "granules" tend to be identical, as if turned out by a mold, each a close replica of its neighbors. By contrast, large neurons are surrounded by far more neuropil, show species likenesses that fall short of being identical, and have long axons extending considerable distances from the somata of origin.

Neurons also occur in a variety of architectonic formations, each of which may be made up of one or a very few cell species. Among them are six-layered cerebral and three-layered hippocampal and cerebellar cortex arrangements, each having its own novel design. Lamellar arrangements are also found at several other sites.

Between the principal basal neuron masses of the cerebrum, neurons vary significantly in amount of neuropil about them, in density of packing, and in group
arrangements.

In brainstem reticular substance, few of the small, short axon neurons are seen.
The principal reticular neurons (see Chapter X) have elongate, scantily branched
dendrites that overlap in longitudinal array passing fore-aft through the tegmentum. There are other neuron assemblies that give rise to the motor components
of cranial nerves. Their dendrites are woven basketlike to surround the neuron
bodies in a closed-field arrangement.

An unexpected difference between larger and smaller neurons was detected
recently. C. J. Herman and L. W. Lapham (1969) examined neuron nuclei as to
their size and DNA (deoxyribonucleic acid, the heredity bearer) content. Comparative values indicate the existence of multiples of the usual diploid amount
of DNA, without, however, implying a doubling of the usual content of chromo-
somes. Large nerve cells, each the standard within its neural environment, show
double the usual amount of DNA. Occasional motoneurons even show four times
the usual amount. Observations suggest subtle differences between neuron species
in their DNA and protein metabolism, which may correlate with other indices
of functioning.

NEURONS ENGAGE IN DELIVERY OF PACKAGED INFORMATION

The number of synapses on a neuron can be incredibly large. A few decades
ago estimates of a hundred or a thousand contact points would have been high.
Yet a study by B. G. Cragg (1967) indicates an average of about 6,000 synapses
for neuron soma and dendrites in a monkey's visual cortex and 60,000 per neuron
in his motor cortex. A. A. Ward, Jr. (1972) has estimated that less than two-tenths
of 1% of the latter immense number of synapse points would need to engage in
epileptic-type, high-frequency bursting to afflict a related neuron with the bursting contagion. In this connection, he comments on the very "compact packaging"
of the information passed on by epileptic bursts, compared with the firing patterns
purveyed over the synapses of neuron circuits engendering normal activity.

Those who believe that the nervous substrate provides the ultimate complexity
in biofunctioning specify as evidence the packaging of information into minute
vesicles within the endbulbs, the large number of synaptic contacts per neuron,
the number of neurons per milligram of tissue, and the totality of neurons in the
brain. But numbers alone may be a specious indicator of complexity for, according to E. D. P. DeRobertis (1971), the electroplaque membrane belonging to but
one electric organ of a torpedo fish may contain 30,000 to 50,000 chemical
synapses, the collective function of which, when massively discharged, is only
to paralyze the fish's prey. Nor can complexity arise solely from the number of
synapses per cell, for in the cerebellum each minute granule cell has but few
synapses with entering axons. Such a cell acts via its own axon to deliver but
a minute amount of information. Yet the very large number of granule cells which

exist provide delivery routes to the Purkinje neurons for exceedingly large amounts of information.

THE ELECTRON MICROSCOPE IN FINE STRUCTURE STUDIES

Current knowledge of fine structure, extensive as it is when compared with that available in the 1890s, still seems slight in view of opportunities offered by contemporary technologies for systematic exploration of the nervous system. Simple, as well as complex, organisms suggest ways of examining the origin of neural processes and how they operate in information gathering, in the control of movement, and in disseminating the paroxysms of epilepsy.

The extraordinary magnifications available to the electron microscopist make his progress seem tantalizingly slow because of the relatively greater ground he has to cover compared with the light microscopist. One small advance may require the slow repetitious study of many ultrathin sections. Proper interpretation requires numerous confirmations.

Ever since the naming of the synapse by Sherrington, it has been presumed that a nexus between two neurons always predicates a useful and continuing role for the connection, either excitatory or inhibitory. In the utilitarian view, if there are 60,000 synapses on a cortical pyramidal cell, must we not use each of them at some time or other, if not repeatedly? Yet E. G. Merrill and P. D. Wall (1972) have described synapses that are effective only if activated by artificial electrical stimulation. These do not respond to the drive of natural activity, reminding one of Volta's reference to Galvani's animal electricity as "weak artificial electricity." Merrill and Wall call such synapses *ghosts*. A concept based on the existence of supernumerary synapses cannot provide a rational base for constructive thinking. So it is consoling to know that although the history of science records many such doubts, it also records the ways in which they have been resolved. Sometimes they have opened new avenues of exploration. Healthy doubt is part of the scientific method. It guards us from being led astray by compelling aspirations.

MODERN KNOWLEDGE CONCERNING THE STRUCTURE OF THE SYNAPSE

In 1915 G. W. Bartelmez was the first to apply the cytological methods of R. R. Bensley to the resolution of problems of synaptic structure. At the suggestion of his peers, Bartelmez selected for his task the Mauthner neurons of a large cell aggregate of the catfish hindbrain. This is a single pair of giant somata, one for each side, lying close to the midline (Fig. 67). Each has the shape of a bent spindle, one principal dendrite extending outward (laterally) into the equilibratory reflex area and the other downward (ventrally) through the reticular core. Bartelmez observed surrounding axons from 12 different sources and also several kinds of synapses contacting the Mauthner cells.

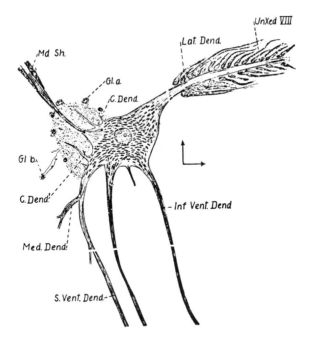

Fig. 67. The pioneer fine structure study of the synapse was carried out on the Mauthner neuron of the catfish hindbrain, illustrated above. A pair of these, of very large size, are situated one on either side of the brainstem. The lateral dendrite, upper right, provides the receptor surface for giant synapses provided by the excitatory terminals of vestibular axons that come from the ear. Those synapses provide equilibrating control over the swimming movements of the fish. The axon leaves the cell at the upper left, surrounded by a cupola of inhibitory terminals called the "cap." (From Bartelmez, 1915.)

A terminal part of each Mauthner lateral dendrite makes direct contact with a group of axons passing inwards from the equilibratory organ of the internal ear. Our concern is with the synapses that exist between the dozen or so equilibratory axon clubs and the lateral dendrite. There Bartelmez identified separate axon and dendrite membranes. In 1933 Bartelmez and N. L. Hoerr repeated these observations, using even better prepared material, and reiterated that each of the elements entering into a synapse has a limiting membrane, although light microscopy may resolve only one at the zone of contact. Four years later, Bodian studied the same synapse in the goldfish, demonstrating the interface membranes of contact.

Early studies of synaptic endbulbs by electron microscopy were carried out by E. D. P. DeRobertis and H. S. Bennett (1955) and by S. Palay and G. E. Palade (1955). They confirmed the existence of a synaptic interface showing separable membranes and also observed a synaptic cleft at the point of fusion. Synaptic vesicles, described by D. Bodian (1971) as the only unique organelles of all neurons, were first observed in the same studies. Several types of synaptic vesicles were identified subsequently. They are concerned with storage and release of chemical transmitters such as acetylcholine (excitatory synapses) and glycine, and gamma-aminobutyric and glutamic acids (inhibitory synapses).

In electron microscopy preparations, "asymmetric" contacts feature in the synapses made by most endbulbs (Fig. 68). The cleft is wide (200 Å) and its pre- and postsynaptic lips are delimited by dense-appearing material that is also present within the cleft. The endbulbs contain mitochondria and one of the three principal types of synaptic vesicles, characterized, respectively, as *round, flat,* and *dense* core. In the prevailing view, round vesicles are associated with excitation, flat vesicles with inhibition, and dense core with aminergic transmission (see Chapter XIII), the latter occurring in both peripheral and central locales of the nervous system (Bodian, 1971). There are also "gap" junctions, spaces of only 20 to 30 Å. These are concerned with rapid electrical conduction (Bennett, 1972) between neurons.

There are various specializations of the synapses described above. E. G. Gray (1959) has distinguished a spine synapse prevalent wherever dendrites are covered with thorny projections. Finally, in the thalamus, there are synaptic nests, or *glomeruli,* that are isolated from their environment by a meshwork of glial processes—glia being both a connective and nutritive tissue of the nervous system and an insulating material. The meshes contain major axonic and dendritic terminals and lesser ones complexly related within the nest (Morest, 1971). Dendrodendritic synapses have been shown in that situation. In cerebellar cortex, glomerular synapses of a different makeup are an outstanding feature.

Experimentally produced degeneration of axonal endbulbs, following sever-

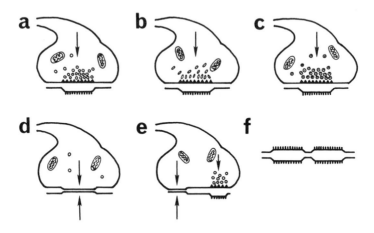

Fig. 68. Terminal axonal endbulbs and other contacts between one neuron and another. Redrawn after Bodian (1972b). Inferences by the present author. **a–e:** Endbulbs that synapse with neuron somata. **a:** Small round synaptic vesicles of excitatory type: **b:** flat vesicles, inhibitory type; **c:** dense core aminergic (?) vesicles; **d:** symmetric junction, gap type, electrical synapse, delayless conduction; and **e:** electrical and chemical synapses, left and right, respectively, made by the same endbulb. **f:** Desmosomal junction type such as occurs between other body cells as well as neurons. They do not conduct signals from one cell to another.

ance from their remote neuronal origins, is one way of identifying their terminal site on the soma and dendrites of a distant neuron. Clustering of remaining synaptic vesicles, their depletion through dissolution, and decay of junctional membranes are identifying features of a degenerating bulb. In some situations, the involved endbulbs also darken appreciably.

WHERE DO PARTICULAR SYNAPTIC BULBS END ON THE NEURON SURFACE?

This is a perplexing problem, which the era of light microscopy passed on to that of electron microscopy (Bodian, 1972a). If there are 60,000 synapses on one pyramidal neuron, it is improbable that they could be arranged haphazardly. It seems more likely that until shortly before birth, space allotments on still naked neuron surfaces are reserved for future occupancy. As phases of a master genetic plan unfold, the areas could be filled by waves of arriving terminals that successively occupy reserved seat sections on the somata and dendrites.

AXONAL TRANSPORT MECHANISMS IN NEURONS

The accumulated evidence of a century of neuroanatomy shows that the neuron somata must be responsible for the synthesis of nutrients and other materials required by the axonal endbulbs in conducting their activities. Until recently, the mechanism by which this took place was unknown. Various theories involving transport were suggested to explain the process.

Axoplasmic flow was first suggested by P. Weiss and H. B. Hiscoe (1948), a fast flow component shown by S. Ochs, M. I. Sabri, and J. Johnson (1969), and a slow flow reported later. B. Droz and C. P. LeBlond (1963) postulated the synthesis of protein within the soma in the course of research on mice, using an autographic process consisting of the injection of an amino acid tagged with a radioactive hydrogen atom (tritiated leucine) and a photographic emulsion as the detector. R. J. Lasek (1970) showed that transport of a radioactive label distally along axons could be used to detect their course and terminus, and W. M. Cowan *et al.* (1972) developed a successful technique for identifying tagged endbulbs within the central nervous system.

Later work turned to ribosomes, cellular constituents that form macromolecules for restitution of the neuron. Whether or not any significant buildup of ribosomes can occur in an endbulb itself is open to question—probably not. The slow transport mechanism, one-fifth of an inch (0.5 centimeters) per day, which follows after the rapid one, 4 inches (10 centimeters) per day, outlines the courses of the axons as well as adding to the accumulation in the terminals. Other proteins destined to reach the terminals are transported at intermediate speeds.

The use of axon transport experiments in plotting synaptic endbulb patterns within the brain may be appraised from reports of studies of specific projects. D. I. Gottlieb and W. M. Cowan (1973) studied the commissural connections between left and right hippocampus of the rat, placing a tritiated leucine injection into the cell layers of one and plotting the distribution of tagged endbulbs in the other. One neuronal subfield of hippocampus (Fig. 69) appears to relate principally to its opposite number, the tagged terminals being densely distributed over both the basal dendrites of the hippocampal pyramids and the middle sectors of their apical shafts. Clearly omitted were the soma surfaces between. In experiments carried out by others, projections from discrete loci of origin in the brainstem could be traced to such endings as cerebellar fibers that climb like ivy over the dendritic ramifications of Purkinje cells.

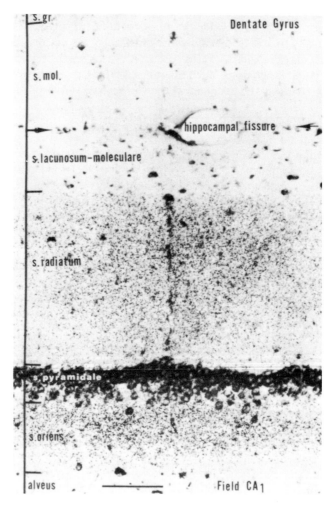

FIG. 69. Tritiated leucine, active transport, hippocampus. Note heavy labeling in *s. oriens* and *s. radiatum,* terminals of commissural axons arising from opposite hippocampus. (From Gottlieb and Cowan, 1973.)

There are still other aspects of identification that can be pursued using the transport principle. For example, horseradish peroxidase enzyme injected into gastrocnemius muscle can be traced inward over the motor axons to those motoneuron somata within the spinal cord that supply muscle terminals. There it is identified in the motoneurons containing it by action of the horseradish enzyme on a proper substrate (Kristensson and Olsson, 1971). Finally, certain fluorescing dyes, such as procion yellow or brown, injected intracellularly into somata and dendrites of a neuron, can be examined as a unit of dye fluorescence under a dark field microscope (Kuffler, 1973). Using tritiated amino acids, dendritic transport also has been shown to occur at a rate of one-eighth of an inch (0.3 centimeters) per hour.

Colchicine is a drug that expressly binds neurotubular protein, interfering with axonal transport by blocking the neuron's internal circulation (neurotubular system) (Schubert, Kreutzberg, and Lux, 1972). Its injection causes a severe reduction in transport along both axons and dendrites. When injected into a neuron through a micropipette, neurotubular staining reveals colchicine involvement over wide areas of neuron somata (Grafstein, McEwen, and Shelanski, 1970; Cuénod *et al.,* 1972). Colchicine-induced changes in the vesicles of the synaptic endbulb depress synaptic activity as measured in electrophysiological preparations (Perísíc and Cuénod, 1972).

NEURON DROPOUTS IN SENSORY CORTEX FOLLOWING POSTNATAL SENSE ORGAN REMOVAL

Experimentally induced instances of degeneration of the several elements of a neuron chain have been rare indeed, although the method was developed in newborn animals by B. A. von Gudden during the heyday of neuron studies a century ago. H. A. Van Der Loos and T. A. Woolsey (1973) observed the occurrence in rat somatosensory cortex of unique neuron formations residing in layer IV, which they refer to as "barrels." After an individual mouse whisker with its associated sense organs is removed, the corresponding cortical "barrel" disappears by the tenth day of life, indicating a clearly transsynaptic deterioration in the infant cortex. This discovery has opened up still another method of tracing the exact composition of neuron chains extending upward through the nervous system from peripheral sense organs to cerebral cortex.

COMMENT

The development of histotechnologies in the late nineteenth century led to the enunciation of the neuron doctrine. That doctrine held that neurons are separated from each other except for connectors called synapses that permit conduction of signals to occur along chains and circuits arranged in series, axosomatic or axodendritic synapses intervening between one neuron and the next.

The large remaining problems of nervous organization—and new ones that have been introduced by the successful exploitation of fine structure by electron microscopy—have been partially identified in this chapter. Emphasized are the vast number of endbulbs deriving from diverse sources that attach to the somata and dendrites of individual neurons, the differing morphologies of these synapses as seen ultrastructurally, the unraveling of synaptic sites occupied by terminals arising from different distant sources, and the utility of axon transport in advancing knowledge of the sites of particular connections between axon terminals and with somata and dendrites.

From the standpoint of the spread of epileptic seizures, it has been shown that neurons are not nearly as insular as once believed. Dendrodendritic, somasomatic, and axoaxonic synapses provide side-by-side junctures between neurons as well as lengthwise ones taking the more circuitous routes involving intersynaptic links consisting of somaaxodendritic successions.

REFERENCES AND BIBLIOGRAPHY

Bartelmez, G. W. Mauthner's cell and the nucleus motorius tegmenti. *J. Comp. Neurol.* 25:87–128, 1915.

Bartelmez, G. W., and Hoerr, N. L. The vestibular club endings in Ameiurus: Further evidence on the morphology of the synapse. *J. Comp. Neurol.* 57:401–428, 1933.

Bennett, M. V. L. A comparison of electrically and chemically mediated transmission, pp. 221–256. In G. Pappas and D. P. Purpura, eds. *Structure and Function of Synapses.* New York: Raven Press, 1972.

Bodian, D. The staining of paraffin sections of nervous tissues with activated protargol. *Anat. Rec.* 69:153–162, 1937.

Bodian, D. Presynaptic organelles and junctional integrity. *J. Cell Biol.* 48:707–711, 1971.

Bodian, D. Synaptic diversity and characterization by electron microscopy, pp. 45–65. In G. Pappas and D. P. Purpura, eds. *Structure and Function of Synapses.* New York: Raven Press, 1972*a*.

Bodian, D. Neuron junctions: A revolutionary decade. *Anat. Rec.* 174:73–82, 1972*b.*

Cowan, W. M., Gottlieb, D. I., Hendrickson, A. E., Price, J. L., and Woolsey, T. A. The autoradiographic demonstration of axonal connections in the central nervous system. *Brain Res.* 37:21–51, 1972.

Cragg, B. G. The density of synapses and neurones in the motor and visual areas of the cerebral cortex. *J. Anat.* 101(4):639–654, 1967.

Cuénod, M., Boesch, J., Marko, P., Perísić, M., Sandri, C., and Schonbach, J. Contributions of axoplasmic transport to synaptic structures and functions. *Int. J. Neurosci.* 4:77–87, 1972.

DeRobertis, E. D. P. Molecular biology of synaptic receptors. *Science* 171:963–971, 1971.

DeRobertis, E. D. P., and Bennett, H. S. Some features of the submicroscopic morphology of synapses in frog and earthworm. *J. Biophys. Biochem. Cytol.* 1:47–58, 1955.

Droz, B., and Leblond, C. P. Axonal migration of proteins in the central nervous system and peripheral nerves as shown by radioautography. *J. Comp. Neurol.* 121:325–346, 1963.

Gottlieb, D. I., and Cowan, W. M. Autoradiographic studies of the commissural and ipsilateral association connections of the hippocampus and dentate gyrus of the rat. I. The commissural connections. *J. Comp. Neurol.* 149:393–421, 1973.

Grafstein, B., McEwen, B. S., and Shelanski, M. L. Axonal transport of neurotubule protein. *Nature* 227:289–290, 1970.

Gray, E. G. Electron microscopy of synaptic contacts on dendrite spines of the cerebral cortex. *Nature* 183:1592–1593, 1959.

von Gudden, B. A. *Experimental-Untersuchungen über das Schaedelwachsthum.* Munchen: Oldenbourg, 1874. 48 pp.

Herman, C. J., and Lapham, L. W. Neuronal polyploidy and nuclear volumes in the cat central nervous system. *Brain Res.* 15:35–48, 1969.

Kristensson, K., and Olsson, Y. Retrograde axonal transport of protein. *Brain Res.* 29:363–365, 1971.

Kuffler, S. W. The single-cell approach in the visual system and the study of receptive fields. *Invest. Ophthalmol.* 12:794–813, 1973.

Lasek, R. J. Protein transport in neurons. *Int. Rev. Neurobiol.* 13:289–324, 1970.

Lehninger, A. L. The importance of cell membranes. *Neurosci. Res. Symp. Summ.* 1:4–6, 1966.

Lehninger, A. L. The neuronal membrane. *Proc. Natl. Acad. Sci. USA* 60:1069–1080, 1968.

Merrill, E. G., and Wall, P. D. Factors forming the edge of a receptive field: The presence of relatively ineffective afferent terminals. *J. Physiol.* 226:825–846, 1972.

Morest, D. K. Dendro-dendritic synapses of cells that have axons: The fine structure of Golgi type II cell in the medial geniculate body of the cat. *Z. Anat. Entwicklungsgesch.* 133:216–246, 1971.

Ochs, S., Sabri, M. I., and Johnson, J. Fast transport system of materials in mammalian nerve fibers. *Science* 163:61–67, 1969.

Palay, S., and Palade, G. E. The fine structure of neurons. *J. Biophys. Biochem. Cytol.* 1:69–88, 1955.

Perišić, M., and Cuénod, M. Synaptic transmission depressed by colchicine blockade of axoplasmic flow. *Science* 175:1140–1142, 1972.

Robertson, J. D. Design principles of the unit membrane, pp. 357–408. In G. Wolstenholme and M. O'Connor, eds. *Ciba Foundation Symposium. Principles of Biomolecular Organization.* London: J. & A. Churchill, Ltd., 1966.

Schmitt, F. O. Brain cell membranes and their microenvironment, pp. 195–325. In F. O. Schmitt, T. Melnechuk, G. C. Quarton, and G. Adelman, eds. *Neurosciences Research Symposium Summaries,* Vol. 4. Cambridge, Mass.: The MIT Press, 1970.

Schmitt, F. O., and Davison, P. F. Role of protein in neural function, pp. 377–398. In F. O. Schmitt, T. Melnechuk, G. C. Quarton, and G. Adelman, eds. *Neurosciences Research Symposium Summaries,* Vol. 2. Cambridge, Mass.: The MIT Press, 1967.

Schubert, P., Kreutzberg, G. W., and Lux, H. D. Neuroplasmic transport in dendrites: Effect of colchicine on morphology and physiology of motoneurones in the cat. *Brain Res.* 47(2):331–343, 1972.

Synaptic ghosts. (News and Views) *Nature* 243:185, 1973.

Van Der Loos, H., and Woolsey, T. A. Somatosensory cortex: Structural alterations following early injury to sense organs. *Science* 179:395–398, 1973.

Ward, A. A., Jr. Basic mechanisms of the epilepsies, pp. 91–96. In M. Critchley, J. L. O'Leary, and B. Jennett, eds. *Scientific Foundations of Neurology.* Philadelphia: F. A. Davis Co., 1972.

Weinstein, R. S., and McNutt, N. S. Cell junctions; current concepts. *N. Engl. J. Med.* 286:521–524, 1972.

Weiss, P., and Hiscoe, H. B. Experiments on the mechanism of nerve growth. *J. Exp. Zool.* 107:315–395, 1948.

Chapter XIII

Neurotransmitters

Acceptance of the neuron theory made it necessary to identify the means of excitatory (and inhibitory) transmission. The evolution of that knowledge began with increased understanding of the neuromuscular endplate and of the autonomic ganglia, the latter containing postsynaptic neurons. Even before the neuron theory had been formulated, R. Koelliker around 1845 had noticed microscopically the discontinuity between nerve and muscle. He foresaw the important bearing this had on corresponding separations between neurons in the central nervous system.

The motor endplate became the prototype of the excitatory synapse. A corresponding one for inhibition had been discovered in 1845 by the brothers E. F. W. and E. H. Weber, who showed that slowing of the heart occurred when the vagus nerve was stimulated. Acetylcholine, which today occupies first rank among the transmitters, was synthesized in 1867, four decades after the initial organic synthesis of urea by F. Wöhler (see Chapter XV). The pharmacological properties of acetylcholine were explained in 1914 by H. Dale, who observed that it mimicked the response to stimulation of autonomic nerves such as the vagus. In 1921 O. Loewi made the important discovery that acetylcholine mediated vagal effects. Acetylcholine was to be recognized later as the transmitter at the motor endplate as well as the principal transmitter of the vertebrate nerve centers.

For spinal reflexes, the central transmission hypothesis can be traced to the central excitatory and central inhibitory states described in 1932 by Sherrington and his associates (Creed et al., 1932). The word *state* implies the action of one or another chemical species released by presynaptic endings to act upon postsynaptic membranes (Lloyd, 1961). In the early stage of transmitter research, chemical mediation seemed too slow and complex to serve the requirements of rapid action, but it had the advantage of producing local effects at separate excitatory and inhibitory endings and even of the segregation of inhibitory endings to the axon hillock, where, by valvelike control, they could interrupt ongoing action of excitatory terminals.

In the decade preceding World War II, there was continuing debate between protagonists of chemical transmission and those of electrical transmission, chiefly related to excitatory processes. Even in autonomic ganglia, the effects described were excitatory. No one at that time could document the existence of chiefly inhibitory synapses. After World War II, J. C. Eccles, B. Katz, and their collaborators proved the occurrence of rapidly mediated chemical transmission, and for a time the pendulum swung to the belief that all transmission was chemically based. It has now swung back to the acceptance of electrical transmission in several varieties of vertebrate synapses (Bennett, 1972).

With the advent of the cathode ray oscillograph and its ultimate development into a flawless recorder of rapid and transient nerve impulses, it was established that both the spike of the presynaptic axon terminus and the postsynaptic cell potential could be recorded, separated by a half a millisecond, representing the interlude of a single synapse. Longer intervals, allowing for central axon conduction and additional time for further synaptic delays, were indicative of conduction proceeding over multisynaptic pathways.

As a result of Eccles' studies after World War II, it became possible to record both excitatory and inhibitory postsynaptic potentials from within neurons. These terms have since been abbreviated to EPSPs and IPSPs, respectively. Recorded inside the cell, the two postsynaptic cell potentials are of opposite electrical sign, the excitatory one resulting from membrane depolarization, the inhibitory one from membrane hyperpolarization.

These discoveries were not made in rapid succession. In addition to electrophysiology, electron microscopy also has played an important role in proving the existence of the synaptic vesicles, which lie in clusters within the individual endbulbs of the axon and are storage sites of acetylcholine. Ultrastructural studies also permitted distinction between the pre- and postsynaptic interfaces of a synapse and the separating cleft that identifies a chemical as opposed to an electrical synapse, the gap in the former amounting to 200 Å.

In chemical mediation, the transmitter diffuses across the gap, attaching to available receptor sites on the postsynaptic membrane, and increases the permeability of the postsynaptic neuron to one or more ions (see Chapter XIV), setting up electrical circuits within it. The circuits, in turn, contribute to the discharge of impulses along the axon of the postsynaptic element (Bennett, 1972). At electrically transmitting synapses, the membranes come together (i.e., they form *gap junctions*). The two neurons are joined by a low resistance that directly connects their interiors. Whereas chemically mediated synaptic transmission shows a half-millisecond delay, electrical transmission is "instant." As well as the chemically and electrically mediated synaptic transmission of polarized axosomatic and axodendritic type, there are dendrodendritic, axoaxonic, and somasomatic synapses as described in Chapter XII. These are of the tight or gap junction types, presumably electrically connected. Some may lack polarization and conduct equally well in either direction.

A chemical transmitter cannot exist in chemical isolation within a neuron. However, during neural activity, it can be formed in surplus amounts that require destruction. A mechanism of replenishment is also required (Hebb, 1970). The details of a transmitter substance's biosynthesis, metabolism, transport along the axon to the terminal, and release have not been examined in detail for central cholinergic (i.e., acetylcholine reactive) neurons, although they have for peripheral terminals. Acetylcholine requires a synthesizing enzyme (acetylcholine transferase) for replacement and a hydrolyzing enzyme (acetylcholinesterase) for its removal.

Using thin sections attached to glass slides and chemical methods, the presence of the latter enzyme can be detected to map the cholinergic paths microscopically as they extend through the nerve centers. The neuronal pathways of another class of transmitters, called *monoamines,* can be similarly mapped using fluorescent (ultraviolet) microscopy. The exploitation of such ancillary methods has been a decided advantage in providing correlations between transmitter type and electrophysiological or electron microscopic evidence concerning the central neuronal pathways. There is a third group of amino acids that provide inhibitory transmitters, but they have yet to be traced by these or related methods.

QUANTAL TRANSMISSION

J. del Castillo and B. Katz (1954) were the first to discover *miniature* endplate potentials. These develop at neuromuscular junctions in a bathing solution that contains a high concentration of magnesium and a low concentration of calcium. Such miniature endplate potentials arise in response to nerve stimulation. They have the same size and shape as other such potentials of the same preparations that appear spontaneously. Accumulating evidence indicates that the tiny potentials are the building blocks of large, fully developed ones that can be evoked in response to a maximal nerve stimulus in an ionically normal bathing solution. One of the large potentials consists of a number of units, which, in response to a nerve stimulus, fire synchronously, adding together as they do. The discovery of the fledgling potentials led to the *quantum* concept of chemical mediation, which emphasizes discontinuity in the release of transmitter quanta. Other support of the quantum hypothesis has come from studies of spinal motoneurons (Kuno, 1971).

Excitatory postsynaptic potentials set up in motoneurons have been shown to present statistical fluctuations in amplitude consistent with transmitter release, increments occurring in quantal steps. (A quantum is a minimum that can be released at one time.) The corollary of this hypothesis is that synaptic vesicles of uniform size contain preformed packets of transmitter substance. This is very probable, but rigorous scientific proof is not yet at hand.

RECEPTOR SITES OF ACETYLCHOLINE

The excitatory action of acetylcholine at the motor endplate involves two stages. The first consists in combining the diffused transmitter with local protein conformations of endplate membrane called *receptor sites.* This increases the permeability of the postsynaptic membranes to ions, with a resultant short-lived depolarization. Certain snake venom components can bind some receptor sites reversibly, others irreversibly. This has parallels in interpretation of the action of neuromuscular blocking agents that serve as models for myasthenia gravis, a human muscle disorder that manifests itself as extreme muscular weakness.

CENTRAL CHOLINERGIC PATHS

Methods for detecting acetylcholinesterase are used to trace the cholinergic paths of the central nervous system. Evidence indicates that acetylcholine is the transmitter at the synapses of the ascending reticular activating system. As outlined in Chapter X, the change from slow-wave sleep to activated sleep increases the liberation of acetylcholine from cerebral cortex (Jasper and Tessier, 1971). Rapidly repeated stimulation of the reticular core also increases the output of acetylcholine. Proof lies in the accumulation of the transmitter at the system terminus during stimulation. The hippocampus, referred to earlier in the discussion of the causation of temporal lobe epilepsy, also gives rise to cholinergic systems. The thalamocortical relays belonging to the specific sensory systems likewise appear to have cholinergic termini.

MONOAMINE TRANSMISSION

The earliest monoamine studies stemmed from investigations of the adrenal gland. With increased understanding of norepinephrine, epinephrine, and dopamine (all adrenal by-products), studies of monoamine distribution passed to the brain because of the possibility of their participation in neurotransmission across cerebral synapses. In addition to the catecholamines, the mammalian brain also can synthesize serotonin (5-hydroxytryptamine, 5-HT) and histamine. The entire group makes up the monoamines (Wurtman and Fernstrom, 1972).

With the exception of the catecholamine-containing cell groups of the hypothalamus (related to the pituitary gland), the neurons containing these amines are located in the tegmentum of the midbrain, the pons, and the medulla oblongata (Fig. 70). From the last site, axons containing norepinephrine or serotonin, as traced by fluorescence microscopy, descend into the spinal cord and ascend to the cerebrum. Others reach various cell groups of the lower brainstem (Hebb, 1970). Few serotonin-transporting axons reach the cerebral cortex, but norepinephrine axons are found throughout its layers. Both the catecholamines and serotonin can be localized by their fluorescence with a high degree of fidelity (Dahlström and Fuxe, 1965; Kety and Sampson, 1967). Dopamine cannot be distinguished from the closely related congener DOPA, but in the brain this is of little importance since DOPA is present there in very low concentration. Dopamine axons and their terminals are principally ascending. Among them is a significant tract extending from the substantia nigra of the midbrain to the striatum, which is one of the large neuron aggregates of the basal ganglia of the cerebrum.

Correlative physiological studies support this evidence concerning monoamine transmitters. Dopamine has been shown to exercise an inhibitory action in the basal ganglia, whereas serotonin has both excitatory and depressor actions. Monoaminergic transmitters play a role in the ascending reticular activating system as well. These exemplify the potential value of the search for monoamine

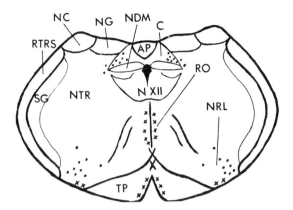

Fig. 70. Transverse section, lower hindbrain, experimental study. Positions of catecholamine neurons indicated in dots (lateral reticular nucleus, NRL). 5-Hydroxytryptamine neurons indicated by crosses (nucleus of the raphe, RO). (From Dahlstrom and Fuxe, 1965.)

paths in understanding brain functioning. Doubtless, many significant connections are yet to be established, some of which could have immense value for epilepsy research.

STORAGE OF CHOLINERGIC AND MONOAMINERGIC TRANSMITTERS

From electron microscopic studies, it is generally agreed that acetylcholine is stored in similar-size, clear, small vesicles having a diameter of 200 Å (Kety and Sampson, 1967). That identification is strongly supported by their occurrence in the motor endplate and in the central endbulbs, known to be cholinergic. Other workers divide the small vesicles into round and flat types, presuming the latter to be inhibitory in function. Another vesicle of significantly larger size (400 to 600 Å) has a dense core. There is strong evidence that it contains catecholamines. Evidence for such a localization has been presented by Bloom and Barnett (1966), based on histochemical studies in which the adrenal medullary granules that contain norepinephrine are made electron dense. Bloom and Barnett have also shown the localization of radioactive norepinephrine to the basal ganglia of animals given intraventricular injections of that compound. In those studies electron-struck photographic silver grains were located around cell bodies and along dendrites, indicating that the associated neurons had picked up the tagged monoamine.

INHIBITORY TRANSMITTERS—NEUTRAL AMINO ACIDS

Many substances have been proposed as inhibitory transmitters. In fact, acetylcholine has been shown to act as one in certain invertebrate nerve circuits. In the mammalian nervous system, however, neutral amino acids seem to have the inside track for possession of transmitter properties—despite the difficulty in invariably distinguishing between the transmitter and the metabolic roles of the same amino acid. In transmitter action, the neutral amino acids would seem subject to the same rules that govern cholinergic and aminergic transmitters, namely, enclosure within vesicles and release into the confined synaptic cleft, where diffusion is limited instead of opening into the extracellular space that winds slitlike between neuronal and glial membranes (Hebb, 1970).

In a group of large neurons in the hindbrain serving the preservation of body balance (vestibular) functions, the neutral amino acid gamma-aminobutyric acid (GABA) seems to have come closest to satisfying the stringent criteria of an inhibitory transmitter. There GABA, applied by microinjection to the cell interior, causes hyperpolarization of the neuron membrane. But the same neurons do not show blocking of inhibition by strychnine, the classic action of that convulsant on spinal neurons. GABA has also received impressive support as the inhibitory transmitter of cerebral cortex (Hebb, 1970).

Much negative evidence has accumulated concerning the previously proposed action of GABA as the spinal inhibitory transmitter, and, conversely, much positive evidence now supports glycine, another amino acid, as the true inhibitor for that region of the nervous system. Glycine is considered the probable transmitter for inhibitory interneurons, and it now seems reasonable to regard it as the principal, if not the only, spinal inhibitory transmitter.

Strychnine, a bitter poisonous alkaloid deriving from *Strychnos nux-vomica,* upon administration in animals produces excessive irritability of the spinal cord and convulsions. It was first synthesized 25 years ago and is said to have the most complex molecular conformation known to science. A. B. Young and S. H. Snyder (1973) used tritiated (radioactive) strychnine sulfate upon membrane fractions containing receptor sites (see Fig. 71), proving that the tritiated (^{3}H) convulsant binds specifically with the postsynaptic receptor sites specific to the neurotransmitter glycine, inactivating them. This dovetails with the theory that strychnine produces excessive excitability through blocking such inhibitory receptor sites.

CRITERIA FOR IDENTIFICATION OF A CENTRAL TRANSMITTER

Agents suspected of being transmitters should be matched to the action criteria demanded of any natural transmitter, the search for which is always underway (Werman, 1966). The existence of an inactivating enzyme close to the site of transmitter action seems to be necessary, since the accumulation of any natural transmitter in large quantities could be expected to poison either animal or man. Another requisite is that the transmitter substance should be contained in those neurons from which it is to be released. If, instead, it is ubiquitous in occurrence, a specific release mechanism must be present at the receptor sites where the transmitter attaches. The transmitter substance should be detectable in the extracellular fluid collected from the activated region. The latter is a difficult criterion to satisfy within the central nervous system, unless the accompanying inactivation process is blocked during analysis. It also is necessary that mechanisms be available both for the local manufacture of the transmitter and for its release.

The most important criterion a test substance must satisfy is its ability to mimic the action of the natural transmitter. The development of microinjection techniques has greatly strengthened the precise applicability of this criterion. Finally, in considering pharmacological identity, it is important to recognize that whatever interacts with physiological synaptic agents should interact with a test substance in the same way, a criterion only applicable to those agents that act on the postsynaptic membrane.

FALSE AMINERGIC TRANSMITTERS

The synthesis, storage, and release of monoamine neurotransmitters is sufficiently nonspecific to permit substitution of other amines for the physiological transmitter. Called *false neurotransmitters,* they are less active than the amines for which they substitute and result in lowering the efficiency of transmission at the nerve endings where they accumulate (Kopin, 1972).

Uptake and retention of serotonin (5-HT) by catecholaminergic neurons has been demonstrated for the central nervous system. Thus, in the brain, as well as in adrenergic neurons of the outlying ganglia, the uptake and storage mechanisms may permit the accumulation of amines other than the natural transmitter. Their accumulation at the sites of activation also could result from nerve stimulation, thus meeting another criterion of transmitters.

TRANSMITTERS AND OTHER NEUROSECRETORY PRODUCTS IN THE TEST TUBE

More than a decade ago, E. DeRobertis (1962) and V. P. Whittaker (1972), with their respective associates, showed that nervous tissue converted into soups (homogenates) by homogenizers and blenders can be further processed in a manner that concentrates the transmitter substances into separate layers. From the soups, particles were extracted in large numbers through the use of density gradient centrifuges, descendents of yesteryear's routine laboratory centrifuges. In the density gradient separation, the synaptosomes (pinched off and resealed nerve endings) were largely restricted to one layer (Fig. 71) and were distinguishable from other subcellular particles. This layer proved to be a much enriched source of neurotransmitters and their related enzymes and storage mechanisms. Since it is a widely accepted belief that other transmitters besides acetylcholine and the catecholamines are stored in vesicle form, the advance promises a new approach to the classification of transmitters and the identification of their storage sites by electron microscopy.

Research uses of the synaptosome preparation are multiplying rapidly. Because isolated synaptosomes are capable of maintaining a high rate of respiration in

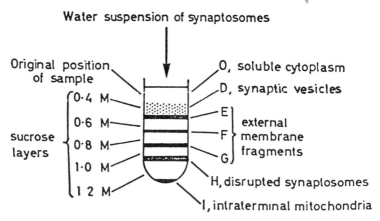

Water suspension of synaptosomes

Original position — O, soluble cytoplasm
of sample — D, synaptic vesicles

sucrose layers:
- 0·4 M
- 0·6 M
- 0·8 M
- 1·0 M
- 1 2 M

E
F } external membrane fragments
G

H, disrupted synaptosomes

I, intraterminal mitochondria

Appearance of gradient after 60 000 g x 2 hr.

Fig. 71. Synaptic vesicles (D) occupy a layer containing synaptic transmitter and associated enzymes after 2 hours of density gradient centrifugation. (From Whittaker, 1972.)

the test tube, it is possible to release the transmitters and amino acids by either electrical stimulation or by exposure to a high concentration of potassium, the latter acting as a membrane depolarizer.

Such synaptosomes also can be used as models for studying neurosecretory processes in the all-important *brain-pituitary axis* system, which provides the generalized control the brain exercises over the body's endocrines. Thus, the method promises a more cohesive effort by neurochemists, neuropharmacologists, and neuroendocrinologists in the study of brain release factors that control the outputs of the several endocrine glands. A splendid spin-off of neuropharmacological research, it offers many new opportunities for system analysis by research psychiatrists.

COMMENT

The various actions of neurotransmitters may appear rather irrelevant to the causative mechanism underlying epileptic attacks. If instant electrical transmission alone could account for the dissemination of seizure activity through brain and spinal cord, only cholinergic or other excitatory synapses would be required to incorporate the massive movements characterizing the convulsive aspect of the generalized attack.

Not discussed previously, however, was the importance of failure of central inhibition, which necessarily involves loss of inhibitory synaptic transmission, at the beginning of seizures. The theory of S. Baglioni concerning the spinal action of strychnine (see Chapter XIV) was the origin of J. R. Hunt's (1922) opinion that seizures result from failure of a generalized central inhibitomotor mechanism, consisting of Golgi type II cells situated at all levels of the nervous system from cortex to spinal cord. Hunt theorized that within the spinal cord the laterobasal cell group of the posterior horn, consisting of Golgi II cells, was the site of the inhibitomotor mechanism, just as the motoneurons were the site of the excitomotor one. In speaking of the action of strychnine, Hunt refers to a paralysis of inhibition that releases the excitomotor mechanism. This concept of strychnine action as due to a blocking of inhibition has been carried over into modern thought by F. Bremer, J. C. Eccles, and others, just as the Golgi II neuron has been restored as the archetype of the inhibitory neuron.

Hence, excitomotor release due to inhibitomotor paralysis still requires serious consideration in explaining the genesis of seizures.

REFERENCES AND BIBLIOGRAPHY

Aghajanian, G., and Bloom, F. E. Electron-microscopic autoradiography of rat brain following H^3-DOPA. *Fed. Proc.* 25:383, 1966.

Bennett, M. V. A comparison of electrically and chemically mediated transmission, pp. 221–256. In G. D. Pappas and D. P. Purpura, eds. *Structure and Function of Synapses.* New York: Raven Press, 1972.

Bloom, F. E., and Barnett, R. J. Fine structural localization of noradrenaline in vesicles of autonomic nerve endings. *Nature* 210:599–601, 1966.

Creed, R. S., Denny-Brown, D., Eccles, J. C., Liddell, E. G. T., and Sherrington, C. S. *Reflex Activity of the Spinal Cord.* Oxford: Clarendon Press, 1932. 183 pp.

Dahlström, A., and Fuxe, K. Evidence for the existence of monoamine containing neurons in the central nervous system. II. Experimentally induced changes in the intraneuronal amine levels of bulbospinal neuron systems. *Acta. Physiol. Scand.* 64 (Suppl. 247):1–36, 1965.

del Castillo, J., and Katz, B. Quantal components of the endplate potential. *J. Physiol.* 124:560–573, 1954.

DeRobertis, E., Pelligrino de Iraldi, A., Rodriguez de Lores Arnaiz, G., and Salganicoff, L. Cholinergic and noncholinergic nerve endings in rat brain. I. Isolation and subcellular distribution of acetylcholine and acetylcholinesterase. *J. Neurochem.* 9:23–35, 1962.

Deutsch, J. A. The cholinergic synapse and the site of memory. *Science* 174:788–794, 1971.

Hebb, C. CNS at the cellular level: Identity of transmitter agents. *Annu. Rev. Physiol.* 32:165–192, 1970.

Hunt, J. R. A theory of the mechanism underlying inhibition in the central nervous system and its relation to convulsive manifestations. *Assoc. Res. Nerv. Ment. Dis.* 7:45–64, 1922.

Jasper, H. H., and Tessier, J. Acetylcholine liberation from cerebral cortex during paradoxical (REM) sleep. *Science* 172:601–602, 1971.

Kety, S. S., and Sampson, F. F. The neural properties of biogenic amines. *Neurosci. Res. Symp. Summ.* 2:399–514, 1967.

Kopin, I. J. False aminergic transmitters, pp. 339–348. In S. H. Snyder, ed. *Perspectives in Neuropharmacology.* London: Oxford University Press, 1972.

Kuno, M. Quantum aspects of central and ganglionic synaptic transmission in vertebrates. *Physiol. Rev.* 51:647–678, 1971.

Lloyd, D. P. C. A study of some twentieth century thoughts on inhibition in the spinal cord, pp. 13–31. In E. Florey, ed. *Nervous Inhibition.* New York: Pergamon Press, 1961.

Martin, A. R. Quantal nature of synaptic transmission. *Physiol. Rev.* 46:51–66, 1966.

Neurochemistry Correspondent. Neurosecretion in the test tube. *Nature* 244:520, 1972.

Werman, R. Criteria for identification of a central nervous system transmitter. *Comp. Biochem. Physiol.* 18:745–765, 1966.

Whittaker, V. P. The use of synaptosomes in the study of synaptic and neural membrane function, pp. 87–100. In G. D. Pappas and D. P. Purpura, eds. *Structure and Function of Synapses.* New York: Raven Press, 1972.

Wurtman, R. J., and Fernstrom, J. D. L-typtophan, L-tyrosine, and the control of brain monoamine biosynthesis, pp. 143–193. In S. H. Snyder, ed. *Perspectives in Neuropharmacology.* New York: Oxford University Press, 1972.

Young, A. B., and Snyder, S. H. Strychnine findings associated with glycine receptors of the central nervous system. *Proc. Natl. Acad. Sci. USA* 70:2832–2836, 1973.

Chapter XIV

Experimental Studies in Epilepsy

Experimental models are the most direct approach available for furthering interpretation of seizure activity. In it also lies the promise of devising more effective and less costly means for screening the efficacy of potentially antiepileptic drugs. Historically, such models have often developed out of neuroscientific efforts to advance understanding of the functioning of cortex and subcortical gray matter. The search for new models, of course, also can increase general neurobiological knowledge and broaden the search for more effective means of treatment.

Experimental investigations of epilepsy must consider the animal species best suited to the pursuit of a specific objective; the physical, chemical, or metabolic excitant most appropriate to a particular study; and the end to be achieved by a model of particular design. The simplest possible epilepsy model is a single cortical neuron impaled by an ultrafine quartz microtubule in an anesthetized animal. Through it, a test drug can be delivered to the unit's interior, and its effect on the neuron's electrical activity can be ascertained. Other models provide important clues concerning the source of epileptic discharge in a community of neurons. Epilepsy can spread rapidly through the brain, and the efficacy of a pharmaceutical product may depend largely on its ability to prevent or retard the spread of seizures.

Given a sufficient state of nervous excitation, in all species—including those of birds, reptiles, fish, and even some invertebrates—either clinical seizures can develop, or the existence of an epileptic state can be detected by the burst discharge of a neuron studied by electrical recording. Common laboratory animals (mouse, rat, guinea pig, rabbit, cat, and monkey) are ordinarily used in experimental investigations. Some members of any species may show a preexisting seizure vulnerability to particular agents, physical, chemical, or metabolic; and statistical methods can be used to establish the prevalence of the predisposition in the population. Thus, species vulnerability must be taken into account in selecting experimental models.

Certain genetic traits of animals can themselves provide valuable experimental models. Audiogenic seizures occur in a variety of mouse, and photogenic ones in a species of baboon from Senegal (Purpura et al., 1972). In rare situations, disembodied neural tissues, such as the head of a turtle or an animal brain in tissue culture, are utilized.

Experimentally produced metabolic derangements also may produce seizures. The oldest effort in this direction was the production of anemia through bleeding. Both hypoxia (oxygen deficiency) and hyperbaric oxygen (at three atmospheres pressure or more) can result in generalized seizures in animals. Hypocarbia (reduced carbon dioxide concentration in the blood) and hypercarbia (increased CO_2 concentration) produce a marked slowing in the electrical activity of the brain, an occurrence that in normal animals can be associated with clonic movements (Purpura et al., 1972). In those humans suspected of having petit mal epilepsy, decreasing the concentration of carbon dioxide in the blood by deep breathing can elicit spike-waves in the electroencephalogram (EEG), sometimes with the coincident activation of a petit mal attack. Seizures can also be brought on in man by a pyridoxine (vitamin B_6) deficiency, or induced in animals by injecting agents that deplete the body's store of that vitamin, and also produced by hypoglycemia.

Several classic electrical seizure patterns of human beings can be activated in animals and used to judge the potencies of antiepileptic drugs. The continuous spike pattern associated with attacks of grand mal epilepsy in man can be produced experimentally in animals by several agents either administered systemically or applied to the cortical surface. True seizures can be set off by somewhat larger doses. Three-per-second spike-waves of petit mal epilepsy were produced in animals by electrical activation of the midline thalamus (Jasper and Droogleever-Fortuyn, 1947). Finally, localized involvement, such as occurs in temporal lobe epilepsy, is simulated by the spread of electrical discharges through the hippocampal formations that lie within each temporal lobe, protruding from the wall into the lateral ventricle (see Chapter XI). A cobalt implant at the site may produce such a result.

HISTORICAL RÉSUMÉ

Early efforts to study experimental epilepsy were quite crude (Dandy and Elman, 1925). Controversial as was Marshall Hall of England (see Chapter VI), his animal experiments excited the attention of others. Human epilepsy was among his interests. In 1830 he published a brief clinical book covering the convulsive complications of bloodletting, a treatment then used widely for a variety of ailments. Seizures that developed as blood was drawn suggested to him and others that cerebral anemia was the causative factor. In 1824 G. Kellie of Scotland and 2 years later P. Piorry of France produced experimental convulsions in animals by depriving the brain of blood through tying off its principal arteries. Others achieved the same results by obstructing the venous return. In 1867 L. Landois of France, for example, produced convulsions in young dogs by compressing the veins in the neck. In 1857 A. Kussmaul and A. Tenner of Germany verified the earlier studies on arterial ligation and also concluded that a convulsive center exists within the hindbrain. In 1896, when L. Hill of England compressed one of his own carotid arteries, a unilateral convulsion followed. Such studies undoubtedly show that cerebral anemia can bring about convulsions, but they give no proof that it causes all the convulsions of human epilepsy.

Studies of the role of brain and spinal trauma in the causation of convulsions began with C. E. Brown-Séquard, who induced them in 1851 in rabbits by injuring various parts of the nervous system. Either lesions or a simple puncture of the spinal cord could produce an injury sufficient to excite seizures; so did damage to nerves (see Chapter VI) or to the midbrain. At that time the cerebrum was still believed to be inexcitable. Brown-Séquard also showed that convulsions can occur after the cerebrum, cerebellum, and upper brainstem had been removed. Mistakenly, he came to the view that epilepsy resulted from loss of control by the hindbrain over excitable spinal reflexes. In his time, normal rabbits were generally believed very susceptible to convulsions. Yet his prestige gave credence to his findings.

In 1868 C. W. H. Nothnagel produced small focal lesions of the brainstem and interpreted the subsequent convulsions as resulting from stimulation of two independent opposed centers, a convulsant and a vasomotor one, impairment of the latter producing the coma that accompanies generalized convulsions.

Of the chemical agents that induce convulsions, absinthe was first used in 1864 by C. Morcé of France and popularized in 1876 by his countryman V. Magnan. Observation of its effect led to the impression that the clonic phase of seizures derives from cerebral cortex, because conversion of clonic to tonic phase ensued immediately upon cortical removal.

The theory that epilepsy was due to autointoxication led to the trial of various biological products as possible local irritants of cerebral cortex. This wave of research came in the wake of the successes of Fritsch and Hitzig on cortical excitability and localization. The enthusiasm these aroused led to applications of creatine and urinary products, bile pigment, and Liebig's meat extract to the cortical surface, one at a time. All of these and other substances were said by some to produce convulsions when applied topically.

In 1900 S. Baglioni of Italy first used strychnine in experiments on the spinal cord of the frog. With G. Magnini, in 1909 he showed that strychnine applied topically also had a specific excitatory effect on the cerebral cortex of the dog, acting on neurons and not on axons of the subcortical white substance. In 1910 J. G. Dusser de Barenne commenced extensive experiments on the sensory mechanisms, also selecting strychnine as his experimental agent. Baglioni, however, deserves credit for priority in introducing it.

In 1878 L. Luciani of Italy began the study of convulsions related to brain trauma in experimental animals. After excising the monkey motor cortex, he observed convulsions following a latent interval lasting from a few days to several months. The convulsions arose locally on the side opposite the lesion.

In 1910 H. Barbour and J. Abel made the interesting observation that after brain injury smaller doses of an injected aniline dye were required to produce convulsions than were needed in normal control animals. As a result of a local lesion, the dye was absorbed more effectively and a deeper blush appeared over the whole brain. It is a wonder that observations of such potential importance, pointing perhaps to damage to the capillary barrier between blood and brain, were not followed up.

Dandy and Elman, previously mentioned, set out to learn if localized brain injury actually renders animals more susceptible to convulsions than their controls and if the site of injury within the cerebrum is an important factor. One-third to one-seventh of the dose of absinthe required to produce convulsions in control animals sufficed to set off seizures in those with motor cortex injury. The threshold dose was also somewhat lower with cerebellar than with occipital lobe injuries. Thus, they at least demonstrated that brain injury is a significant factor in increasing susceptibility to convulsions.

EARLY RUSSIAN AND POLISH INVESTIGATORS

M. A. B. Brazier (1973) has discovered several early studies made in eastern Europe that are of historical significance in experimental epilepsy. Commencing with Caton's report on the electrical manifestations of brain activity made at the Ninth International Medical Congress, Washington, D.C., in 1887 (see Chapter VIII), his work became more widely known than it had been earlier, chiefly among Russian and Polish workers. In 1904 P. Y. Kaufman, working under V. M. Bechterev and I. P. Pavlov, decided to repeat the earlier experiments of Caton using the more refined recording equipment then available. He especially wanted to test the postulate that an epileptic attack might be associated with abnormal brain discharges. His attempt in 1912 to record from the brain during seizures was probably the first. By curarizing his animals, he showed that during a seizure abnormal electrical activity arose from the brain and not from the muscles, which in the curarized state could not contract. Thus, he undid the work of Gotch and Horsley of England, who believed, according to Brazier, that the abnormal electrical activity occurring in a seizure is due to evoked potentials arising from sensory endings in contracting muscle. Since Kaufman had no camera for recording his results, records of his experiments do not exist. He changed his name thereafter, entered the Russian army, and, alas, did not again contribute to the scientific literature.

Kaufman evidently had been in communication with A. Beck and N. Cybulski of Poland, who were conducting similar studies. The former was discussed in Chapter VIII. The latter, in cooperation with Jelenska-Macieszyna, undertook to induce seizures in dogs and monkeys. Overcoming the many technical difficulties that resulted from interference by muscle activity, they took the first photographic records of brain activity during experimental seizures. With the onset of seizure, they noted a marked increase in amplitude and frequency of brain waves. Spikes were not recorded, due to the inadequacy of the galvanometer used. World War I broke out the same year.

ELECTRICAL STIMULATION IN THE EXPERIMENTAL STUDY OF EPILEPSY

As discussed previously, Fritsch and Hitzig showed that the cerebral cortex is electrically excitable, and Caton demonstrated that electrical activity could be recorded from the brains of living animals. The consequences were manifold, but here, first of all, is a brief consideration of electrically activated seizures.

In describing the electrical events that characterize seizures, the word *potential* will be used repeatedly in referring to the high-amplitude wave or spike processes that occur repetitively during the seizure state. It is used elsewhere to cover all bioelectric processes, but the magnitude and wave shapes of the convulsive potentials are their distinguishing feature in this context.

Today there is much versatility in electrical brain recording, and both *unit potentials* of neurons and *field potentials* deriving from masses of neurons can be recorded simultaneously. The recording of unit potentials requires extremely fine saline-filled quartz microtubules mounted on a microdrive that permits deliberately slow and nondamaging entry to a cell's interior. Such units also can be recorded from the cell's exterior as well, but with the chance of complicating the unit potential with those of similar units recorded from neighboring cells. Field potentials are recorded by means of much larger-tip electrodes and constitute the summed discharges of neuron masses. The scalp electrode of the EEG records a field potential from outside the cranium—as alpha rhythm. In experimental studies on animals, it is more likely that the electrode tip will be in immediate contact with the neuronal aggregate whose records are to be studied. Even when large and tiny electrodes lie in the same neighborhood, it is impossible to identify a unit potential as contributing to the field potential unless they recur again and again simultaneously.

Related to the succession of spikes or spike-waves that characterize grand or petit mal epilepsy in the human EEG is an underlying slow potential shift such as accompanies the experimentally driven activation of thalamocortical recruiting patterns (see Chapter X). Slow shifts are also field potentials. Elicited in an animal brain, for example, by a quick succession of electrical stimuli, a recruiting wave follows each stimulus of a succession, the shift underlying the whole recruiting sequence.

To record slow potential shifts requires Du Bois-Reymond type nonpolarizable electrodes to minimize other baseline shifts of nonbiological (i.e., physical) origin. The equipment of the pioneer electroencephalographers was ideal for such a purpose. Followers of Du Bois-Reymond, they exercised maximal care in making their electrodes nonpolarizable. The galvanometers used for recording were the equivalent of today's electronic amplifiers without condenser coupling. Thus, it is entirely probable that, as in Caton's results, potentials evoked by visual stimulation from the animal brain were slow potential shifts and not the sinelike alpha waves or evoked potentials we recognize today.

In present experimental work it has not been possible to attribute all such slow potentials to a neuronal origin. Glial cells, closely associated with neurons, may contribute a significant share.

Seizures of brief duration can be activated by repetitive electrical stimulation of the cortex. Such rapidly successive stimuli have been designated tetanizing currents (after the repetitive output of the Du Bois-Reymond inductorium) and are so defined in the subsequent explanation. To distinguish between tetanizing (rapidly repetitive) currents, as picked up by an electroencephalograph during stimulation, and the repetitive seizure activity with which it may be mixed during a stimulus period, it is well to recall Volta's suggestion that Galvani's frog muscle twitches were due to "weak artificial electricity," as opposed to the animal electricity that Galvani thought he was recording. The tetanizing current in our experimental model is a weak artificial electricity delivered by a stimulator, whereas the brain waves with which it is mixed represent animal electricity. After the stimulus is turned off, the brain continues to produce epileptic spikes for a time. These are called *after-discharges* and consist *only* of animal electricity. This will become important somewhat later, when we talk of experimental situations that utilize tetanizing currents for activation and provide a description of the ensuing after-discharges in terms of unit and field potentials.

In the hippocampus, as studied by E. R. Kandel and W. A. Spencer (1961), after-discharge can be produced experimentally in animals by tetanizing axons of pyramidal neurons as they leave the gray to enter the white matter. In that instance the artificial electricity stimulates the bodies of a whole field of neurons, setting up a massive epileptic-type discharge that outlasts the stimulus period.

R. M. Crowell and C. Ajmone-Marsan (1972) similarly studied tetanizing currents applied locally to the surface of the cerebral cortex, recording from neuron units both inside and outside. Units in the neighborhood of the stimulating electrodes were often active during after-discharge. Recorded at a distance from the stimulating electrodes, that was unusual. At the stimulus locus, neurons discharging when the stimulus was applied were sometimes inactivated instead of activated, but that was never the case when the actively discharging units were at a distance. As used here, activation implies the excitation of epileptic burst discharges.

G. V. Goddard, D. C. McIntyre, and C. K. Leech (1969) permanently implanted stimulus electrodes in another epilepsy model of animals to be used for study of electrical activity afterward. They recorded the routine EEG daily during stimulation, starting 1 week following implantation and using identical stimulus currents and frequency for each test. On the first trial there was no behavioral change, but on the seventh, 1 week later, minimal convulsive movements were observed and after-discharges akin to those described earlier were recorded. The initial bilateral convulsion occurred at the end of the second week, and thereafter convulsions occurred on trials made on successive days. They called this the "kindling" effect, because animals refractory to seizures at first developed them regularly as the trials progressed. In a general way, their results parallel those of Dandy and Elman (1925) with absinthe.

Tetanizing current also has been used in animals to examine seizure threshold by a method akin to electroshock therapy in man. Such a model was first used to test the potency of a new antiepileptic drug as a prelude to human trials in epileptics. The drug in this instance was diphenylhydantoin; the investigators were T. J. Putnam and H. H. Merritt in 1937; the drug's clinical success is discussed in Chapter XV.

ALKALOID MODELS IN ANESTHETIZED PREPARATIONS

Alkaloids comprise a large group of organic basic substances found in plants. Many are useful in preparing human medicaments. A few of them have convulsant properties. Strychnine, bicuculline, and veratrine have been used in experimental models of epilepsy. Strychnine in a weak solution applied in a minute amount to an animal's anesthetized motor cortex produces opposite-side seizure-jerks and induces seizure-discharges in the EEG. Bicuculline, given intravenously to anesthetized animals, can produce a status epilepticus in which a seizure-discharge continues over long intervals. It is an antagonist of gamma-aminobutyric acid (GABA), an inhibitory transmitter (see Chapter XIII), and acts to abolish the inhibitory cortical activity, one of whose functions is to prevent the nervous system from developing excesses of excitation.

Used in anesthetized animals in which evoked potentials are being recorded from visual or other sensory cortex, the first alteration to be detected after the application of a dilute strychnine solution is a significant exaggeration in the size of the evoked potentials. Next, the much exaggerated evoked potentials repeat themselves following a light flash or other sensory stimulus. Finally, such spikes develop independently, having the same shape as the evoked response but showing further increase in size. Recurring spontaneously, they are called strychnine spikes and are indistinguishable from the grand mal spikes of human epileptic attacks.

Similarly applied in much higher dilution, veratrine also produces spontaneous spikes of considerable amplitude, but of a polarity opposite to that of strychnine spikes. The difference in polarity may stem from their origin deep in the cortex rather than near its surface. The effect of veratrine on the steady (or slow) potentials of cerebral cortex is akin to that of an electrical phenomenon of cerebral cortex called "spreading depression," in which a marked slow-potential shift sweeps slowly along the brain from front to back, accompanied by a corresponding loss in spontaneous activity. That sweep is reversible (see Purpura et al., 1972, pp. 174–196) and can occur repeatedly during an experiment.

Studying unit discharges of cortex in cats, following the application of convulsant agents, T. F. Enomoto and C. Ajmone-Marsan (1959) showed brief slow-potential shifts, often capped by a burst of high-voltage spikes in the intraneuronal record (see Fig. 73, lower traces). The shift also can be reflected in the field potential simultaneously, as recorded from the cortical surface. These brief shifts occur in the quiet intervals between runs of an epileptic discharge of high voltage. H. Matsumoto and C. Ajmone-Marsan (1964) designated them as *paroxysmal depolarizing shifts,* and they have since been verified by many other workers.

TOPICAL METAL APPLICATIONS

In 1942 L. M. and N. Kopeloff and S. E. Pacella introduced the experimental use of alumina gel to establish a chronic epileptogenic focus within cerebral cortex. At the site of application a scar develops over ensuing months that of itself could not account for the seizure-activating character of the lesion. The EEG, however, becomes increasingly abnormal, more so over the side on which alumina gel was applied. The peak of brain wave abnormality occurs from the fifth to ninth week after application of the gel. Thereafter, removal of the scar reduces both brain wave abnormality and seizure frequency. Producing a scar alone, without the application of alumina gel, was unlikely to produce seizures under the condition of these experiments.

A. A. Ward, Jr. (1961) studied abnormal patterns of electrical discharge in neuron units neighboring on sites of alumina gel application. Such "epileptic neurons" gave rise to bursts of high-frequency spike discharge, such as those seen by Enomoto and Ajmone-Marsan.

L. M. Kopeloff (1960) was the first to report that implantation of pure cobalt metal on mouse cortex would induce seizures. Since then it has been used often, because epileptogenic foci develop more rapidly than with alumina gel. R. J. Grimm et al. (1970) reported a short-lived focus in squirrel monkey cortex with rare spread to involve the cortex generally and without evident loss of awareness by the animal. R. Mutani (1967) implanted cobalt in the amygdala and ventral hippocampus, producing the behavior of temporal lobe seizures comparable with those occurring in humans with psychomotor epilepsy.

EPILEPTOGENIC LESIONS PRODUCED BY FREEZING

In 1833 E. Openchowski observed that dogs suffered generalized seizures after a small spot of cerebral cortex was frozen. More than a century later, F. M. Nims, C. Marshall, and A. Nielsen (1941) used dry ice or an ethyl chloride spray (which evaporates rapidly) for freezing and saw characteristic convulsoid changes in the EEG, occurring with or without bodily seizures. The electrical discharges were not unlike those that occur in man during an epileptic attack. F. Morrell (1961) used a fine ethyl chloride spray on the dural covering of the animal brain, producing the same discharges without accompanying bodily seizures. He also studied mirror foci (identical points in the two cerebral hemispheres connected by commissural paths that carry the mirror seizure patterns from one hemisphere to the other) in the opposite cerebral hemisphere. These produced discharges that were secondary to the discharges that recur at the seizure site. Mirror foci were not evident immediately, but developed within 3 days after application of ethyl chloride, and they vanished after removal of the frozen cortical area. In other experiments, F. Morrell, F. Proctor, and D. A. Prince (1965) used a probe designed especially to freeze points within the subcortical gray matter, including the thalamic nuclei. Depth electrodes penetrating other sites within the thalamus and basal ganglia showed that secondary discharges corresponding to the cortical mirror focus could be established from frozen areas in the brain's interior.

THE PENICILLIN FOCUS

A. E. Walker and H. C. Johnson (1945) were first to observe that the widely used antibiotic penicillin has convulsive properties. This is not nearly as dangerous to patients as one might surmise, for the brain is protected from clinically administered penicillin by a constantly vigilant blood-brain barrier. Yet the observation should not be overlooked by the practicing neurosurgeon.

Applied directly to the cortical surface in animals, penicillin causes spikes and slow waves to appear in the related EEG. This led to its widespread use as an experimental model that could further the understanding of events that transpire both inside and outside the neuron during an epileptic attack. Penicillin injected intraneuronally has been shown to increase the neuronal firing rate within motor cortex, producing its result by causing marked reduction of GABA-mediated inhibition (see Chapter XIII). Penicillin also has been microinjected into the neuron interior at many sites within the cortex. Burst firing, described previously as resulting from the application of epilepsy activators, occurs in this instance also (Dichter and Spencer, 1969; Ayala et al., 1971).

THE HIPPOCAMPAL MODEL

The hippocampus (see Chapter XI, Fig. 63) has been used as an experimental model for exploring simultaneously the intra- and extraneuronal events that occur during interseizure intervals in which the trace is quiescent except for random spike discharges that signal overexcitability. Seizure-discharges were explored from the perspective of a microelectrode used to record from within the membrane covering a neuron body and also from that of a larger electrode used to monitor the field potential in the extracellular environs that occur coincidently. Penicillin was the epileptogenic agent, placed in the neighborhood of the external field potential electrode (Kandel and Spencer, 1961; Dichter and Spencer, 1969; Ayala et al., 1973). The general schemata of such a neuron, showing excitatory and inhibitory synapses, are represented in Fig. 72, and the electrical records of their excitatory and inhibitory postsynaptic potentials (Fig. 72) are followed by corresponding seizure records (Fig. 73) of the same.

The seizures induced in a nontreated hippocampal preparation by tetanizing its axonal outflow (see Chapter XI, Fig. 62) and recording the extraneuronal field potential trace are of the excitatory type, showing evidence of widespread neuronal seizure involvement in the environs of the electrode. The unit trace recorded from the interior of a single neuron also is principally excitatory (DEPOLARIZING OR EXCITATORY CHANGE in the neuron membrane; see Glossary) in its membrane shift. Thus, in this instance, both inside and outside electrodes give identical reports of what the neuron is doing.

Deafferentation, by interruption of the pathways of incoming axons, changes the picture materially. The trace from the interior of a neuron may now show hyperpolarization, indicating that it has lost its excitatory synapses through the deafferentation process. But it does retain those inhibitory synapses that arise from recurrent collaterals of the axons of neighboring pyramidal cells, and thus it behaves in an inhibitory fashion. Seizures in man that are inhibitory in nature are sometimes observed, and this bit of electrophysiological evidence may offer an explanation for their occurrence.

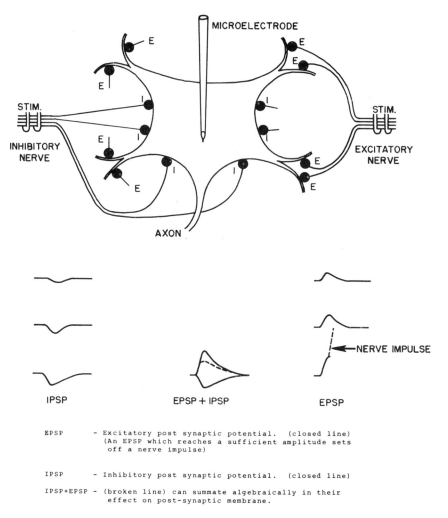

Fig. 72. Sketch of excitatory (E) and inhibitory (I) synapses converging on a neuron; Stim. (stimulating electrodes). Records of EPSPs and IPSPs are of opposite polarity and increase with increasing stimulus strength in top-bottom sequence. Note that bottom EPSP is of sufficient magnitude to excite a conducted nerve impulse *(broken line)*. IPSP and EPSP (center) sum algebraically. (From Goldring, 1963. Published in 1963 by the University of California Press; reprinted by permission of the University of California Press.)

LEAKAGE OF POTASSIUM AND THE GLIAL MEMBRANE POTENTIAL

Slow-potential shifts have been referred to previously as a third type of brain potential. Evident in many examples of nervous activity, the shifts are particularly noticeable during convulsive activity (Goldring, 1963; Karahaski et al., 1966; Castellucci and Goldring, 1970). Some shifts take place abruptly; others develop

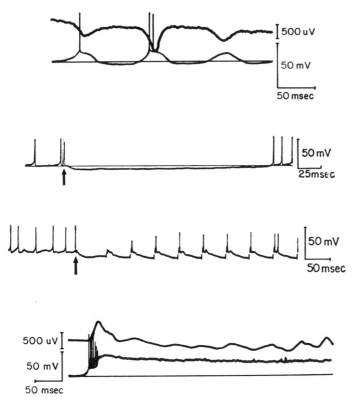

FIG. 73. *Top traces:* (Upper) Electrocorticogram during seizure, recorded from large electrodes. (Lower) Intracellular traces, microelectrode. Note that of three successive seizure transients, the first and second show synchronized EPSPs, the third does not. ***Middle traces:*** Seizure trace, EPSPs. Note prolonged IPSP beginning at arrow following EPSP in upper member of middle pair. In lower member, firing rate slows and each EPSP is followed by an IPSP. ***Lower traces:*** (Upper) Derives from surface electrocorticogram. (Lower) A *paroxysmal depolarizing shift* recorded intracellularly. The last two derived simultaneously from a lesser animal injected with Metrazol and were recorded in an interseizure period. (From Goldring, 1963. Published in 1963 by the University of California Press; reprinted by permission of the University of California Press.)

slowly. It has been shown by these authors that under certain conditions glial depolarization will explain the slow-potential shifts.

Glia in leech, amphibia, and mammalian cerebral cortex recently has been shown to be exquisitely sensitive to potassium. Taken with the rather continuous coupling of glial processes through tight junctions, this could result in current being drawn from neighboring unaffected glia, moving potassium away from sites of intensive neuronal activity such as seizure. In fact, glial membrane might be permeable only to potassium, and not to sodium. Therefore, in the experimental model described, one could speculate that glia might contribute significantly to preventing a seizure or reducing its severity. An increase in extraneuronal potassium is known to depolarize neuronal membrane, and excessive depolarization is epileptogenic.

Such problems have no simple solution, such as changing the balance of sodium or potassium in the diet. In the metabolism of the body, these salts are generally distributed and regulation is systemic. Dietary excesses are readily excreted. It is the glial implications for the brain's functioning that afford the fascinating outlook, and it is comfortable to have evidence of a tangible function for glia other than those of holding together the neurons and playing a role in the reaction of the nervous system to injury.

COMMENT

The experimental approach to the causes of epilepsy began inauspiciously in the early nineteenth century. Knowledge of the nervous system was still too rudimentary to support more than the crudest efforts to get at the underlying factors. At the start, cerebral anemia was used to provoke seizures in animals, even though the relationship to the seizures of human epilepsy was obscure. Then it was believed that convulsions are only a symptom of hyperexcitability of nervous tissue, and that they could arise from defective tissue oxygenation, from ingestion of exotoxins, or from disordered systemic metabolism and the accumulation of toxic breakdown products. All of these were classed by late nineteenth-century investigators as intoxicants. Trauma, especially that associated with birth defect, was proved to be another precipitant of seizures. Seizures also are associated with several specific brain diseases. In historical progression, autointoxication took the place of anemia, and trauma of intoxicants, in the logic of the early experimentalists.

Absinthe was the first convulsant drug to be used in animal trials. It served several purposes, including study of the comparative effects of lowering the convulsive threshold in normal as compared with previously traumatized animals. Its experimental use, along with that of thujone, continued into the twentieth century.

Strychnine was the first convulsant that proved efficacious in minute amounts. Its origin can be traced to the pharmacological investigations of F. J. Magendie in the early nineteenth century. S. Baglioni recognized its value in central nervous system investigations. Starting with studies on spinal sensory mechanisms, he proceeded to its cortical application and produced convulsions localized to the musculature of the opposite side of the body. By recognizing the importance of dilution in gauging the potency of a convulsant, he originated the use of experimental trials of a series of dilutions directed at observing threshold effects.

The really important experimental projects were developed after the advent of electroencephalographic and, later, sophisticated electrophysiological recording. The recognition that either strychninization of cortex, or its tetanization by electrical currents, produces a generalized dysrhythmia with a pattern akin to the EEG traces of some epileptics, led to further experiments. These centered on surface applications of certain alkaloids such as strychnine, electrical tetanization, contact of brain with such metallic substances as alumina gel and cobalt, freezing, and penicillin. Dysrhythmias (abnormal electrical seizure patterns) developed earlier and persisted longer than did bodily seizures. Thus, cerebral dysrhythmia became a sensitive detector of the imminence of seizure.

The most successful adaptations of routine electroencephalography to the study of experimental epilepsy came with the use of stable direct-coupled amplifiers and nonpolarizable electrodes, which permitted simultaneous recording of the steady potential changes associated with seizure-discharge. Certain epilepsy models also required the use of micropipettes for external and internal unit recording and the introduction of convulsants into the neuron interior. For successfully recording unit potentials, development of a cathode ray oscillograph was essential.

Recent studies using experimental models have opened up significant new avenues of research. They have established the premise that depolarization of neuron membrane is a prime factor in the development of a seizure. In the hippocampal model de- and hyperpolarization evidently can be brought about through positive and negative feedbacks. This is initiated over recurrent axon collaterals of hippocampal neurons, each half of such a synaptic mechanism contributing in its own way to build-up and cessation of seizure. Increase of potassium in extracellular space is known to depolarize neuronal membrane, and excessive depolarization is shown to be epileptogenic. Excessive potassium is drawn away by the neighboring glia through a spatial buffering mechanism. Finally, the "epileptic" neuron can be thought of as a pathologic entity that is subject to abnormal spike electrogenesis.

REFERENCES AND BIBLIOGRAPHY

Ayala, G. F., Spencer, W. A., and Gumnit, R. J. Penicillin as an epileptogenic agent: Effect on an isolated synapse. *Science* 171:915–917, 1971.

Ayala, G. F., Dichter, M., Gumnit, R. J., Matsumoto, H., and Spencer, W. A. Genesis of epileptic interictal spikes. New knowledge of cortical feedback systems suggests a neurophysiological explanation of brief paroxysms. *Brain Res.* 52:1–17, 1973.

Baglioni, S. M., and Magnini, M. Azione di alcune sostanze chimiche sulle zone eccitabili della corteccia cerebrale del cane. *Arch. Fisiol.* 6:240–249, 1909.

Barbour, H. G., and Abel, J. Tetanic convulsions in frogs produced by acid fuchsin and their relation to the problem of inhibition in the central nervous system. *J. Pharmacol. Exp. Ther.* 2:167–199, 1910–1911.

Brazier, M. A. B. Historical introduction: The role of electricity in the exploration and elucidation of the epileptic seizure, pp. 1–9. In M. A. B. Brazier, ed. *Epilepsy: Its Phenomena in Man,* UCLA Forum in Medical Sciences, No. 17. New York: Academic Press, 1973.

Castellucci, V. F., and Goldring, S. Contribution to steady potential shifts of slow depolarization in cells presumed to be glia. *Electroencephalogr. Clin. Neurophysiol.* 28:109–118, 1970.

Crowell, R. M., and Ajmone-Marsan, C. Topographical distribution and patterns of unit activity during electrically induced after discharge. *Electroencephalogr. Clin. Neurophysiol.* (Suppl.) 31:59–73, 1972.

Curtis, D. R., Game, C. J. A., Johnston, G. A. R., McCulloch, R. M., and Maclachlan, R. M. Convulsive action of penicillin. *Brain Res.* 43:242–245, 1972.

Dandy, W. E., and Elman, R. Studies in experimental epilepsy. *Johns Hopkins Hosp. Bull.* 36:40–49, 1925.

Dichter, M., and Spencer, W. A. Penicillin-induced interictal discharges from the cat hippocampus. II. Mechanisms underlying origin and restriction. *J. Neurophysiol.* 32:663–687, 1969.

Enomoto, T. F., and Ajmone-Marsan, C. Epileptic activation of single cortical neurons and their relationship with electroencephalographic discharges. *Electroencephalogr. Clin. Neurophysiol.* 11: 199–218, 1959.

Goddard, G. V., McIntyre, D. C., and Leech, C. K. A permanent change in brain function resulting from daily electrical stimulation. *Exp. Neurol.* 25:295–330, 1969.

Goldensohn, E. S., and Purpura, D. P. Intracellular potentials of cortical neurons during focal epileptogenic discharges. *Science* 139:840–842, 1963.

Goldring, S. Negative steady potential shifts which lead to seizure discharge, pp. 215–236. In M. A. B. Brazier, ed. *Brain Function: Cortical Excitability and Steady Potentials; Relations of Basic Research to Space Biology.* UCLA Forum in Medical Sciences, No. 1. Berkeley: University of California Press, 1963.

Grimm, R. J., Frazee, J. G., Kawasaki, T., and Savić, M. Cobalt epilepsy in the squirrel monkey. *Electroencephalogr. Clin. Neurophysiol.* 29:525–528, 1970.

Jasper, H. H., and Droogleever-Fortuyn, J. Experimental studies on the functional anatomy of petit mal epilepsy. *Res. Publ. Assoc. Nerv. Ment. Dis.* 26:272–298, 1947.

Kandel, E. R., and Spencer, W. A. The pyramidal cell during hippocampal seizure. *Epilepsia* 2:63–69, 1961.

Karahashi, Y., Sheptak, P., Moossy, J., and Goldring, S. Intracellular potentials from experimental glial tumors. *Arch. Neurol.* 15:538–540, 1966.

Kopeloff, L. M. Experimental epilepsy in the mouse. *Proc. Soc. Exp. Biol. Med.* 104:500–504, 1960.

Kopeloff, L. M., Barrera, S. E., and Kopeloff, N. Recurrent convulsive seizures in animals produced by immunologic and chemical means. *Am. J. Psychiatr.* 98:881–902, 1942.

Matsumoto, H., and Ajmone-Marsan, C. Cortical cellular phenomena in experimental epilepsy: Interictal manifestations. *Exp. Neurol.* 9:286–304, 1964.

Morrell, F. Microelectrode studies in chronic epileptic foci. *Epilepsia* 2:81–88, 1961.

Morrell, F., Proctor, F., and Prince, D. A. Epileptogenic properties of subcortical freezing. *Neurology* 15:744–751, 1965.

Moruzzi, G. *L'Épilepsie Expérimentale.* Paris: Hermann et Cie., 1950. 139 pp.

Mutani, R. Cobalt experimental hippocampal epilepsy in the cat. *Epilepsia* 8:223–240, 1967.

Nims, L. F., Marshall, C., and Nielsen, A. Effect of local freezing on the electrical activity of the cerebral cortex. *Yale J. Biol. Med.* 13:477–484, 1940–1941.

Purpura, D. P., Penry, J. K., Tower, D. B., Woodbury, D. M., and Walter, R. D., eds. *Experimental Models of Epilepsy. A Manual for the Laboratory Worker.* New York: Raven Press, 1972. 615 pp.

Putnam, T. J., and Merritt, H. H. Experimental determination of the anticonvulsant properties of some phenyl derivations. *Science* 85:525–526, 1937.

Sugaya, E., Goldring, S., and O'Leary, J. L. Intracellular potentials associated with direct cortical response and seizure discharge in cat. *Electroencephalogr. Clin. Neurophysiol.* 17:661–669, 1964.

Tower, D. B. Neurochemical mechanisms, pp. 611–638. In H. H. Jasper, A. A. Ward, Jr., and A. Pope, eds. *Basic Mechanisms of the Epilepsies.* Boston: Little, Brown and Co., 1969.

Walker, A. E., and Johnson, H. C. Convulsive factor in commercial penicillin. *Arch. Surg.* 50:69–73, 1945.

Ward, A. A., Jr. The epileptic neurone. *Epilepsia* 2:70–80, 1961.

Chapter XV

ANTIEPILEPTIC DRUGS

The latter half of the nineteenth century was a period of progress in the understanding of epilepsy. It witnessed the use of the first effective antiepileptic drug by C. Locock in 1857 and the description of salaam attacks by W. J. West (see Chapter III). Hughlings Jackson, and later W. R. Gowers, made important steps toward explaining seizures and the march of epilepsy across the cortex (see Chapter VI). Studies of focal seizures provided the most rewarding information. Their enduring fruitfulness is documented by modern classifications that devote more space to focal than to generalized attacks, even though the latter afflict a much larger segment of the epileptic population. A late version of the International Classification of Seizures, for which the Section on Epilepsy of the National Institute of Neurological and Communicative Disorders and Stroke is the source, is provided below:

International Classification of Epileptic Seizures

I. Partial Seizures (seizures beginning locally).
   A. Partial seizures with elementary symptomatology (generally without impairment of consciousness).
      1. With motor symptoms (including Jacksonian seizures).
      2. With special sensory or somatosensory symptoms.
      3. With autonomic symptoms.
      4. Compound forms.
   B. Partial seizures with complex symptomatology (generally with impairment of consciousness). Also called temporal lobe or psychomotor seizures.
      1. With impairment of consciousness only.
      2. With cognitive symptomatology.
      3. With affective symptomatology.
      4. With "psychosensory" symptomatology.
      5. With "psychomotor" symptomatology (automatisms).
      6. Compound forms.
   C. Partial seizures secondarily generalized.
II. Generalized seizures (bilaterally symmetrical and without local onset).
      1. Absences (petit mal).
      2. Bilateral massive epileptic myoclonus.
      3. Infantile spasms.
      4. Clonic spasms.
      5. Tonic seizures.
      6. Tonic-clonic seizures (grand mal).

    7. Atonic seizures.

    8. Akinetic seizures.

III. Unilateral seizures (or predominantly so).

IV. Unclassified epileptic seizures (due to incomplete data).

From a different and quite valuable perspective, J. R. Reynolds (1861) emphasized the importance of examining statistically various aspects of the natural history of *idiopathic epilepsy*. He said, sensibly, that to obtain a numerical estimate of symptoms and signs, case material should be selected in which epilepsy occurs in its purest form, that is, "apart from all other recognizable pathological conditions." This grouping of idiopathic, or "centric," epilepsy continues to have much importance today. Cases drawn from the epileptic population to test the efficacy of newly developed drugs, for example, are ordinarily representative of idiopathic epilepsy. They are the cases that are least likely to show complicating structural defects, gross or microscopic. The idiopathic group also has the highest hereditary predisposition. The symptomatology of centric epilepsy is often protean in its manifestations, so it can be presumed that its causes are also varied. Yet recent studies point toward a single cause, a disturbance in the neural inhibitory mechanism. The prototype of this condition is the experimental action of strychnine, a convulsant drug that blocks inhibition and simultaneously releases excitatory action. Against this conceptual background, modern antiepileptic therapy has evolved.

The first effective antiepileptic to be discovered was not a synthetic organic chemical as are today's standard remedies. Rather, it was the salts of bromine, called *bromides*. The element bromine was isolated at about the time of Friedrich Wöhler's (1800–1882) synthesis of organic urea from inorganic ammonium cyanate in 1827. The bromides found their first medical use 10 years later. Before Locock introduced them for epilepsy, Indian hemp, alkaloids derived from plants (such as hyocyamus), and salts of tin and zinc were in use.

Electrical-machine treatments also were popular. In all probability they began with the use of static electricity; then galvanic and finally faradic currents were used. F. J. Magendie and C. E. Brown-Séquard were special devotees of electrotherapeusis for epilepsy (see Chapter VI).Phenobarbital, first of the synthesized compounds found useful in the treatment of epilepsy, was introduced as an anesthetic in 1912. In the same year, A. Hauptmann of Freiburg, Germany, called attention to its value in epilepsy. The bromides were chiefly useful for treating grand mal seizures, whereas phenobarbital had a wider effective range. J. E. P. Toman (1970) rated it as the most widely used, the cheapest, and the most potent of the antiepileptics. Its marked sedative effect, however, tends to restrict the dosage. Now phenobarbital is used effectively in combination with diphenylhydantoin (Dilantin®). When used in combination, lower dosages of each minimize the untoward effects possible when administered separately. For a quarter of a century after it became a recognized antiepileptic, phenobarbital had little competition from other drugs. But, by the time of H. H. Merritt and T. J.

Putnam's researches in the late 1930s, it had become apparent that phenobarbital should share the stage with other compounds, if they could be developed.

THE RESEARCHES OF MERRITT AND PUTNAM

Unlike the bromides and phenobarbital, the discovery of diphenylhydantoin stemmed from a deliberate search for other organic compounds that might prove effective as antiepileptics. Using an electric-shock device on laboratory animals (Fig. 74), Merritt and Putnam tested promising synthetics chemically related to phenobarbital. They selected those that combined the least sedative effect with the greatest antiepileptic effect, the latter gauged by ability to suppress electro-shock convulsions.

Diphenylhydantoin was first synthesized in 1908 by J. Blitz of Germany. Prior to its study by Merritt and Putnam, it had been screened for them by Parke Davis and Company, because it was chemically related to phenobarbital and had a lower sedative effect than the latter. It proved quite effective in suppressing seizures in cats. In later human testing, it also proved successful. Diphenylhydantoin has been in use since 1938, preventing or lessening seizures in countless individuals. It is particularly effective in grand mal and to a lesser extent in temporal lobe epilepsy. With phenobarbital and primidone, it shares the urea moiety that had

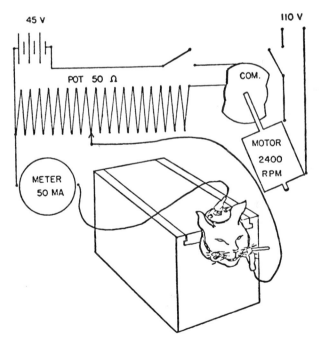

Fig. 74. Experimental equipment used for testing electroshock thresholds in diphenylhydantoin development. (From Putnam and Merritt, 1937.)

been synthesized long before by Wöhler (see Chapter III) from ammonium cyanate, an inorganic compound. Because at that time urea already was a well-known excretory product of the animal body, Wöhler's synthesis had much significance. It firmly rebutted the vitalistic view that a special class of substances exists belonging exclusively to living things.[1]

Electrophysiological studies on lesser animals clarified the antiepileptic efficacy of diphenylhydantoin. Toman has summarized those findings (1970). It seems that the drug promotes sodium ion efflux from neurons, tending to stabilize their threshold of excitability and protect them against overexcitation. Experimentally, it also reduces the tetanic effects of rapidly stimulating the postsynaptic membrane, another index of neural stabilization. Diphenylhydantoin also stabilizes the axon membrane that extends over the endbulbs, adding a presynaptic stability.

Toxic reactions rarely interfere with diphenylhydantoin treatment. Hyperplasia of the gums may be troublesome in about one-fifth of the patients. Hirsutism is not uncommon. Blood disorders are quite infrequent, but may include the complication of a rare anemia. Unsteadiness of gait (called *ataxia*) is a troublesome complication that may indicate overdosage, but it should disappear when the level of medication is reduced. In extremely rare instances, when the use of high dosages over a long period has been imperative, the Purkinje cells of the cerebellum can be lost and ataxia then becomes permanent. Two such cases were reported recently (Selhorst, Kaufman, and Horwitz, 1972).

TRIMETHADIONE

Trimethadione, brought out by the Abbott Chemical Company, represents an important step in the development of new antiepileptics. Initially, trimethadione was developed as an analgesic, but its antiepileptic properties were soon recognized. They were investigated by R. K. Richards, G. M. Everett, and K. L. Pickrell (1946). It was found that the compound is highly specific for the treatment of petit mal epilepsies as first reported by M. A. Perlstein (Richards and Perlstein, 1946). According to E. A. Swinyard and L. S. Goodman (1972), its discovery emphasized the fruitfulness of the systematic search for new antiepileptics on the basis of a well-designed battery of laboratory tests. The successful outcome of trimethadione research also established the principle that specific clinical effects may reside in related specificities of chemical structure, diphenylhydantoin being effective in grand mal and trimethadione in petit mal epilepsy. Trimethadione has a chemical nucleus differing materially from that of diphenylhydantoin, phenobarbital, and primidone. Its success stimulated the synthesis of many new compounds, each having possible antiepileptic value.

Trimethadione acts chiefly within the cell groups of the thalamus and the cortical fields to which they are related by interexchange of signals, providing inhibitory control (Toman, 1970). The unique petit mal, spike-wave discharge (see Fig. 49) could relate to disordered action within such a loop of circulating signals, cortex and thalamus reexciting each other.

A sister compound, paramethadione, has a trivial structural difference from trimethadione, and its therapeutic use, dosage, and toxicity manifestations are similar to those of the related drug. The principal troublesome side effects of trimethadione are sedation and dimming of vision in bright light, the former tending to diminish as medication is continued and the latter to be controlled by the use of dark glasses. Rarely, more serious toxicity manifestations occur, including skin rashes and kidney, liver, and blood cell ailments. Appearance of a rash may suggest discontinuation of medication. Grand mal seizures are sometimes activated by trimethadione in those afflicted with epilepsy.

PRIMIDONE

Introduced by the Ayerst Pharmaceutical Company, primidone is a phenobarbital congener in which there is a substitution at one link in the urea moiety. Because of the substitution, it is sometimes necessary to use significantly higher dosages than would be used for phenobarbital (Toman, 1970). The area of chief usefulness includes the temporal lobe epilepsies. Side effects of drowsiness, ataxia, and nausea occur in some subjects. Reduction in white cells of the blood may occur, but liver and kidney damage is said to be rare if it occurs at all. The special anemia mentioned in connection with diphenylhydantoin also develops rarely.

OTHER ANTIEPILEPTICS

The drugs mentioned above, all currently in use, are historical examples of the development of safe, effective control of epileptic seizures. A listing of all antiepileptics marketed in the United States at this time is given in Table 2, with trade name, generic name, company of origin, and year introduced. For other data see Goodman and Gilman (1970) and D. M. Woodbury, J. K. Penry, and R. P. Schmidt (1972).

THE TESTING OF NEW ANTIEPILEPTIC DRUGS

The earliest testimonials for an antiepileptic remedy were those of grateful relatives of patients, and they still are the best. The clinical trials of phenobarbital in 1912 were sketchy, and it was not until the studies by Merritt and Putnam (1937, 1938) that animal trials for efficacy and safety preceded human investigations. Even today, antiepileptic agents present many problems that make their value difficult to assess. One of them is reluctance to remove a patient from a medication of proven efficacy to enter him into a series planned to appraise an unknown product. Yet, while it is difficult to evaluate the overall efficacy of antiepileptics now in use, rough figures do indicate that 2,000,000 of the world's

TABLE 2. *Anticonvulsants marketed in the United States*

Year introduced	Trade name	Generic name	Company
1912	Luminal	phenobarbital	Winthrop
1935	Mebaral	mephobarbital	Winthrop
1938	Dilantin	diphenylhydantoin	Parke-Davis
1946	Tridione	trimethadione	Abbott
1947	Mesantoin	mephenytoin	Sandoz
1949	Paradione	paramethadione	Abbott
1950[a]	Thiantione	phenphenylate	Lilly
1951	Phenurone	phenacemide	Abbott
1952	Gemonil	metharbital	Abbott
1952[b]	Hibicon	benzchlorpropamide	Lederle
1953	Milontin	phensuximide	Parke-Davis
1954	Mysoline	primidone	Ayerst
1957	Celontin	methsuximide	Parke-Davis
1957	Peganone	ethotoin	Abbott
1960[c]	Elipten	amino-glutethimide	Ciba
1960	Zarontin	ethosuximide	Parke-Davis
1968[d]	Valium	diazepam	Roche
1974	Tegretol	carbamaxepine	Geigy

Source: Section on Epilepsy, Applied Neurologic Research Branch, Collaborative and Field Research, National Institute of Neurological Diseases and Stroke.
[a] Withdrawn, 1952.
[b] Withdrawn, 1955.
[c] Withdrawn, 1966.
[d] Approved by FDA as adjunct.

epileptics and 200,000 of those in the United States have not been aided materially by available drugs. This shows the need for continuing the effort to improve the products, for the lot of the uncontrolled epileptic is a most difficult one.

What should an ideal antiepileptic drug have to offer? Toman (1970, p. 206) answers as follows:

> The ideal antiepileptic drug should be capable of complete suppression of seizures at a dosage level that does not cause sedation or other undesired central toxicity. Since it must be used continuously for months or years, it should be well tolerated by the oral route, inexpensive, long-acting, and incapable of inducing tolerance or withdrawal signs. It should be devoid of systemic toxicity, and free of even occasional idiosyncratic effects on skin or bone marrow of sensitized patients. Preferably, it should have such a wide margin of safety that lethal amounts could not be ingested by suicidally inclined patients. Ideally, one drug would control all types of clinical seizures, and would exert its actions directly upon the seizure focus.

Shortly after World War II, the Judiciary Committee of the American Medical Association recommended restrictions on the use of human subjects in investigating new drugs and requirements of prior animal investigation and proper medical management. Since these recommendations were not approved, the matter of controls covering drug testing remained unregulated until 1962, at which time the Kefauver-Harris drug amendments were adopted by Congress. They gave deserved emphasis to the technique of clinical investigation, assessment of probable efficacy of the drug to be tested, and patient safety.

Sponsors of new drugs, under these amendments, must provide the Food and Drug Administration (FDA) with requested information on a form entitled "Notice of Claimed Investigational Exemption for a New Drug" (IND). Complete chemical and manufacturing information is required, with the results of preclinical (including animal) investigations, showing that an undue hazard would not result from the institution of human studies. Also required are credentials of the investigators and copies of informational material provided by each, including an agreement to notify the FDA of adverse effects experienced, submission of informed consent forms obtained from the patients, and annual progress reports (Cereghino and Penry, 1972).

To summarize the test procedures before and after the IND, a drug is first screened for biological activity in laboratory animals. If it shows evidence of useful pharmacological or therapeutic activity, the toxic effects are then determined in other laboratory animals. Obviously, the toxic effects should be minimal or nonexistent and their assessment takes into consideration the requirement that the same dose of drug per body weight should reach the drug receptors in the test animal as in man, who would be the chief benefactor of successful trials. The evaluation is complex, as shown in the following example. In the case of diphenylhydantoin, between ingestion and arrival at receptor sites in nervous tissue, the drug must be transported across no less than 16 membranes, each involving contacts with many enzyme systems, the effects of any one of which could differ significantly between animal and man. Thus, comparative toxicities must be weighed carefully before undertaking human trials.

The same cautious attitude should be adopted in evaluating antiepileptic drug efficacy in animals. The test battery should include at least electrical stimulation as used by Merritt and Putnam (1938), induction of audiogenic and photogenic seizures, and the use of convulsant and irritant agents as determinants of seizure threshold. Comparisons should be undertaken with and without prior dosage of the test substance.

Metabolic testing is another *sine qua non* of animal trials. On it rests much of the basic information which must be extrapolated to metabolic evaluation in man. Where possible, electrophysiological testing should be undertaken for evidence of tangible protective effects engendered at the receptor sites in the nervous system.

In human testing (Coatsworth and Penry, 1972), it is important to select a patient group having a size and case distribution calculated to produce statistically analyzable data. Even the human volunteers required for Stage I testing must be screened for convulsions, for it is known that 7% of our population will have had at least one convulsion during their lives. In selecting Stage II and III groups, it is important that they be as homogeneous as possible for the seizure type under investigation (see International Classification at beginning of chapter), but they should not be so homogeneous as to exclude, for example, the well-adjusted and prosperous patient as well as severe epileptics with difficult economic and social problems.

Patients already well controlled on an antiepileptic drug of known efficacy should not participate in a test group at the risk of breaking a seizure control that is already effective; if it seems necessary to add the new product to existing medication, the interacting factors should be appraised carefully and kept to a minimum. Blind studies, in which the patient is not told whether he is taking the test drug or a placebo, and double-blind permutations of the studies, in which both the patient and the physician are in ignorance of whether the test substance or a placebo is being taken and records are kept by a third party, should be undertaken as an important aspect of the evidence collected.

ELECTROENCEPHALOGRAPHY AND DRUG EFFICACY TESTS

Used properly, electroencephalography should offer an important addition to drug test protocols. It must not be forgotten that abnormal rhythms will be found in the pretest tracings of some normal individuals. Even so select a group as airplane pilot candidates will contain one or two persons per thousand showing convulsive activity in the brainwave trace. Such findings in presumed normal persons must be weighed carefully in assessing drug control data. Electroencephalography offers decided advantages in selecting a pool of patients with petit mal epilepsy if the processing includes a 20-minute electroencephalogram (EEG) with a 2- to 3-minute period of controlled overbreathing to activate the spike-wave forms that are a usual accompaniment of this form of epilepsy. The disappearance under therapy of such spike-wave sequences, together with corresponding loss of the petit mal "absences," would be convincing evidence that the test agent could be effective in controlling such seizures.

WHAT HAPPENS TO INGESTED DRUGS?

Of necessity, most information concerning ingestion, distribution, biotransformation, and excretion of ingested drugs must be based on data from laboratory animals. Yet there are many indications that similar mechanisms exist in man. Biotransformation can be defined as an enzyme-dependent degradative process that terminates the effectiveness of an ingested dose of any synthetic product. Drugs are metabolized by enzymes, which may serve other purposes in the bodily economy to which drug detection is incidental. Diphenylhydantoin, for example, is broken down by a microsomal enzyme in the ergastoplasm of liver cells (see Fig. 65). The microsomes handle the biotransformation of many other drugs as well. Significantly, the drug may enhance its own metabolism as well as that of other drugs taken coincidentally. It does this by stimulating the action of drug-metabolizing enzymes. Through inhibition of certain enzymes, particular drugs that have almost no pharmacological action of their own can increase the actions of diverse families of other drugs. The mechanism of such inhibition remains unknown. Finally, it should be remembered that drugs are not usually metabolized in the organ on which they act. This is especially true for antiepileptic drugs, whose seat of action is the central nervous system.

Ordinarily, drugs are excreted by the kidneys, being eliminated either unchanged or as metabolites to which they have been degraded by enzyme action. Some such metabolites may retain pharmacological activity. The path of elimination of a drug may also be less direct than indicated above. By radioactive carbon labeling, diphenylhydantoin given in a single intravenous dose to animals may be detected afterwards in many visceral organs, lesser concentrations appearing in brain, fat, and muscle. Even when using this reliable labeling technique, the drug is not detected in the animal after 24 hours following injection. The liver is its chief site of detoxification, the metabolite being excreted in the urine (Woodbury and Swinyard, 1972). Much information on what happens to ingested drugs will be found in Brodie, Cosmides, and Rall (1965), Fingl and Woodbury (1965), and Woodbury and Swinyard (1972).

PLASMA CONCENTRATIONS OF ANTIEPILEPTIC DRUGS

One of the principal difficulties in controlling seizures in patients and lesser animals lies in maintaining an effective blood plasma concentration of the selected antiepileptic. Cumulatively, the forgetfulness of the patient may produce a significant disparity between dosage and antiepileptic effect seen by the physician. Blood plasma levels consistent with the dosage prescribed are evidence that absorption has been normal. For diphenylhydantoin, the method of choice to monitor the concentration in the blood may be spectrography, thin-layer chromatography, benzophenone extraction, or gas-liquid chromatography. Other conditions being equal, the plasma level required for seizure suppression relates to the severity of the convulsive problem for which control is required.

Phenobarbital concentrations in the blood can also be measured, as can those for primidone and trimethadione. The metabolite of trimethadione, dimethadione, is excreted slowly, appearing in the blood serum in ratios of 20 to 1 by comparison with the trimethadione ingested. This suggests that the metabolite is more active as an antiepileptic agent than is the ingested trimethadione.

The estimation of plasma levels of diphenylhydantoin has indicated that there is no difference in drug concentration between taking the prescribed daily medication in a single or several divided doses (Buchanen et al., 1972). The single-dose schedule seems easier for the patient to adhere to.

COMMENT

Commencing with phenobarbital in 1912, synthetic agents with antiepileptic properties have been used almost to the exclusion of all others. Proof by Merritt and Putnam of the antiepileptic efficacy of diphenylhydantoin, which is a close kin of phenobarbital but with a much lower sedative effect, showed the importance of investigating all chemically related products and synthesizing others as well. The hydantoin experience also led to the development of a battery of tests for assaying the antiepileptic efficacy of any drug under study for whatever purpose.

In 1946 the antiepileptic action of trimethadione was discovered through the use of such a test battery for screening purposes. It already was known to have analgesic properties. Trimethadione's molecular structure was significantly different from either phenobarbital or diphenylhydantoin; it was found to be successful for treating petit mal, instead of grand mal, epilepsy. This led to a flurry of investigation in the pharmaceutical industry, and to FDA approval of a dozen other antiepileptic compounds between 1946 and 1960. Since then interest has waned in the planned synthesis of new compounds, and their systematic testing has fallen off appreciably. Some of the reasons for this are discussed in the final chapter.

The fact that 10% or more of epileptics cannot be effectively treated with the presently approved drugs is sufficient cause to cite the need for strenuous efforts to regain the momentum lost in the early 1960s. Restoration of momentum is always difficult, particularly in this instance, since more stringent regulations for drug development plus economic inflation have raised the estimated cost of marketing a new product.

The development of new techniques for examining blood plasma levels of antiepileptic drugs has added an important control factor to antiepileptic therapy. All of the principally used agents now can be controlled in this manner in the security that the drug ingested has been properly absorbed and distributed and that the patients are not missing frequent doses through absentmindedness.

Significant advances have been made in understanding the mechanisms by which drugs are absorbed, distributed, detoxified, and excreted and in understanding how the drug action takes place. The field of pharmacological therapeutics has expanded rapidly. These factors emphasize the crucial necessity for storage and retrieval of information on the biological effects of chemicals, on satisfying the needs for drug information, and the collection and analysis of information about adverse drug reactions. There also is a need to establish centers of research and training in pharmacology and toxicology and, by expansion of training, to correct the growing manpower shortage in these specialties (Brodie et al., 1965).

NOTE

[1] Temkin (personal communication) has called to my attention the article of McKie (*Nature* 153:608–610, 1944) who points out that Wöhler obtained cyanate actually from animal matter so that his urea synthesis was not from inorganic material.

REFERENCES AND BIBLIOGRAPHY

Bogoch, S., and Dreyfus, J. *The Broad Range of Use of Diphenylhydantoin. Bibliography and Review.* New York: The Dreyfus Medical Foundation, 1970. 169 pp.

Brodie, B. B., Cosmides, G. J., and Rall, D. P. Toxicology and the biomedical sciences. *Science* 148:1547–1554, 1965.

Buchanan, R. A., Kinkel, A. W., Goulet, J. R., and Smith, T. C. The metabolism of diphenylhydantoin (Dilantin) following once-daily administration. *Neurology (Minneap.)* 22:126–130, 1972.

Cereghino, J. J., and Penry, J. K. Testing of anticonvulsants in man, pp. 63–73. In D. M. Woodbury, J. K. Penry, and R. P. Schmidt, eds. *Antiepileptic Drugs.* New York: Raven Press, 1972.

Coatsworth, J. J., and Penry, J. K. Clinical efficacy and use, pp. 87–96. In D. M. Woodbury, J. K. Penry, and R. P. Schmidt, eds. *Antiepileptic Drugs.* New York: Raven Press, 1972.

Fingl, E., and Woodbury, D. M. General principles, pp. 1–36. In L. S. Goodman and A. Gilman, eds. *The Pharmacological Basis of Therapeutics,* 3rd ed. New York: The Macmillan Co., 1965.

Gastaut, H. Clinical and electroencephalographical classification of epileptic seizures. *Epilepsia* 11: 102–113, 1970.

Goodman, L. S., and Gilman, A., eds. *The Pharmacological Basis of Therapeutics,* 4th ed. New York: The Macmillan Co., 1970. 1794 pp.

Merritt, H. H., and Putnam, T. J. Sodium diphenylhydantoinate in the treatment of convulsive disorders. *JAMA* 111:1068–1073, 1938.

Putnam, T. J., and Merritt, H. H. Experimental determination of the anticonvulsant properties of some phenyl derivatives. *Science* 85:525–526, 1937.

Reynolds, J. R. *Epilepsy: Its Symptoms, Treatment, and Relation to Other Chronic Convulsive Diseases.* London: John Churchill, 1861. 360 pp.

Richards, R. K., and Perlstein, M. A. Tridione: A new experimental drug for treatment of convulsive and related disorders. *Arch. Neurol. Psychiatry* 55:164–165, 1946.

Richards, R. K., Everett, G. M., and Pickrell, K. L. Pharmacological and clinical studies of tridione with special reference to its analgesic action. *Anesth. Analg.* 25:147–151, 1946.

Selhorst, J. B., Kaufman, B., and Horwitz, S. J. Diphenylhydantoin-induced cerebellar degeneration. *Arch. Neurol.* 27:453–455, 1972.

Sieveking, E. H. Analysis of fifty-two cases of epilepsy observed by the author. *Lancet* 1:527–528, 1857.

Swinyard, E. A., and Goodman, L. S. Introduction, pp. 1–5. In D. M. Woodbury, J. K. Penry, and R. P. Schmidt, eds. *Antiepileptic Drugs.* New York: Raven Press, 1972.

Toman, J. E. P. Drugs effective in convulsive disorders, pp. 204–225. In L. S. Goodman and A. Gilman, eds. *The Pharmacological Basis of Therapeutics,* 4th ed. New York: The Macmillan Co., 1970.

Woodbury, D. M., and Swinyard, E. A. Diphenylhydantoin: Absorption, distribution and excretion, pp. 113–123. In D. M. Woodbury, J. K. Penry, and R. P. Schmidt, eds. *Antiepileptic Drugs.* New York: Raven Press, 1972.

Woodbury, D. M., Penry, J. K., and Schmidt, R. P., eds. *Antiepileptic Drugs.* New York: Raven Press, 1972. 536 pp.

Chapter XVI

ROLE OF NEUROLOGICAL SURGERY IN THE TREATMENT OF EPILEPSY

Opportunity-to-learn walks into the operating room with any surgeon who has unanswered questions in his mind.

W. Penfield
(1969, p. 781.)

Today's surgery for epilepsy is carried out in an operating room environment that would have astonished the neurosurgical pioneers. Conditions necessary to maintain sterility are rigorously maintained. The most delicate instruments, which would be damaged by the usual steam autoclaving or antiseptic solutions, can be safely gas sterilized. Bacterial content of room air is kept at a minimum by regulating circulation of air through high-volume laminar flow and superfiltration, an innovation engineered by NASA. In some operating theaters, the surgeon even wears protective glasses and a hood while operating under ultraviolet lighting, which further sterilizes the air. The lighting is remarkable. Aside from overhead lights, which are designed to provide focal illumination and minimize glare, light can be transmitted through malleable glass fibers (diameters as small as one-twenty-fifth of an inch or 1 millimeter) to permit resolution of fine anatomical detail in deep surgical exposures, outside the range of ceiling-mounted lights. Many neurosurgeons now operate with a microscope. Structures are magnified 6 to 25 times, improving the safety of the dissections and permitting surgical accomplishments hitherto impossible. *Pari passu* microsurgical instruments have been developed that enable the handling of the small delicate structures revealed by the extra magnification. Anesthesia has become remarkably safe, and prompt recovery of consciousness after procedures lasting many hours is taken for granted. No longer must the surgeon race against time to avoid an anesthetic death. Also, modern anesthetic methods, which are constantly being improved by advances in cardiorespiratory physiology, have greatly reduced the serious complication of brain swelling during surgery. Monitoring of vital signs is routine, with continuous visual display of blood pressure, pulse, respiratory rate, and electrocardiogram for the surgeon.

In operations for epilepsy, where knowledge of the brain's electrical activity and of muscle reactions provide important information, additional spin-offs from modern technology prevail. Through televised monitoring the surgeon can observe movements (convulsive and otherwise) of the subject's limbs and face directly. Without it, the surgeon has to receive such information indirectly from an assistant since, except for the operative field of the brain, the patient is hidden from direct observation by drapes. Equipment of sophisticated electronic design permits facile recording of the brain's intrinsic rhythms and responses to stimulation, both used in assessing the boundaries of an epileptogenic lesion. Even the epileptogenic discharge of a single neuron can be observed. Computers facilitate identification of the cerebral convolutions concerned with motor control and sensation that the surgeon needs to avoid in his excision of an epileptogenic lesion.

HOW IT ALL BEGAN

In 1828 Benjamin Dudley, professor of anatomy and surgery at Transylvania University in Lexington, Kentucky, reported five cases of posttraumatic epilepsy in which he had trephined the skull to alleviate seizures. He effected a favorable outcome for each (Cutter, 1930). After the trephining, either bone fragments were removed or a residue of old blood (called a subdural hematoma) was evacuated. In that pioneer epoch of American medicine, his success was remarkable. During the last half of the nineteenth century, long after Dudley's report, the mortality in similar cases was still 50% in the urban areas of the Eastern seaboard and in the surgical capitals of Europe. Dudley attributed his success to the general good health of his patients. He wrote:

> The great authorities of Europe and of our own country have laid down certain principles by which practitioners are generally governed in the treatment of injuries done on the scalp, cranium and brain. *Since the publication of Mr. Abernethy's [John Abernethy (1764–1831), an English surgeon] invaluable paper on injuries of the head, it might seem that little remains to be done in that department of surgery, while it is more than probable that under the present organization and management of the crowded hospitals of the large cities in Europe, no interesting and salutary innovations will be suggested:* whereas in the United States, and especially in the valley of the Mississippi, where there is comparatively no human misery, no remarkable excesses in luxury, no crowded manufactories, and no large cities: where every individual partakes of nourishment equally healthy and invigorating, the fairest prospect is offered of giving new and increasing interest to the subject. (Cutter, 1930, p. 190.)

There is a strong probability that Dudley's excellent results were due to his low incidence of infection because his patients were not cared for in "overcrowded hospitals in populous cities." Also implicit in Dudley's writings was the thought that wherever trephination could be accomplished without an infectious complication, the ultimate in surgical management of posttraumatic epilepsy would have been achieved. The surgeon would have gone as far as he could go. Limited to knowledge of the brain then extant, Dudley's view was correct. Without the forward strides in knowledge of brain structure and function that occurred during the remainder of the nineteenth century, further improvement in the surgical management of epilepsy could scarcely have been accomplished.

In Dudley's time, the prevailing rationale of trephination was decompression of the locale of the injury and that alone. Pressure by pooled blood or depressed fragments of skull, however, was not believed to exert its deleterious effect through compression of the immediately underlying cerebrum. Rather, the existing pressure was thought to be transmitted to either the cerebellum or the medulla oblongata, both hindbrain parts, one or the other of which was deemed the true initiator of convulsive movements (see Chapters VI, VII, and XIV). Those of Dudley's time who thought otherwise attributed a successful trephination to the evacuation of evil air or humors. It had occurred to no one that convulsions could arise from irritative lesions within a cerebral convolution, or that the cerebral gray matter played a major role in controlling the body's movements. Paraphrasing Hughlings Jackson, the universal neuroscientific view of those times was that the cerebral hemispheres were the repository of ideas, not movements. Indeed, before 1870 the convolutions were presumed to be totally inexcitable to mechanical or electrical stimulation. Pierre Flourens (1794–1867), whose writings dominated the thought of physiologists for much of the nineteenth century, said in 1823 about cerebral functioning: "There are no different sites for the different faculties nor for the different sensations . . . the cerebral lobes are the exclusive seat of sensations, perception, and volition" (Clarke and O'Malley, 1968, p. 481).

Yet within a few decades after Dudley all this was changed. Several unrelated discoveries converged to launch the era of epilepsy surgery and to define the discipline of neurological surgery as we know it today.

In 1846 J. C. Warren demonstrated the safety of ether anesthesia before his skeptical colleagues of the Massachusetts General Hospital in Boston. Twenty years later Joseph Lister (1827–1912) reported the use of antisepsis in the management of surgical and traumatic wounds. He declared that infection was not the result of oxygen or other gases of the air, but as Louis Pasteur (1822–1895) had shown earlier, was due to microorganisms. By liberal application of carbolic acid to surgical and traumatic wounds, Lister virtually eliminated the triad of dreaded complications—suppuration, putrefaction, and infection.

At about that time Hughlings Jackson, who has since become an immortal among neurologists, commenced to challenge those who denied the localization of separate functions within the cerebral hemispheres. From many careful observations of the onset and spread of seizures in epileptics, and correlation of seizure patterns with the sites of related cerebral lesions found at autopsy, he concluded, contrary to Flourens, that the cerebral hemispheres, besides their other functions, dealt with the organization of movements. He also saw irritative lesions in the pre-Rolandic convolutions as the cause of convulsions in many instances. Meanwhile, in a case showing motor aphasia as its dominant symptom, Paul Broca (1824–1880) of France had brought forth unequivocal evidence for a motor speech center in the third left frontal convolution, with autopsy verification of the site of the lesion.

The stage was set for the studies of Gustav Fritsch and Eduard Hitzig in 1870 and David Ferrier in 1876. Hitherto, experimental studies on animals had shown cerebral cortex to be inexcitable, mechanically or electrically. The German team used galvanic stimulation of canine cortex to prove electrical excitability of the anterior cerebrum, producing therewith convulsions of the opposite extremities.

Later Ferrier selected monkeys as his principal experimental animals and faradic current for cortical stimulation. Activation of cortex near the midline of the pre-Rolandic convolution produced movements in the opposite-side lower limb, arm, and face centers positioned successively laterad. He also undertook ablative studies, producing hemiplegic monkeys by removal of the opposite pre-Rolandic cortex. So reproducible were Ferrier's findings and so low his mortality in experimental operative studies that he often asserted the feasibility of attempts to remove brain tumors in man by trephining over the area that controlled the initiating movement of a subject's convulsion. A convulsion commencing in the left hand, for example, would suggest exposure of the right side of the brain about 2 inches from the midline and centered on a plane passing across the head just in front of the ears.

In the autumn of 1884, Hughes Bennett, a neurologist, diagnosed the existence of such a tumor during life, localized its situation, and approximated its size and shape, based entirely on the signs and symptoms presented. The site was exposed, and the tumor was found and excised by a surgeon, Rickman J. Godlee, while Jackson and Ferrier, who were in attendance at the operation, looked on. Later, the case was presented at a meeting of the Royal Medical and Chirurgical Society, where they, along with Horsley and William Macewen (1848–1924), a pioneer British neurological surgeon, discussed the case. Not long thereafter, Horsley reported three other cases he had operated on for focal epilepsy. In one, he identified the thumb area of pre-Rolandic motor cortex by electrical stimulation and, even though it appeared normal, excised it along with the neighboring pathologic process. Horsley and Jackson had had the foresight to consider that possibility prior to the operation, and it was their prejudgment to remove the epileptogenic site in any event, even though it only neighbored on the expected scar or tumor and was not included in it. In other words, if epilepsy were to be arrested, the cortical site of seizure onset, even if normal in appearance, would have to receive prime consideration. Although handicapped by a lack of prior experience, they had envisioned the crux of a perplexing problem that recurs time and again during epilepsy surgery as performed today.

During his surgical procedures, Victor Horsley used electrical stimulation extensively to identify cortical motor points. This practice was followed by Fedor Krause (1856–1937) and Otfrid Foerster (1873–1941) of Germany. The latter operated on his epileptic subjects under local anesthesia to facilitate cortical mapping. Also, he explored the brain's surface, area after area, by electrical stimulation, with the view of identifying a cortical locus that would reproduce the subject's clinical convulsion. The maps of human cortical localization, published by Foerster, were constructed on systematic data derived from many individual patients.

One more discovery, however, was required before epilepsy surgery, as carried out today, could commence its steady evolution. Although feeble electrical currents had been recorded from the surface of the rabbit's brain in 1875 by Richard Caton of England, it was not until 1929 that Hans Berger of Germany obtained corresponding records from man. He first recorded rhythmic electrical activity in subjects having skull defects resulting from past head injuries and later did the same through intact skull and scalp (see Chapter VIII). The latter was the origin of the electroencephalogram (EEG), which was to prove invaluable in identifying epileptics having focal lesions by use of a harmless diagnostic procedure. The method yields evidence concerning both focal brain wave disturbances associated with known focal seizure onsets and those that appeared unexpectedly in subjects of generalized seizures. In 1939 Sachs, Schwartz, and Kerr were the first American neurological surgeons to record such activity directly from the surface of the human brain.

Later writings on surgical treatment of epilepsy have been largely the labor of Wilder Penfield of Canada, an eminent neurological surgeon, working with a succession of collaborators, among whom Herbert H. Jasper, neurophysiologist and electroencephalographer, has been a frequent coauthor. Penfield and Jasper commenced the use of the EEG as a routine preoperative method to establish that abnormal activity arose from a single focus on one side of the brain in contrast to the diffusely distributed abnormal discharges of the generalized epileptic attack. They also recorded abnormal focal activity directly from the brain during surgery (the electrocorticogram, ECG). However, the early excisions did not include areas of the cerebrum that generated abnormal focal activity but otherwise appeared normal. Then, Penfield favored limiting the excision to the lesion (often a scar) and its borders. Later he came to excise with the lesion all surrounding areas from which abnormal electrical activity was recorded, provided such excision did not encroach on an area known to have a vital function, such as speech.

Before proceeding further, it is of value to recapitulate the random but connected discoveries that preceded the launching of both epilepsy and other neurological surgery, for the two came into specialty practice through the same door. The discoveries were each necessary antecedents to the solution of some clinical problems. A Parisian bacteriologist (Louis Pasteur) proved that the septic effect of air is due to the minute organisms it contains. An English surgeon (Joseph Lister) concluded that wound infection results from the growth of organisms within wounds, hospital crowding contributing to the spread of lethal infections from one patient to another and carbolic acid solution proving an effective deterrent. An unusually gifted London neurologist (Hughlings Jackson) hypothesized the representation of movements within specific local regions of the human cerebrum. Experimental proof for the thesis was provided by two young German physiologists who used electrical stimulation of localized areas of the dog's cerebral cortex to produce opposite-side convulsions.

None of those workers was motivated initially by a desire to find a way to manage epilepsy or remove brain tumors surgically. In several cases, their interests lay far removed from those of the neurological surgeon, yet each made an integral contribution to the important series of scientific developments that launched brain surgery. At the beginning, had significant grant support been available for establishing epilepsy or brain tumor centers, many of these men might not have applied, considering their own interests irrelevant to the disease. Had any applied, his project, judged by standards of the time, might not have been considered appropriate for funding.

WHAT KINDS OF EPILEPTICS BENEFIT FROM BRAIN SURGERY?

Surgical treatment is helpful to only a small percentage of the total epileptic population. In the majority, antiepileptic medication (see Chapter XV) either controls seizures completely or reduces them to a frequency that does not interfere with usual life pursuits. True, 25% of epileptics have attacks that are very difficult to control by available medication. Only a low percentage of those, however, have seizures that might benefit from the surgical removal of an abnormal area of the brain.

To be considered for surgery, a subject of intractable epilepsy must have seizures that arise invariably from a circumscribed area of one side of the brain, do not respond to medical management, and present evidence that the condition will become permanently disabling. It is also important that the brain area involved not be concerned with such vital functions as speech or motor control. There may be instances, however, in which a hemiparesis (weakness of a side of the body) is preferable to a chronic convulsive state that either keeps the patient home-bound and family-dependent or relegates him to institutional care. Such cases are rare indeed. Even when subjects of focal seizures are difficult to control medically, surgery may be deferred for several years, while available antiepileptic drugs, used in different combinations, are given an adequate opportunity to control the seizures. Especially in children, surgical treatment is commonly delayed, since the possibility must be entertained that the seizures will disappear with increasing age. Epilepsy itself is seldom a threat to life in the sense that a progressively growing brain tumor is. With seizures alone, there is always the promise that an effective new drug will emerge from laboratory research.

Frequent convulsions over extended intervals and lowered mental activity, attributable in part to excessive doses of antiepileptic agents, however, may render a child uneducable, just as they make an adult unfit for work and dependent on his family or society. Thus, in the epileptic with seizures of focal origin, the time may come when the quality of life, present and future, must be weighed against both the surgical risk and the probability that the surgery undertaken may effect seizure control. Theodore Rasmussen, former director of the Montreal Neurological Institute, has analyzed the results of 1,456 patients who underwent surgery at his institution between 1926 and 1968. Of 1,044 in whom the epilepsy was of nontumoral origin and who had been followed for at least 2 years, 61% either remained seizure-free or showed a marked reduction in seizure frequency. There was but a 1% mortality rate, and in only half of 1% did surgery result in hemiparesis. Speech impairment and difficulty with recent memory occurred in a few isolated instances in which resection of the dominant anterior temporal lobe was required to eradicate the epileptogenic focus. It is against such risks, and the lack of complete assurance that seizures can be controlled surgically, that the subject or his parents must decide for or against surgery. If the decision is to risk surgery, it is important that it be accepted confidently, because such motivation is necessary to assure cooperation during the many diagnostic tests and the lengthy surgical procedure that may be necessary.

CAUSES OF FOCAL EPILEPSIES AMENABLE TO SURGICAL TREATMENT

Usually, a long-standing epileptogenic lesion is a residual of a head injury incurred at birth or postnatally. Past inflammatory processes (brain abscess or chronic encephalitis) and anoxia (deprivation of oxygen) also play roles in causation. In 20% of cases, the cause in unknown. Of the focal epilepsies considered for surgery, psychomotor attacks are the commonest variety. This group made up 50% of the epileptics treated surgically at the Montreal Neurological Institute during the 40 years covered by the survey.

Lesions producing psychomotor attacks are usually found in the medial inferior gyrus of the temporal lobe and its hippocampal adnexa (See Figs. 7 and 60). There, neurons are lost and replaced by glia. Glial cells, unlike neurons, retain their proliferative capacity and are transformed into scars as a reaction to brain injury. Such a scar is referred to as *medial sclerosis*. It has been estimated that 50% of institutionalized epileptics who die of natural causes will show such medial sclerosis (Falconer and Taylor, 1968).

Finally, some cases of cerebral tumors and of congenital blood vessel anomalies should be included in a general discussion of epilepsy surgery. Intractable seizures may be the only symptom, and the most highly specialized X-ray procedures ordinarily used in surgical diagnoses of tumor may prove negative. In such cases, when least expected, a tumor may be found at operation, or the growth is recognized by the pathologist through microscopic examination of tissue excised from the brain as a presumed scar.

SURGICAL PROCEDURE EVOLVED BY PENFIELD AT MONTREAL

In 1928 Penfield (Fig. 75) joined the staff at McGill University as Head of the Department of Neurology and Neurosurgery. Subsequently, with the aid of generous grants from the Rockefeller Foundation, he established and became first director of the Montreal Neurological Institute. Unlike his contemporaries, his training did not include a year or more spent in one of the early neurosurgical clinics, then the usual preparation for a career in neurological surgery. Rather, he entered upon his new appointment after having acquired expertise in neurophysiology and neuropathology, especially the latter. As a Rhodes Scholar at Oxford in 1919, he studied under Sir Charles Scott Sherrington. His neuropathologic training came under Pio Del Rio-Hortega in Madrid. Between 1926

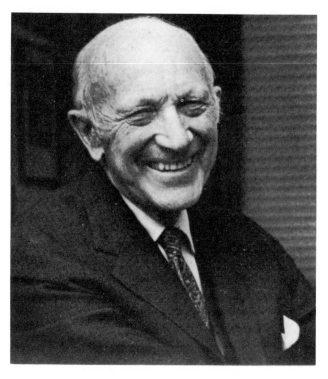

FIG. 75. Wilder Penfield, pioneer of modern epilepsy surgery.

and 1928, while a member of Alan Whipple's surgical clinic at the Presbyterian Hospital in New York, he founded and directed a neurocytology laboratory. Later he studied under Otfrid Foerster in Breslau, Germany, and much of his time there was spent in microscopic examination of the brain scars that Foerster removed from his epileptic patients. Penfield's initial surgical procedures for epilepsy were patterned upon those he observed in Foerster's clinic.

The evidence that shows a seizure state to be of focal origin derives largely from the sequence of development of the attacks. Does the seizure commence with a twitching of the left thumb and then spread to involve the entire left side, indicating a focus in the thumb area of the right pre-Rolandic motor cortex? Or does the subject develop a bland stare, lose contact with his surroundings, and fumble with his clothes, behavioral features of a psychomotor seizure originating from one or the other temporal lobes? In either instance, EEG confirmation of the existence of a focus is required before proceeding with surgery.

This is especially true with a temporal lobe seizure, where the character of the attack often fails to provide a clue to the side of the brain involved. In some cases, EEG tracings, even a series of them, will not provide information as to location because they derive from the scalp and hence register most clearly the events that occur at the brain's surface and not in the depth of the temporal lobe, the usual site of the involvement. Such deep-lying abnormalities are reflected fuzzily, if at all, in scalp records. In these cases, properly spaced electrodes inserted through the nasopharynx to the base of the skull may reveal focal spiking. Getting the tips even closer to the medial inferior gyrus by guiding an electrode under X-ray visualization to the sphenoid bone (Rovit et al., 1961*b*) may provide even sharper localization.

There is yet another limitation on use of the EEG to localize a seizure focus. In routine waking traces, scalp or other leads may not show focal discharges, whether seizure activity arises near the brain surface or not. In such instances, various means are used for "activating" latent abnormalities, which also can indicate an epileptogenic focus. Recordings during sleep, or as a consequence of the injection of seizure activating agents by vein, may be successful when routine recordings are negative. In temporal lobe epilepsy, ethyl-methyl glutamic acid or sodium thiopental is used. In other forms of epilepsy, pentylenetetrazol is given or the seizure may be activated by having the subject gaze at a light that flashes intermittently at 3 to 16 per second, so-called photic driving.

In a few instances, neither the EEG abnormality nor the character of the attack is localizing or lateralizing. Instead, the subject may have generalized seizures and show a diffusely disordered EEG. Yet, the seizures may have a focal origin, usually in the frontal lobe. Then, advantage may be taken of the fact that the blood irrigating each anterior half of the brain is largely supplied by a single carotid artery. An anesthetic agent injected into one carotid at a time will abolish the abnormal electrical activity on both sides if injected on the side containing the locus. Conversely, when the carotid supplying the innocent hemisphere is injected, the abnormal activity will only be affected on that side (Rovitt, Gloor, and Rasmussen, 1961a). The same discrepancy will arise during the activation of electrical seizure discharge by carotid injection of a convulsant agent.

A similar method (Wada and Rasmussen, 1960) is used to decide the dominant side of the brain, that which controls both speech and the dextrous hand. This always is important preoperative information for the surgeon, who must gauge the indications for undertaking remedial surgery, especially if an anticipated brain exposure neighbors on the speech area. The test utilizes the intracarotid injection of sodium amobarbital. Dominant-side injections produce transient loss, both of the ability to speak and to move the limbs opposite the side of injection. By contrast, delivered to the nondominant hemisphere, sodium amobarbital occasions only a transient weakness of the opposite side of the body.

Other information also is necessary before deciding on surgery. Patients require special X-ray examinations to exclude the possibility of a tumor or a congenital nest of abnormal blood vessels (technically, an arteriovenous malformation) as a cause of the epileptic attacks. Shadows of both the ventricles and the spaces surrounding the brain can be obtained after replacing some of the brain's cerebrospinal fluid with air inserted through a small needle that penetrates the base of the spine below the end of the spinal cord. Intra-arterial injections of a radio-opaque substance into the carotid arteries permit visualization of much of the intracranial blood supply through a procedure called arteriography. The combined appraisal of the results of the two methods can give the surgeon advance understanding of the conditions to be encountered during a contemplated procedure. Brain scans provide similar information. These are made by injecting a radioactive substance into the blood through an arm vein. In regions of abnormal vascularity or damaged areas of brain, increased diffusability through the vascular walls causes the injected substance to remain in these sites a sufficient time to permit detection by appropriate sensors that pick up changes in distribution of radioactivity.

The most recent technological innovation available to the neurosurgeon is a truly remarkable one, a milestone in diagnostic advance. It utilizes a computer to resolve fine differences in absorption of X-rays as they pass through the normal tissues of the head, i.e., scalp, bone, brain, and any pathologic ones that might also be present. The technique, known as *computerized transaxial tomography* (CTT), is painless and does not require injections or other manipulations of the patient. The subject rests comfortably for 20 minutes while the head is scanned with X-rays and the data are computed. A two-dimensional view of the brain results, revealing any abnormality that might exist.

Surgery is usually carried out under local anesthesia of scalp, muscle, and the blood vessels of the encasing dural membrane. These are the only cranial tissues that contain pain-sensitive receptors. The brain itself, amazing as it may seem for an organ that responds so sensitively to the intolerable pains generated in other organs, is totally insensitive to damage involving itself. Given a well-motivated patient, and a surgeon attentive to his needs and comfort, the operative procedure is tolerated well, even though it may be prolonged. General anesthesia is avoided whenever possible, because it suppresses the abnormal electrical activity that is so useful in identifying the boundaries of epileptogenic cortex.

Under anesthesia, responses to electrical stimulation of the convolutions may become difficult or impossible to elicit. Anesthesia elevates the stimulus-threshold for eliciting bodily movements. Identification of the somatosensory area is impossible to elicit because it requires the patient to report a tingling or similar sensation in a body part when the appropriate cortical area is stimulated. However, special purpose computers have made it possible to identify the somatosensory area in anesthetized subjects (Fig. 76).[1] Neither can the speech area be localized under anesthesia because the only reliable method of identifying it is by its suppression. A conscious subject can be asked to count from 1 to 10 as an electrode is applied to the area under test. If it is indeed the speech area, the count stops at once. Such functional identification is critical because these are the only clues that provide the surgeon with a precise geographic awareness of the vital regions. Otherwise, one area of the brain's cortex within the operative field looks much like any other. Local electrical stimulation is another means of identifying an epileptogenic focus, a stimulus effective in eliciting after-discharge (see Chapter XIV) only in the epileptogenic area, being unable to do so outside that area. Production of after-discharge is especially significant as an indication of epilep-

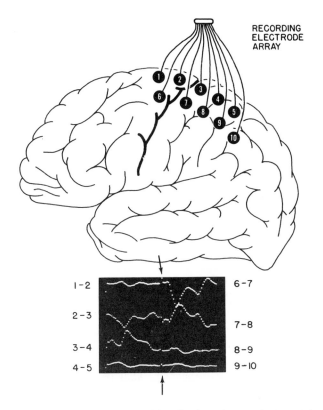

Fig. 76. Electrode display for computerized localization of sensorimotor region, left human cerebrum, above. The record combinations indicated below correspond to positions on the brain surface. Two columns, left and right, separated by arrow positions, consist of four records each. Only in records from electrode combinations that include cortical sites 3 and 7 does a response to sensory nerve stimulation appear. The responses identify the convolution in which they occur as somatosensory. The heavy-branched, black line separates that convolution from the pre-Rolandic motor cortex.

togenicity when accompanied by the partial seizure with which a naturally occurring convulsion begins.

After the limits of the cortex to be removed are mapped and the vital areas are identified, the involved tissue is excised and the electrical recordings are repeated along the margins of the removal, seeking residuals of epileptogenic tissue. If abnormal activity still exists, these areas, too, are excised, provided they do not encroach upon the source of a vital function.

SPECIAL CONSIDERATIONS IN EPILEPSY SURGERY

Temporal Lobe Epilepsy

Temporal lobe epilepsy is the commonest variety of the disorder treated by the neurological surgeon. A temporal lobe seizure may consist only in a brief loss of orientation and lapse of consciousness, or the episode may last longer and be accompanied by automatic behavior, such as chewing, fumbling with clothes, walking or running aimlessly, phrasing incoherent speech, or performing aggressive and asocial acts. For these events, the subject is amnesic. Less frequently, the seizure consists of or includes perceptual illusions (objects looking brighter, larger, or smaller; sounds seeming louder; a *déjà vu* recall of what is past and very familiar). Vague feelings of impending doom or of unreality also may arise, and for many of these perceptual experiences there is recall. Finally, a seizure may have hallucinatory aspects. These may include odors, sights, sounds, or combinations of visual and auditory perceptions. When such special sense seizures relate to a focus in one or the other temporal lobe, the hallucination, if visual, may be experienced only in the opposite half-field of vision. For example, a subject, who proved later to have a glial tumor of the right temporal lobe, complained of recurring episodes in which a herd of sheep was being led across the road. The sheep always entered at the margin of his field of vision to the left of his body. Because of the frequent psychic accompaniments of temporal lobe seizures, they are called *psychomotor.*

Penfield and Flanigin (1950), Morris (1956), Bailey and Gibbs (1951), and J. R. Green, R. E. H. Duisberg, and W. B. McGrath (1951) were among the first to remove parts of the temporal lobe to alleviate such seizures. Bailey and Gibbs (1951) resected the laterally placed temporal gyri, the resections being based on EEG findings. Penfield and Flannigan introduced the operation of temporal lobectomy, now elected most frequently. That resection includes the medially placed amygdala and hippocampus.

In the currently used procedure, 2 to 3 inches of the anterior temporal lobe are removed. Since the actual focus usually lies deep in the medial inferior region of the lobe, the resection must include brain tissue not involved in the epileptogenic process. Such a liberal resection is permissible since the region involved is relatively silent insofar as known brain functions are concerned. Brenda Milner (1958) of the Montreal Neurological Institute has shown that in the nondominant hemisphere such removals have little effect on mentation, except that they reduce understanding of pictures. A corresponding resection within the dominant hemisphere is associated with word-recall difficulties. The losses in mentation indicated are of debatable significance in any case because in temporal lobe epileptics they usually exist before a lobe's removal.

Whereas a unilateral temporal lobectomy can be carried out with relative impunity, bilateral removals produce marked impairment of recent memory. Because of this, special consideration must be given a subject who shows abnormal electrical discharges that arise independently from the two temporal lobes, but in whom seizures can be shown to develop in only one. Since electrical events may be the sign of more widespread abnormality, either temporal lobe, alone, may be incapable of normal function as it relates to memory. In such cases, unilateral resection of either temporal lobe carries the same risk as a bilateral one. Fortunately, however, it is possible to evaluate the status of preoperative memory, one side at a time. Sodium amytal, injected into one carotid artery, transiently inactivates the recent memories residing in the temporal lobe belonging to that side. Before each injection, the subject is given simple memory tests that have predictive value concerning the impairment that might ensue if the lobe were removed.

In recent years temporal lobe epilepsy has been a major interest of Murray Falconer (1967, 1968, 1970) of the Guy-Maudsley Neurosurgical Unit in London. His observations have emphasized the importance of asphyxia during infancy as a cause of medial sclerosis, such episodes occurring in conjunction with status epilepticus, febrile convulsions, severe infections, and head injury. His results with anterior temporal lobectomies are similar to those reported from Montreal. Relief from attacks was recorded in 62% of subjects followed 2 to 12 years after surgery.

Before leaving this topic, it is necessary to comment on personality disorders associated with temporal lobe conditions. About 50% of Falconer's patients had a history of episodes of aggression, neuroticism, or even psychosis. A. Earl Walker (1957, 1965), former professor and head of Neurological Surgery of the Johns Hopkins University School of Medicine, lucidly describes such deviations from normal behavior:

> These interpersonal aberrations are continuously manifested by withdrawal, seclusiveness, anxiety, paranoia, insecurity, fanatic pseudoreligiosity, or paroxysmal outbursts of temper, which lead to a personality label of queer. One of the most frequently encountered behavioral deviations is a modification of aggression expressed in all modalities of conduct. In temporal lobe epilepsy, aggressivity is typically "impulsive irritable behavior," characterized by relatively unmotivated, paroxysmal outbursts of episodic anger, abusiveness or assaultiveness, quite in contrast with the patient's usual behavior. Between those outbursts, the individual usually is good-natured. Close associates often can recognize dysphoric moods characterized by increasing irritability and hypersensitivity, lasting hours or days, which may herald an outburst of anger or a seizure. After such an episode, the irritable patient regains his normal more pleasant disposition. (Walker, 1973, p. 73.)

The effect of surgical removal of the temporal lobe on the aggression mentioned by Walker holds special interest here. In both Falconer's and Walker's experiences, the majority of subjects whose epilepsy was relieved by surgery also showed marked lessening of aggressive behavior after operation. Walker also noted a similar salutary effect of surgery on the hyposexuality that characterized about 70% of his patients having intractable temporal lobe epilepsy. Before surgery they had little or no heterosexual interest or outlet. Thereafter, sexual drive improved in about one-third, the improvement correlating positively with relief from psychomotor seizures.

In neither Falconer's nor Walker's subjects was surgery done merely because of the existence of a behavior disorder, but solely for the relief of seizures. Partial operations, such as amygdalectomy, have been carried out to correct intractable aggressive behavior with or without the coexistence of epilepsy. Although the reports suggest that most patients so treated are helped, there is disagreement among neurological specialists concerning the indications for and the benefits to be derived from such procedures. This subject has been studied recently by a panel of experts appointed by the National Institute of Neurological and Communicative Disorders and Stroke. The following conclusion was reached:

> Operative treatments for patients suffering from severe psychiatric or neurological illnesses or both, with intractable violence and aggression, have been performed by many neurosurgeons. Many responsible neurosurgeons believe that withholding such therapy from individuals with otherwise uncontrollable violence and aggression may be depriving them of their only chance for assistance and relief. Though most of these surgical procedures are reported as successful, the evaluation of the outcome is made difficult because of the following reasons: the diversity of symptoms in patient selection; the lack of information regarding the preoperative evaluation; a lack of detail concerning the degree, character, and thoroughness of the follow-up; ambiguities in regard to additional therapeutic factors, i.e., drugs, psychotherapy, institutionalization, and change in the environmental situation. (Goldstein, 1974, p. 32.)

Epilepsy Associated with Infantile Hemiplegia

Victims of epilepsy associated with infantile hemiplegia either were born with complete paralysis of one side of the body (hemiplegia) or acquired that defect in infancy. Later they may develop epilepsy and frequently show mental retardation, asocial behavior, or both. Although called "infantile," such persons may reach adult life and present severe problems in control of seizures, asocial behavior, and need for continuous, often institutional, care. The asocial behavior of the infantile hemiplegic is usually characterized by episodic, aggressive outbursts and unprovoked temper tantrums. The convulsions are usually focal in origin, later becoming generalized, or may be generalized from the start. Psychomotor seizures also occur. The unique feature is a pathologic process that is limited to one hemisphere which becomes shrunken and shows many regions of neuron replacement by reactive glial tissue. Large hemispheral areas are also replaced by cysts that may or may not communicate with the ventricular system.

The causes are various: birth injury, occlusion of a major cerebral artery, hemorrhage, trauma, and focal infection. In some instances the etiology remains unknown. The badly deteriorated hemisphere serves *no* purpose. All useful motor and mental activities have to be instigated from the uninvolved half of the brain. A damaged hemisphere, however, is not simply a missing one. Rather, its remaining action is excessively positive, its effect being expressed in repeated convulsions and episodic abnormalities in behavior. It is because the hemisphere contributes nothing that is useful and much that is injurious to brain and mind that the diseased hemisphere can be entirely removed without incurring additional disability.

In 1938 K. G. McKenzie of Toronto was the first to perform such a hemispherectomy in a young woman who had a spastic hemiplegia and intractable convulsions that stemmed from a severe childhood head injury. The surgical commitment at first seemed so overwhelming to others that his lead was not followed up for more than a decade. Then R. A. Krynauw (1950) of Johannesburg, South Africa, reported excellent results in 12 subjects, and others commenced to carry out hemispherectomies in similarly disabled individuals. The procedure has since become an established treatment for many intractable epilepsies associated with infantile hemiplegias. Review of a large series of cases (Wilson, 1970) shows that following hemispherectomy, 82% of the subjects either had no further seizures or showed a substantial reduction in number of attacks and their severity. Improvement in behavior has been equally gratifying. Ninety-three percent show disappearance or marked improvement of abnormal behavior. The aggressive episodes cease. In a significant number, the I.Q. improves, and some subjects become educable. There are examples, admittedly not many, of those who have completed a college education after having had such a hemispherectomy.

In a large number of subjects, it is the left hemisphere that is involved. Even though the left side is usually dominant for speech, that function is not affected because the damage had been done prior to the time that the child learned to talk, and during early infancy either hemisphere can develop into the repository for speech function. It is of added significance that one-third of subjects also show improved motor function on the paralyzed side, due, in all probability, to lessening of the disabling spasticity of the paralyzed limbs. In other words, the rigidity of the affected arm and leg lessens, and their gross movements, at least, are more readily achieved. In walking, the affected leg moves more freely, and arm movements are accomplished with less difficulty. Inability to perform finger movements persists, however. Many such subjects have now been followed for 20 years after hemispheric removal. In the majority, the results are lasting and excellent, but in about one-quarter of the cases, hydrocephalus develops later, or repeated episodes of bleeding occur into the part of the cranial cavity that harbored the removed hemisphere. If the latter complication develops, it usually happens quite late, occurring as long as 12 years after surgery. In many instances these complications are remediable, and the possibility of their occurrence is not a deterrent to hemispherectomy.

Prevention of Seizure Spread

Those who have studied human epilepsy prior to surgery through use of implanted recording electrodes have repeatedly observed localized seizure-discharges that occur unaccompanied by clinical manifestations (Fig. 77). Such an abnormal discharge probably occurs in a silent area (an area not yet completely explored) of the brain. The clinical seizure state only becomes manifest as it spreads to involve a discrete critical region or a brain volume of sufficient size to cause loss of consciousness and convulsion. This suggests that an alternative

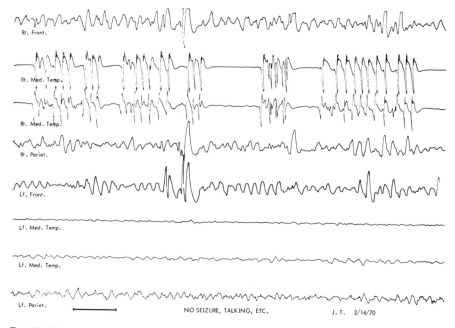

Fig. 77. Direct brain recording from subject of temporal lobe epilepsy. A localized seizure-discharge occurs during normal behavior. Front. and Pariet. refer to surface cortical areas of the frontal and parietal lobes. Med. Temp. relates to the medial temporal lobe in the region of the amygdala. The electrical seizure-discharge evident in the right medial temporal region endured for more than a minute. During this time, the subject carried on normal conversation, performed calculations, etc.

method of dealing with drug-resistant epilepsies might be the interruption of paths of preferential spread of seizure-discharge. Such an approach would be especially useful in those cases of intractable epilepsy in which no epileptogenic focus can be demonstrated, or where it is ill-defined, or located in a vital area where a surgical attack would represent a calculated risk of some magnitude.

Such a rationale prompted W. P. Van Wagenen and R. Y. Herren (1940) to section the corpus callosum, the major link (commissure) connecting the two cerebral hemispheres (see Chapter III, Fig. 4), in subjects of generalized convulsions. They theorized that in some individuals such seizures originate in one or the other of the two hemispheres, but not both. Thus, by commissurectomy intractable generalized convulsions could be contained within one hemisphere and converted into partial ones, if not prevented entirely. Some of Van Wagenen's subjects improved, but the beneficial results were not sufficiently convincing to prompt more than occasional use of callosal section for surgical treatment of intractable epilepsy. More recently, a relatively large experience with this procedure has been reported by Bogen, Sperry, and Vogel (1969). In addition to dividing the corpus callosum, they disconnected the anterior commissure that relates the two temporal lobes. Of 10 subjects in whom "generalized" convulsions had been occurring with high and increasing frequency before surgery, the seizures of 9 of them were largely abolished for 7, 6, 5, 5, 4, 4, 3, 3, and 2 years.

Of special interest is the minor functional impairment that is caused by a total cerebral commissurectomy. Special psychological tests have revealed, however, that disconnecting the cerebral hemispheres have effects on highest level functioning. An example is the inability of blind-folded, right-handed subjects to name objects placed in their left hand, information regarding size, shape, and texture of the object felt with that hand being registered only in the right hemisphere. A commissurectomy prevents such information from being transferred to the dominant left hemisphere, a prerequisite for verbal recognition of the object held. A long, flat object with teeth becomes a comb only after the dominant hemisphere thinks of the word for it and its use.

STEREOTAXIC EPILEPSY SURGERY

Some paths that spread from an epileptic focus lie within the brain's interior and cannot be approached directly by surgery without excessively damaging the brain. But a strategic site can be reached and explored by recording electrodes directed by stereotaxic techniques. As noted in Chapter VII, one can use skull landmarks to construct a tridimensional grid of the cerebral interior that permits placement of an electrode tip within any millimeter cube of the brain's interior. Such electrodes can record electrical activity from known sites in the depth of the brain, or, if used for electrical stimulation, they can sometimes reproduce the functional role of the area or activate seizure-discharges, using still stronger pulses of current. Substituting a heat-generating radio frequency current, or using some other form of energy, small spots of brain in the immediate vicinity of the electrode can be destroyed. It is of considerable historical interest that Horsley, who first excised an epileptogenic focus along with R. H. Clarke, played an important role in establishing the stereotaxic instrument as a neurological tool of great utility in epilepsy surgery (see Chapter VII).

The first Clarke-Horsley equipment in the United States was brought from England by Ernest Sachs, a Horsley fellow in neurological surgery who in 1911 became a neurosurgeon at Barnes Hospital, St. Louis.[2] Later he was appointed Professor of Neurological Surgery at the Washington University School of Medicine which is associated with the hospital. The instrument was observed in Sachs' laboratory by S. W. Ranson. On becoming head of the Institute of Neurology at Northwestern University Medical School, Ranson had a duplicate made which he used in his researches on the hypothalamus. Ralph Gerard of the University of Chicago had another model made from Ranson's design, and use of the instrument spread widely from their laboratories.

First to use the stereotaxic technique in treating intractable seizures were E. A. Spiegel and H. T. Wycis (1950) of Temple University School of Medicine, Philadelphia. At the 1949 American Neurological Association meeting, they reported on two patients having drug-resistant petit mal epilepsy. The electrode tips had been guided stereotaxically to the center of the thalamus. The choice of that target was influenced by the earlier animal studies of H. Jasper and J. Droogleever-Fortuyn (see Chapter X), who showed that episodes resembling petit mal and grand mal could be initiated in freely moving cats by electrical stimulation of the medial thalamic neuron aggregates.[3] To Spiegel and Wycis the result suggested that generalized seizures might have a focal origin in the medial thalamus. Recordings were made after introducing the electrodes; thereafter, direct current was used to coagulate the tissue in the immediate neighborhood of their electrode tips. The results were inconclusive, and no further lesions were made there. But in 1958 they reported on an additional group of patients in whom lesions were made in a neighboring area of subcortical gray matter (see Chapter IV) called globus pallidus, either singly or in combination with the amygdala. Earlier experimental studies by A. Walker, G. Poggio, and O. Andy (1956) had demonstrated preferential spread of seizure-discharge from cerebral cortex to the globus pallidus, as well as to other subcortical neuron aggregates, and this prompted the Spiegel-Wycis choice of the pallidus as a site of interruption. The observation that cortical seizure-discharges appear to invade the pallidus rather than travel over more direct descending routes for the propagation of movements (pyramidal fibers) suggested it as a strategically placed small site at which to interrupt the spread of seizure activity without causing paralysis. The subjects selected had both salaam (see Chapter III) and grand mal attacks. They were observed for many years after undergoing surgery, and Wycis, Baird, and Spiegel (1966) reported a follow-up on the group. The results are somewhat difficult to evaluate, but it appears that the salaam attacks were favorably influenced in 6 of 10 patients who exhibited such seizures. All six were freed of such attacks or had only sporadic occurrences after surgery.

Other surgeons have placed lesions in the lateral neuron aggregates of the thalamus, posterior internal capsule, or subthalamus. The reports are few in number, and each such series is small. The follow-up intervals are also too short to permit a conclusive statement concerning the percentage of successes. One of the larger series of stereotaxic lesions placed for this purpose is that of D. Jannai, a neurological surgeon of Osaka, Japan, who made lesions in the subthalamus for both generalized and focal epilepsy, the latter term excluding temporal lobe epilepsy. At the Third Mexican Congress of Neurological Surgery, J. Mukawa, Jannai's collaborator, reported on 43 subjects who had been followed for 1 to 9 years. Twelve showed complete relief from seizures, and seven were improved. Of those relieved completely, four had had generalized seizures. Lesions in the subthalamus have not proved effective in temporal lobe epilepsy.

Temporal lobe seizure problems have also been managed stereotaxically by placing lesions in amygdalar neuron aggregates. The reason these limited, targeted destructions have been effective is probably that expressed by Walker, who says that "the preferential pathways for discharge from temporal cortex is the amygdala and hippocampus, and from these medial structures to mesencephalic and diencephalic centers, whereby the external manifestations of the epileptic discharge is mediated" (Walker, 1965, p. 16). The fact that only small areas of brain have to be destroyed in this instance would render it the obvious procedure of choice if it were as effective as removal of the entire anterior temporal lobe. Yet, the results, so far, do not appear to be as enduring as those that follow anterior temporal lobectomy. Nevertheless, stereotaxic amygdalectomy may prove to have a lasting place in managing some cases of temporal lobe epilepsy, especially those complicated by independent epileptogenic foci in the two temporal lobes. Until the present time, such cases have been considered inoperable because, as noted, bilateral temporal lobectomy can cause profound memory impairment, as well as other serious behavioral changes. In contrast, memory impairment has not been observed to follow bilateral amygdalar lesions.

Although the collective experience with stereotaxic surgery has been insufficient to assess its ultimate role in the surgical treatment of epilepsy, the stereotaxic placement of electrodes for chronic recording is used increasingly and has added a new dimension to epilepsy surgery. It has become even more clear that the most reliable evidence for localizing an epileptogenic focus is that which occurs in electrical recordings made during a *spontaneously occurring* convulsion. Abnormal electrical discharges recorded interictally have too frequently proved inaccurate in identifying the focus.

The implanted electrodes must be strategically distributed on the cortical surface and/or in cerebral depth (if indicated) to permit a valid sampling from many sites. They must be fixed rigidly so that they are not affected by convulsive movements that could render the record useless. Also, since spontaneously developing seizures are random in their occurrence, reliable recordings must continue uninterruptedly over long time intervals if the electrical seizure-discharge accompanying the convulsion is to be recorded. Chance dictates the occurrence of a seizure during a routine scalp EEG, even when recording time is increased beyond the 20 to 30 minutes usually allotted to it. The same applies to recordings made directly from the brain in the limited time that can be allowed during surgery. Frequently, no seizure occurs during routine presurgery recordings, forcing reliance on the interpretation of interictal electrical abnormalities alone or on seizure-discharge activated by convulsant drug or electrical stimulation.

The shortcomings of interictal records for specifying the location of an epileptogenic focus has been emphasized by the French neurosurgeon J. Talairach, working with the epileptologist J. Bancaud:

> In other words, the classical exploratory methods (*EEG* and *ECG*—surface recording from brain during surgery) ruling surgical therapy in epilepsy are unable to specify the origin of a paroxysmal discharge if a spontaneous epileptic seizure is not recorded. No interictal electrical discharge can be a sure sign of the paroxysmal activity. (Talairach and Bancaud, 1966, p. 93.)

In this country Paul H. Crandall, a neurosurgeon, among others, arrived at the same conclusion (1973). To facilitate the recording of spontaneous seizures, he has used radiotelemetry for continuous monitoring of brain waves. The patient wears a telemetry pack (approximately 6 X 3 X 1 inches) incorporated into a head dressing or in a special helmet. The pack amplifies and broadcasts the brain waves to a remote receiver, from which they are recorded on tape. The subject, unhampered by trailing wires, is free to move about. Nurses note the occurrence of any seizures together with the tape location at the time it develops. Each morning the activity from the segments of tape associated with a seizure are transferred to an EEG machine for write-out and interpretation.

EPILEPSY SURGERY: A UNIQUE OPPORTUNITY FOR GAINING NEW INSIGHTS INTO BRAIN FUNCTION

When assessing brain functioning by electrical stimulation or recording, animals cannot report how or what they feel, nor can they perform tasks—even simple ones—on command without elaborate and lengthy prior conditioning. Consider, then, that during most epilepsy operations, the patient is of necessity awake and able to communicate freely with the surgeon. Also by necessity, electrical stimulation and recording are integral steps in the surgical procedure. These are circumstances that cannot be simulated in any experimental laboratory; and, provided the patient's welfare and comfort are the primary consideration, the opportunities for accumulating knowledge are considerable.

Penfield took full advantage of this unique situation with the result that many aspects of normal and abnormal functioning of the human brain have been explained. The activation of neuronal mechanisms by electrical stimulation of the epileptic human temporal lobe, with the reproduction of perceptual illusions and auditory or visual hallucinatory responses, aroused worldwide interest. The role of the medial temporal structures in memory, the refined localization and interrelationships of the cerebral speech area, the relations of somatosensory and motor function in the human pre- and post-Rolandic convolutions, and the identification of the second somatosensory area in the lower central region and of the supplemental motor area on the medial aspect of the intermediate frontal region are other well-known contributions arising from Penfield's meticulously documented electrical stimulation studies carried out as aspects of the special field of neurological surgery (Rasmussen, 1972).

More recent discoveries have been made possible by a burgeoning technology that includes solid-state electronics and special purpose computers. A. A. Ward, Jr., professor of Neurological Surgery at the University of Washington, in Seattle, a former Penfield student, using microelectrodes, has recorded the activity of single nerve cells in human epileptogenic foci. Such cells show high-frequency bursting activity, which Ward considers to be the characteristic discharge pattern of "epileptic neurons." The writer has recorded the activity of single neurons involved in the execution of voluntary movements (Fig. 78). M. Brazier (1973), a neurophysiologist, has used a computer to map normal and abnormal (epileptogenic) neural paths of the amygdala and hippocampus of Crandall's patients. Similar studies have been carried out by a French team (Buser, Bancaud, and

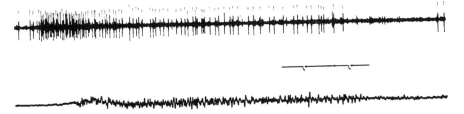

Fɪɢ. 78. Discharge from a single cortical neuron of man during hand closure. The upper record shows unit activity from a neuron in the hand area of motor cortex. The lower trace is of electrical activity of muscles that flex the fingers. Time markers shown between neuronal and muscle records indicate 1 second. At the beginning of the records, the subject was instructed to close his hand. Observe that the neuron begins its discharge before the muscle activity commences and continues to fire until the subject opens his hand several seconds later. Such neurons have been called *command cells.*

Talairach, 1973) and in Italy by the neurosurgeon G. F. Rossi. A. and M. Scheibel (1973), anatomists, and W. J. Brown (1973), neuropathologist, have used light and electron microscopy, respectively, to describe minute changes in neurons of the epileptogenic specimens removed by Crandall. In particular, they have noted loss of dendritic spines, nodular changes on dendrites, shrunken somata, and a windblown appearance of dendritic arbors of the gyrus dentatus, an adnexa of the hippocampus.

NOTES

[1] Recently, special purpose computers have made it possible to identify the somatosensory area with assurance even in anesthetized subjects. From animal experiments, it long has been known that stimulation of nerve evokes a localized electrical disturbance (evoked potential) in the related somatosensory region, even in anesthetized subjects. Such responses in man are frequently difficult to distinguish, however, from features of the spontaneous electrical rhythms of the EEG. The computer is programmed to add the electrical activities, both evoked and spontaneous, that follow each stimulus of a repetitive sequence. The sum of the evoked potential (which are nonrandom events) increases directly with the number of responses added, while the sum of random EEG waves increases as the square root of the number of samples obtained. Thus, the two activities grow at a disproportionate rate, and the evoked response is exposed above the spontaneous background rhythms. This technique is known as "averaging." In practice, one uses a grid of recording electrodes spaced over the presumed Rolandic region and its environs. The computer adds over time the successive disturbances (evoked potentials) induced by slowly repetitive electrical stimulation of the opposite side of the face, hand, or foot. In about 1 minute (25 to 50 stimuli delivered at one per second), records from electrodes resting on the somatosensory area show an evoked response, while others do not.

[2] Sachs later presented this instrument to H. W. Magoun, Ranson's former associate at Northwestern University Medical School, and Magoun in turn presented it to the Medical Library of the University of California at Los Angeles.

[3] Medial thalamic neuron aggregates in this instance include "the lamina medullaris interna-level of the commissura media" of the original Spiegel-Wycis report. They are literally at the center of the whole subcortical thalamic mass.

REFERENCES AND BIBLIOGRAPHY

Bailey, P., and Gibbs, F. A. Surgical treatment of psychomotor epilepsy. *JAMA* 145:365–370, 1951.
Bailey, P., Green, J. R., Amador, L., and Gibbs, F. A. Treatment of psychomotor states by anterior temporal lobectomy. Report of progress. *Assoc. Res. Nerv. Ment. Dis. Proc.* 31:341–346, 1953.

Baldwin, M., and Bailey, P. *Temporal Lobe Epilepsy.* Springfield, Ill.: Charles C Thomas, 1958. 581 pp.

Bancaud, J., Angelergues, R., Bernouilli, C., Bonis, A., Bordas-Ferrer, M., Bresson, M., Buser, P., Corvello, L., Morel, P., Szikla, G., Takeda, A., and Talairach, J. Functional stereotaxic exploration (SEEG) of epilepsy. *Electroencephalogr. Clin. Neurophysiol.* 28:85–86, 1970.

Bennett, A. H., and Godlee, R. J. Excision of a tumor from the brain. *Lancet* 2:1090–1091, 1884.

Bennett, A. H., and Godlee, R. J. Case of cerebral tumour. The surgical treatment. *Br. Med. J.* 1:988–989, 1885.

Berger, H. Über das Elektrencephalogramm des Menschen. *Arch. Psychiatr. Nervenkr.* 94:16–60, 1931.

Bogen, J. E., Fisher, E. D., and Vogel, P. J. Cerebral commissurotomy. A second case report. *JAMA* 194:1328–1329, 1965.

Bogen, J. E., Sperry, R. W., and Vogel, P. J. Addendum: Commissural section and propagation of seizures, pp. 439–440. In H. H. Jasper, A. A. Ward, Jr., and A. Pope, eds. *Basic Mechanisms of the Epilepsies.* Boston: Little, Brown and Co., 1969.

Brazier, M. A. B. Regional activities within the human hippocampus and hippocampal gyrus. *Exp. Neurol.* 26:254–268, 1970.

Brazier, M. A. B. The human amygdala: Electrophysiological studies, pp. 397–420. In B. E. Eleftheriou, ed. *The Neurobiology of the Amygdala.* New York: Plenum Press, 1972.

Brazier, M. A. B. Electrical seizure discharges within the human brain: The problem of spread, pp. 153–170. In M. A. B. Brazier, ed. *Epilepsy: Its Phenomena in Man.* (UCLA Forum in Medical Sciences, No. 17.) New York: Academic Press, 1973.

Broca, P. Remarks on the seat of the faculty of articulate language, followed by an observation of aphemia (1861), pp. 49–72. In W. W. Nowinski, ed. *Some Papers on the Cerebral Cortex.* (Trans. from the French and German by G. von Bonin.) Springfield, Ill.: Charles C Thomas, 1960.

Brown, W. J. Structural substrates of seizure foci in the human temporal lobe, pp. 339–374. In M. A. B. Brazier, ed. *Epilepsy: Its Phenomena in Man.* (UCLA Forum in Medical Sciences, No. 17.) New York: Academic Press, 1973.

Buser, P., Bancaud, J., and Talairach, J. Depth recordings in man in temporal lobe epilepsy, pp. 67–97. In M. A. B. Brazier, ed. *Epilepsy: Its Phenomena in Man.* (UCLA Forum in Medical Sciences, No. 17.) New York: Academic Press, 1973.

Clarke, E., and O'Malley, C. D. *The Human Brain and Spinal Cord.* Berkeley: University of California Press, 1968. 1926 pp.

Crandall, P. H. Developments in direct recordings from epileptogenic regions in the surgical treatment of partial epilepsies, pp. 287–310. In M. A. B. Brazier, ed. *Epilepsy: Its Phenomena in Man.* (UCLA Forum in Medical Sciences, No. 17.) New York: Academic Press, 1973.

Cutter, I. S. Benjamin W. Dudley and the surgical relief of traumatic epilepsy. *Int. Abstr. Surg.* 50:189–194, 1930.

Faeth, W. H., Walker, A. E., and Warner, W. A. Experimental subcortical epilepsy. *Arch. Neurol. Psychiatry* 75:548–562, 1956.

Falconer, M. A. Surgical treatment of temporal lobe epilepsy. *N. Z. Med. J.* 66:539–542, 1967.

Falconer, M. A. Significance of surgery for temporal lobe epilepsy in childhood and adolescence. *J. Neurosurg.* 33:233–252, 1970.

Falconer, M. A., and Taylor, D. C. Surgical treatment of drug-resistant epilepsy due to mesial temporal sclerosis. Etiology and significance. *Arch. Neurol.* 19:353–361, 1968.

Ferrier, D. Functions of the cerebrum, pp. 124–137. In D. Ferrier, *The Functions of the Brain.* London: Smith, Elder and Co., 1876.

Foerster, O., and Penfield, W. The structural basis of traumatic epilepsy and results of radical operation. *Brain* 53(2):99–119, 1930.

Fritsch, G., and Hitzig, E. On the electrical excitability of the cerebrum (1870), pp. 73–96. In W. W. Nowinski, ed. *Some Papers on the Cerebral Cortex.* (Trans. from the French and German by G. von Bonin.) Springfield, Ill.: Charles C Thomas, 1960.

Gastaut, H., Jasper, H., Bancaud, J., and Waltregny, A. *The Physiopathogenesis of the Epilepsies.* Springfield, Ill.: Charles C Thomas, 1969. 316 pp.

Goldstein, M. Brain research and violent behavior. *Arch. Neurol.* 30:1–35, 1974.

Green, J. R., Duisberg, R. E. H., and McGrath, W. B. Focal epilepsy of psychomotor type, a preliminary report of observations on effects of surgical therapy. *J. Neurosurg.* 8:157–172, 1951.

Horsley, V. Brain-surgery. *Br. Med. J.* 2:670–675, 1886.

Horsley, V. Remarks on ten consecutive cases of operations upon the brain and cranial cavity to illustrate the details and safety of the method employed. *Br. Med. J.* 1:863–865, 1887.

Horsley, V. An address on the origin and seat of epileptic disturbance. *Br. Med. J.* 1:693–696, 1892.

Horsley, V. The Linacre lecture on the function of the so-called motor area of the brain. *Br. Med. J.* 2:125–132, 1909.

Jinnai, D. Clinical results and the significance of Forel-H-tomy in the treatment of epilepsy. *Confin. Neurol.* 27:129–136, 1966.

Jasper, H. H., Ward, A. A., Jr., and Pope, A., eds. *Basic Mechanisms of the Epilepsies.* Boston: Little, Brown and Co., 1969. 835 pp.

Kennard, M. A., Fulton, J., and Mahoney, C. G. Otfrid Foerster, 1873–1941, an appreciation. *J. Neurophysiol.* 5:1–17, 1942.

Krause, F. *Surgery of the Brain and Spinal Cord,* Vol. II. New York: Rebman Co., 1912. 819 pp.

Krynauw, R. A. Infantile hemiplegia treated by removing one cerebral hemisphere. *J. Neurol. Neurosurg. Psychiatry* 13:243–267, 1950.

Lister, J. On the antiseptic principle in the practice of surgery. *Lancet* 2:353–356, 1867.

Marshall, C. Surgery of epilepsy and motor disorders, pp. 288–307. In A. E. Walker, ed. *A History of Neurological Surgery.* Baltimore: William & Wilkins Co., 1951.

Milner, B. Psychological defects produced by temporal lobe excision. *Assoc. Res. Nerv. Ment. Dis.* 36:244–257, 1958.

Morris, A. A. Temporal lobectomy with removal of uncus, hippocampus, and amygdala. *Arch. Neurol. Psychiatry* 76:479–496, 1956.

Mullan, S., Vailati, G., Karasick, J., and Mailis, M. Thalamic lesions for the control of epilepsy. A study of nine cases. *Arch. Neurol.* 16:277–285, 1967.

Narabayashi, H., and Uno, M. Long range results of stereotaxic amygdalotomy for behavior disorders. *Confin. Neurol.* 27:168–171, 1966.

Penfield, W. Epilepsy and surgical therapy. *Arch. Neurol. Psychiatry* 36:449–484, 1936.

Penfield, W. Epilepsy, neurophysiology, and some brain mechanisms related to consciousness, pp. 791–805. In H. H. Jasper, A. A. Ward, Jr., and A. Pope, eds. *Basic Mechanisms of the Epilepsies.* Boston: Little, Brown and Co., 1969.

Penfield, W. The mind and the highest brain-mechanism. *American Scholar* 43:237–246, 1974.

Penfield, W., and Baldwin, M. Temporal lobe seizures and technic of subtotal temporal lobectomy. *Ann. Surg.* 136:625–634, 1952.

Penfield, W., and Erickson, T. C. *Epilepsy and Cerebral Localization. A Study of the Mechanism, Treatment and Prevention of Epileptic Seizures.* Springfield, Ill.: Charles C Thomas, 1941. 623 pp.

Penfield, W., and Flanigin, H. Surgical therapy of temporal lobe seizures. *Arch. Neurol. Psychiatry* 64:491–500, 1950.

Penfield, W., and Jasper, H. Electroencephalography in focal epilepsy. *Trans. Am. Neurol. Assoc.* 66:209–211, 1940.

Penfield, W., and Jasper, H. *Epilepsy and the Functional Anatomy of the Human Brain.* Boston: Little, Brown and Co., 1954. 896 pp.

Rasmussen, T. Surgical therapy of focal epilepsy, pp. 101–107. In M. Critchley, J. L. O'Leary, and B. Jennett, eds. *Scientific Foundations of Neurology.* Philadelphia: F. A. Davis Co., 1972.

Rovit, R. L., Gloor, P., and Rasmussen, T. Intracarotid amobarbital in epileptic patients. A new diagnostic tool in clinical electroencephalography. *Arch. Neurol.* 5:606–626, 1961a.

Rovit, R. L., Gloor, P., and Rasmussen, T. Sphenoidal electrodes in the electrographic study of patients with temporal lobe epilepsy. *J. Neurosurg.* 18:151–158, 1961b.

Sachs, E., Schwartz, H. G., and Kerr, A. S. Electrical activity of the exposed human brain. *Trans. Am. Neurol. Assoc.* 65:14–17, 1939.

Scheibel, M. E., and Scheibel, A. B. Hippocampal pathology in temporal lobe epilepsy. A Golgi survey, pp. 311–337. In M. A. B. Brazier, ed. *Epilepsy: Its Phenomena in Man.* (UCLA Forum in Medical Sciences, No. 17.) New York: Academic Press, 1973.

Schwab, R. S., Sweet, W. H., Mark, B. H., Kjellberg, R. N., and Ervin, F. R. Treatment of intractable temporal lobe epilepsy by stereotactic amygdala lesions. *Trans. Am. Neurol. Assoc.* 90:16–19, 1965.

Spiegel, E. A., and Wycis, H. T. Thalamic recordings in man with special reference to seizure discharges. *Electroencephalogr. Clin. Neurophysiol.* 2:23–27, 1950.

Spiegel, E. A., Wycis, H. T., and Baird, H. W., III. Pallidotomy and pallido-amygdalotomy in certain types of convulsive disorders. *Arch. Neurol. Psychiatry* 80:714–728, 1958.

Talairach, J., and Bancaud, J. Lesion, "Irritative" zone and epileptogenic focus. *Confin. Neurol.* 27:91–94, 1966.

Trotter, W. A landmark in modern neurology. *Lancet* 2:1207–1210, 1934.

Van Wagenen, W. P., and Herren, R. Y. Surgical division of commissural pathways in the corpus callosum; relation to spread of epileptic attack. *Arch. Neurol. Psychiatry* 44:740–759, 1940.

Wada, J., and Rasmussen, T. Intracarotid injection of Sodium Amytal for the lateralization of cerebral speech dominance. Experimental and clinical observations. *J. Neurosurg.* 17:266–282, 1960.

Walker, A. E. Stimulation and ablation. Their role in the history of cerebral physiology. *J. Neurophysiol.* 20:435–449, 1957.

Walker, A. E. Discussion. (R. S. Schwab, W. H. Sweet, B. H. Mark, R. N. Kjellberg, and F. R. Ervin. Treatment of intractible temporal lobe epilepsy by stereotactic amygdala lesions.) *Trans. Am. Neurol. Assoc.* 90:16–17, 1965.

Walker, A. E. Man and his temporal lobes. John Hughlings Jackson lecture. *Surg. Neurol.* 1:69–79, 1973.

Walker, A. E., Poggio, G. F., and Andy, O. J. Structural spread of cortically-induced epileptic discharges. *Neurology (Minneap.)* 6:616–626, 1956.

Walter, R. D. Tactical considerations leading to surgical treatment of limbic epilepsy, pp. 99–119. In M. A. B. Brazier, ed. *Epilepsy: Its Phenomena in Man.* (UCLA Forum in Medical Sciences, No. 17.) New York: Academic Press, 1973.

Ward, A. A., Jr. The epileptic neurone. *Epilepsia* 2:70–80, 1961.

White, H. H. Cerebral hemispherectomy in the treatment of infantile hemiplegia, review of the literature and report of two cases. *Confin. Neurol.* 21:1–50, 1961.

Wilson, P. J. Cerebral hemispherectomy for infantile hemiplegia. A report of 50 cases. *Brain* 93: 147–180, 1970.

Wycis, H. T., Baird, H. W., and Spiegel, E. A. Long range results following pallidotomy and pallidoamygdalotomy in certain types of convulsive disorders. *Confin. Neurol.* 27:114–120, 1966.

Wycis, H. T., Lee, A. J., and Spiegel, E. A. Simultaneous records of thalamic and cortical (scalp) potentials in schizophrenics and epileptics. *Confin. Neurol.* 49:264–272, 1949.

Chapter XVII

RESEARCH PLANNING IN EPILEPSY

Many of the findings made by neuroscientific research during the last two centuries have had much significance for the interpretation of seizures. Before World War II epilepsy research was done largely by individuals who had responded to the appeal of science, working singly or in small groups. For the most part they were supported by medical schools affiliated with universities and in some instances aided by private philanthropists and foundations. Where intimate associations developed between clinicians and basic scientists, the efforts undertaken usually prospered. Outstanding American examples are the epilepsy studies of W. Lennox, F. and E. Gibbs, H. H. Merritt, and T. J. Putnam, which were aided greatly by contact with the basic science laboratories of Alexander Forbes, Hallowell Davis, Robert S. Morison, and E. Dempsey at Harvard Medical School. A similar development at the McGill University Medical School in Montreal linked Wilder Penfield, working on the neurosurgical therapy of epilepsy, with Herbert Jasper in electroencephalography.

Since 1945, a new era of science and technology has developed. Nationwide liaison between basic and clinically oriented scientists has occurred on a markedly increased scale, and greatly improved research opportunities exist thanks to funding by the government. Industry and the space effort also have contributed largely to the development of a much more diversified technology. Government funding also has encouraged specialization within the traditional university departments and has fostered the utilization of new technologies to an extent undreamed of in the past. Such specialization has become so fruitful that important new working associations have been formed between scientists, based on a commonality of interests in special problems, such as the use of computers in the conduct of investigations.

This approach has enriched especially the opportunities for investigation of the nervous system, and new departments of neurobiology are being organized in universities. These contain an assortment of specialists adept at fine structure analysis, membrane electrophysiology, neuropharmacology, behavioral science, radioautography, and neurogenetics, the last field including, besides "reeler" and other mutant mice, epileptic states in animals that are inheritable and deserve intensive study. All this holds great promise for advances in epilepsy, the soil of which is best cultivated by a multicategorical approach carried out by small communities of specialists, each having brain structure and function as shared interests. Let us review some of the opportunities that exist.

The focus of fine structure analysis is now on the organization of the synapse. It includes the classification of synapses with respect to their chemical or electrical transmitting nature; the typing of synaptic vesicles, each a packet of neurotransmitter substance; the survey of synapses found on neurons in all parts of the nervous system; and the investigations of invertebrate as well as vertebrate neurons. Can some synapses conduct by chemical transmission in one situation, by electrical in another? Do they all obey the law of dynamic polarization formulated by Ramón y Cajal and certainly applicable to the chemically transmitting synapses, or are somasomatic and dendrodendritic synapses found in sufficient numbers to account for spread of excitation laterally from soma to soma under conditions that promote the explosion of epileptic attacks? The search for new excitatory and inhibitory transmitters must continue. Knowledge about the mode of action of known transmitters requires expansion, including the solution of problems related to receptor sites, storage, and the interferences occasioned by false transmitter agents.

The existence of cholinergic and aminergic paths has been established within the reticular core of the brain, and such paths have been followed lengthwise using isotope tags attached to transmitter agents. The possibility of accomplishing this would have seemed remote a decade ago. This problem also relates to that of axonal flow, where tritiated proline has been added to tritiated leucine as another amino acid injectable into regions containing neuron somata as tags amenable to detection in axonal terminals some distance away. This will aid the unraveling of devious paths of the nervous system, the functions of which remain obscure. The question also arises whether aminergic and cholinergic synapses can activate the same neuron, or whether the paths using one transmitter or another are rigidly selective in their functions. Another query of significance concerns the essentiality to metabolism of an amino acid used for following axonal transport. Evidently proline and leucine differ in this respect.

Neuropharmacology has the opportunity—indeed the obligation—to develop explicit criteria for measuring antiepileptic action effectively. More reliable and less time-consuming methods are required for testing newly synthesized pharmaceutical products for their potency as antiepileptic agents. This is a bottleneck in the development of new drugs, for the organic chemist can, with few exceptions, undertake a synthesis and complete it within a reasonable time. If an effective new product could be singled out quickly and surely for safe and productive animal testing, leading to human investigation, development time would be shortened materially and the cost factor in development would be proportionately reduced.

Another important matter requiring full evaluation by the interested agencies is the reluctance of the pharmaceutical industry, considering the economic risks involved, to engage in the development of new drugs. It is estimated that 50% of all epileptics can become seizure-free under treatment when placed on some combination of currently available drugs. Another 25% may benefit materially. The remainder, including those whose attacks occur in clusters, may not improve significantly. It is this group that has the most at stake in the matter of the development of new, effective drugs. Estimating the epileptics of the U.S. population at 2,000,000, about a half million fall into the group for whom a maximal effort is not being made; and this number increases daily.

From the economic perspective, it has been estimated that the total antiepileptic product sold in the United States yields little more than $23,000,000 annually, a figure that must be balanced by the pharmaceutical companies against the presently estimated cost of $5,000,000 to bring one promising antiepileptic drug through the entire gamut of its development and testing, including human investigation. If successful in getting Food and Drug Administration (FDA) approval, the sponsoring company must then meet the competition of established products.

S. Peltzman (1973), an economist researching the costs and benefits of new drug regulation under a grant from the Center for Policy Study, University of Chicago, has recently studied the effects on new drug development of consumer protection legislation designed to prevent wasteful consumer expenditures. The project undertaken relates to a major theme of the Kefauver Antitrust and Monopoly Subcommittee—that in 1962 many new drugs of dubious efficacy were being marketed at unusually high prices. The study by Peltzman sought to determine "whether, and to what degree consumers have succeeded in obtaining a more valuable flow of new drugs under the regulatory system engendered by the 1962 amendments" (1973, p. 1051). His observation, which has special relevance to our subject, is that there has been a precipitous decline in the flow of new drugs since 1962—less than half the prior level. Of course, Professor Peltzman is considering all new drugs, not just those having value in epilepsy. Nevertheless, his findings should be viewed with alarm by those concerned with improving medical treatment for epileptics.

Throughout the neurosciences, wise planning should open up new avenues of research on the problems of epilepsy. However, there always must be readiness to acknowledge shots wide of the mark, and duplications of effort need be avoided where possible. Critical overview of lines of investigation should recognize existing gaps in knowledge and encourage research to fill them. These are matters for continuing communication among leaders in the field and not merely for the cursory attention of those who attend annual society meetings.

A national—even an international—program of clinical investigation with the goal of improving epilepsy therapy is desirable. A good beginning would be the establishment of a nationwide pilot group of outpatient clinics. Such clinics would require subsidy, no doubt, so expansion from a limited beginning should await justification of the operation over a reasonable trial period. The clinic operations should have definite, restricted goals.

At present there is no classification of the epilepsies that is fully acceptable to the clinicians of the Western world, let alone those caring for the remainder of the world's population. The proposed clinics, if successful in their operations, could make a start in that direction, for it would be necessary to provide extremely accurate clinical records as a basis for the cooperative studies that require development.

Current estimates of the efficacy of antiepileptic drugs are in most instances based on reports from the literature and largely presume that the prescribed drugs are taken regularly. A cooperating clinic group, covering areas representative of the entire U.S. population, could not only provide more authentic statistics, but under proper overview, it might also make possible careful long-term reevaluation of the efficacy of drugs currently used in the control of seizures, scoring the seizure frequency of each subject to determine the response to medication. Plasma drug concentrations could also be charted on a regular basis and correlated with changes in seizure frequency. Appearance and disappearance of toxicity manifestations could likewise be charted, and the possible deleterious effects of long usage of the principal antiepileptic medicaments systematically surveyed. Much information also would become available from comparison of treatment practices in the U.S., and perhaps later through international cooperation. Such comparisons also might shed light on the more general problem of the distribution of medical care. The participating clinics could develop listings of patients who have become seizure-free on a single antiepileptic agent, or a simple combination of them, to furnish a basis for future statistical studies. Other listings could provide a pool of subjects, ineffectually treated on current drugs, for consideration for use in testing investigational drugs that might prove more effective.

Planners should also consider the problem of encouraging adequate research and development programs in the pharmaceutical houses. These have declined in the last decade for reasons mentioned and because of mounting costs and the extensive preliminary testing required before products are approved for human investigation.

The high cost of research and development must be reduced if we are to widen the choice between antiepileptic agents that may be used in different permutations to treat patients in whom seizure control is not now adequate. So far, only pharmaceutical houses are geared to large-scale animal testing, so they may have to be subsidized, preferably under contracts that provide a return to the government when a new product proves profitable. The only alternative lies in putting all pharmaceutical research and development in the hands of the government. Surely, it should not depend almost exclusively on the venturesomeness of investors.

COMMENT

There hardly can be a more fitting conclusion to this review of scientific progress in the diagnosis and treatment of epilepsy than the statement made by Ralph W. Gerard[1] in a symposium entitled "Physiological Basis of Epileptic Discharge" at the annual meeting of the American Electroencephalographic Society in 1948 and published in a then new journal, *Electroencephalography and Clinical Neurophysiology:*

> Just as the creative effort of an individual mind starts with the conscious positing of a problem, is followed by the really crucial unconscious work which reveals its answer, and ends in a final conscious period of examination and checking; so the collective effort in solving clinical problems is in the public eye . . . when the doctor triumphantly applies the new remedies to his patients. During the great labor of reaching the fruitful result, the process fades from sight

into the quiet laboratory. The consequence is that people identify such progress with practicing physicians rather than with research biologists; and public support, when marshalled for new attacks, becomes funnelled through clinical rather than laboratory channels. (Gerard, 1948.)

Warm as our gratitude to the bedside doctor is bound to be, we cannot afford to forget that the relief that he or she dispenses has been made possible by the thoughtful and persevering labor of the men and women in the laboratories, the quiet people seeking the knowledge that makes possible the conquest of pain and affliction.

NOTE

[1] It is with sorrow that the Subcommittee engaged in the development of this endeavor acknowledges the recent death of Dr. Ralph W. Gerard. He did much to establish the accuracy of the facts presented and to keep us apprised of the wishes of the parent committee concerning the content and orientation of this document.

REFERENCES

Gerard, R. W. Opening remarks; physiological basis of epileptic discharge; closing statement. *Electroencephalogr. Clin. Neurophysiol.* 1:2, 53–56, 1949.
Peltzman, S. An evaluation of consumer protection legislation: The 1962 drug amendments. *J. Polit. Econ.* 81:1049–1091, 1973.

Glossary

ABNORMAL SPIKE ELECTROGENESIS: Increased irritability at the axon hillock of a neuron causes excessive discharge of signals along the axon.

ABSENCE: Abrupt loss of consciousness of brief duration.

ACETYLCHOLINE: Excitatory neurotransmitter substance.

ADRENAL: Gland situated above each kidney. The adrenal medulla produces epinephrine (adrenaline) and norepinephrine (noradrenaline), the latter a neurotransmitter of the catecholamine group. The adrenal cortex produces steroid hormones, i.e., cortisol, involved in metabolism of protein and glucose, and in inflammatory reactions; aldosterone, involved in salt and water metabolism; and androgenic and estrogenic hormones.

AFFERENT: Conducting toward the brain and spinal cord in the peripheral nervous system; upstream toward cortex in the central nervous system.

AFTER-DISCHARGE: In experimental seizures resulting from repetitive electrical (tetanic) stimulations, the convulsive electrical pattern persists after the stimulus is stopped.

AKINESIA: Loss of power in motor functioning; akinetic seizure, a drop attack. Characterized by falling and lack of motility. Also may be applied to slowness of movement, as in parkinsonism (paralysis agitans).

ALPHA RHYTHM: A sine-like electrical rhythm at 8 to 13 per sec recorded from the relaxed human subject with eyes closed.

AMINERGIC: Activated by the biogenic amines.

AMNESIA: Loss of memory.

ANASTOMOSIS: Network of nerves, as within a plexus.

ANGSTROM (Å): One ten-thousandth of a micron. A minute measurement used in electron microscopy.

ANOXIC: Lacking oxygen.

ANTIEPILEPTIC: (1) Preventing or arresting epileptic seizures, or used to treat epilepsy. (2) A drug that prevents or stops convulsive or nonconvulsive epileptic seizures.

APHASIA: Loss of expression by speech or writing. Includes also loss of ability to name, i.e., nominal aphasia.

ARCHITECTONICS: Pertains to structural design, as lamination of cerebral cortex.

ARTERIOGRAPHY: X-ray film of the skull taken during temporary filling of cerebral arteries with opaque material, which outlines their relative positions in cerebral tumors and detects aneurysms.

ASCENDING: Tracts that rise through the nervous system, usually sensory.

ASTATIC GALVANOMETER: A device for detecting weak electric currents which has two needles with opposite polarities to reduce the effects of the earth's magnetism.

AUDIOLOGY: The science of hearing, including the process of end-organ activation, central conduction along axons, and central processing.

AURA: Sensory experience, usually occurring as an early phase of a seizure, of which the patient is aware. It warns some epileptics of an impending attack.

AUTOMATISMS: Complex, nonreflex behavior that occurs over brief spans of time without awareness of the subject. (In its simplest form it can be a staring spell).

AXON: The core conductor of a nerve fiber; a hair-thin extension of a neuron that provides the mechanism through which neurons communicate.

AXON HILLOCK: Site of departure of axon from soma of a neuron.

AXONOLOGIST: A pre-World War II name for an investigator concerned exclusively with the electrical properties of axons.

BASAL GANGLIA: Large aggregates of gray matter lying deep in the cerebrum. Designation usually applies to caudate nucleus, globus pallidus, and putamen.

BASELINE SHIFT: In direct current electronic amplification the baseline may shift due to electrical artifacts or biopotentials introduced into the input.

BIOELECTRICITY: Animal electricity in its varied manifestations.

BIOPOTENTIALS: Animal electricity. Potentials that are produced during the functioning of the body. Nerve and muscle are prime producers.

BIOTRANSFORMATION: Breakup of a drug within the body through enzymatic action.

BLOCKING: In electroencephalography, refers to disappearance of alpha rhythm during repetitive electrical stimulation.

BOUTONS TERMINAUX: French for axonal endbulbs.

BRAIN SCAN: Intravenous injection of a radioactive carrier such as phosphorus (^{32}P), iodine (^{131}I), or technetium (^{99}Tc). A special device scans the cranium revealing differentials in radioactive shadow between abnormal and normal structures. Display takes place on a fluorescent tube face.

BRAINSTEM: The conically shaped portion of the nervous system that connects cerebrum with cerebellum and spinal cord.

BROAD FREQUENCY RESPONSE: Electroencephalographic tracing in which amplification is the same over a wide frequency range.

BROWN-SÉQUARD SYNDROME: Neurological deficit deriving from hemisection of spinal cord in animals and man. In man it consists of same-side paralysis of leg (and arm as well, if in cervical region). It also includes loss of position and vibratory sense on the side of the lesion and loss of pain and temperature on the opposite side. The entire loss occurs below the level of the lesion.

CATECHOLAMINE: Compound of a chemical grouping that stimulates action of autonomic nervous system.

CAUDAL AND ROSTRAL: In four-footed animals, caudal is toward tail, rostral toward snout. By convention, the same directions can be applied to the human nervous system.

CELL AGGREGATE: Collection of nerve cells of related function. *See* NUCLEUS.

CENTRAL NERVOUS SYSTEM (CNS): Brain and spinal cord.

CEREBRAL CORTEX: The mantle of gray matter that covers the cerebrum. Occupied largely with highest level function.

CEREBRAL LOCALIZATION: Cerebral cortex contains areas of specialized function, such as motor, general sensory, visual, auditory, and olfactory. Several areas have been mapped into subareas bearing consistent relations to brain topography.

CEREBRECTOMY: Removal of a part or parts of one or both cerebral hemispheres.

CEREBRUM: The left and right cerebral hemispheres with their connecting parts.

CERVEAU ISOLÉ: Transection of brain at midbrain level in deeply anesthetized animal.

CHOLINERGIC: Activated by acetylcholine.

CHOROIDAL ARTERY, ANTERIOR: A branch of the internal carotid, chief arterial supply of the upper cranial contents. The branch reaches the tip of the temporal lobe and swings around it to enter the inferior horn of the lateral ventricle, supplying its choroid plexus.

CLONIC: The phase of seizure showing rhythmically interrupted spasm.

COLLAGEN DISEASE: A disease involving collagen, a main component of the connective tissue of the body.

COMMISSURE: Path that crosses directly from one side of the nervous system to the other.

CONGENER: One of the same kind in nature or action.

CONVOLUTION: Tortuous elevations of surface of the cerebrum caused by in-folding of cortex. Synonymous with gyrus.

CONVULSION: Any involuntary contraction of the body musculature. Such contractions may be tonic or clonic, local or generalized (according to whether they are continuous or paroxysmal), and of either cerebral or lower origin.

CRANIAL NERVES: The 12 specialized nerves that arise from the base of the cerebrum or brainstem.

CRANIOFACIAL: Pertaining to cranium and face.

CRANIOTOMY: Any operation on the cranium.

CRYOGENIC: Pertaining to production of low temperatures.

DEFACILITATION: The opposite of facilitation. Elevation of the stimulus threshold required to produce an effective response.

DÉJÀ VU: An aura that precedes some epileptic attacks, particularly those of the temporal lobe, characterized by a feeling that something seen or experienced before has recurred. It may exist as an independent experience.

DEMARCATION: Term used in electrophysiological experiments to denote cut surface boundary of nerve or muscle. The electricity recorded from a cut surface is called "current of injury."

DENDRITES: Arborizing processes of neurons that markedly increase the receptive surface with which synapses are made.

DEPOLARIZATION: Decrease in the potential difference across a nerve cell membrane. Its dynamic effect is to excite a cell to discharge nerve impulses.

DESCENDING: Refers to tracts or impulses (usually motor) that descend from the highest level of the brain.

DIPHENYLHYDANTOIN: DPH, Dilantin. An antiepileptic.

DORSAL ROOT GANGLION: A bulge on each dorsal root of the 31 pairs of spinal nerve roots. Neurons contained therein are sensory, specialized for conduction of stimuli from body and skin receptors into the nervous system.

DURA: Outer tough membrane that encases the central nervous system.

DYSRHYTHMIA: A disordered electrical rhythm of the brain with irregularity in amplitude and frequency. In *paroxysmal dysrhythmia* spikes or spike-waves of convulsive nature occur.

EFFERENT: Conduction downstream from cortex to spinal cord in the central nervous system and outward from spinal cord and peripheral nerves toward the muscles.

ELECTRICAL LOBE: Extensions from the lower hindbrain of a torpedo (electric fish) from which the nerves innervating the electric organs arise.

ELECTROCORTICOGRAM (ECG): Direct electrical recording from the surface of cerebral cortex.

ELECTROENCEPHALOGRAM (EEG): An on-line, graphic recording of the electronically amplified electrical activity of the brain, usually recorded through skull and scalp (*see* Chapter VIII).

ELECTROMAGNETIC FIELD: A field of force made up by associated electrical and magnetic components.

ELECTRON MICROSCOPY: An electron beam is substituted for the light beam of usual microscopy. Permits enormous magnification and great resolving power.

ELECTROPHORESIS: Movement of charged particles in a fluid, such as is contained in the barrel of a recording microelectrode, under the influence of an electric field.

ELECTROPHYSIOLOGY: A specialized aspect of neurophysiology that relates to electrical methods of tracing nerve paths and of investigating synaptic and other aspects of central and peripheral nervous systems, heart, skeletal muscle, and other organs.

ELECTROPLAQUE: The homologue of the presynaptic structure that occurs in the electric organs of fish. Contains synaptic vesicles as do motor endplates of muscle and synaptic endbulbs of the central nervous system.

ELECTROSCOPE: An instrument used for detecting presence of static electricity.

ELECTROTHERAPEUSIS: Physiotherapy by a static, galvanic, or faradic current.

ELECTROTONUS: Longitudinal spread of current in a nerve excited by a current sub-threshold in its stimulus value.

EMBEDDING: Preparing tissue for microscopic study by thin sectioning after dehydration, clearing, and infiltrating with celloidin or paraffin.

ENCÉPHALE ISOLÉ: Transection between brain and spinal cord made in the deeply anes-thetized animal.

ENDBULB: Any terminus of any axon branch. Contains synaptic vesicles and has a surface of presynaptic membrane.

ENDPLATE: Terminus of motor axon in fiber of striated (skeletal) muscle.

ENZYME: An organic compound of protein composition, capable of catalyzing a change in substrate for which it is specific. It may aid the synthesis or the degradation of substrate components.

EPIDIASCOPE: A projector of images of both opaque and transparent objects.

EPILEPSY, IDIOPATHIC: Any type of epilepsy that cannot be linked to an obvious cerebral cause or a recognized metabolic disturbance.

EPILEPTIC CRY: A loud scream that may occur at the outset of an epileptic attack.

EPILEPTIC STATUS: A condition characterized by an epileptic seizure that is sufficiently prolonged, or repeated at sufficiently brief intervals, so as to produce an unvarying and enduring seizure state.

EPILEPTOGENIC FOCUS: A group of neurons involved in a focal epileptic discharge.

EPILEPTOGENIC LESION: Cortical or subcortical lesion characterized microscopically by cell dropout, gliosis, windblown look, and shrivelling of the dendrites.

EPILEPTOGENIC ZONE: A cutaneous zone from which an epileptic attack may be precipi-tated by stimulation.

EVOKED POTENTIAL: In man and experimental animal, an electrical signal of characteris-tic form evoked from the related field of cerebral cortex by stimulation of a skin sense organ, peripheral nerve, eye, or ear.

EXCITATION: The action-producing component of neural mechanism. Uses such choliner-gic transmitters as acetylcholine in its synaptic transfer processes.

EXCITATORY-INHIBITORY BALANCE: The moment-to-moment change in excitatory or inhibitory dominance in the activities of particular neurons. The balance is maintained by relative change in synaptic bombardment from connecting systems having the two kinds of effects.

EXOTOXIN: A toxic substance produced by bacteria and found outside them.

EXPERIMENTAL MODELS IN EPILEPSY: Mechanical, electronic, mathematical, and chemical technologies to develop new information concerning epilepsy, using experi-mental animals.

FACILITATION: A train of subthreshold shocks increases the excitability of neurons so that they overrespond to an effective stimulus.

FARADIZATION: Use of the inductorium to produce a tetanizing current by repetitive stimulation.

FEEDBACK: Return of some of the output of a system to input.

GALENICAL: Medicines (vegetable extracts) prepared according to or like the formulas of Galen.

GALVANOSCOPIC FROG PREPARATION: A frog preparation used to detect the presence of a feeble electrical current. Also called rheoscopic frog.

GAP JUNCTION: A slender cleft that can be distinguished at the fusion point of what otherwise would be a tight junction. "Electrical" synapses are of this kind. *See* TIGHT JUNCTION.

GASTROCNEMIUS: The muscle in the calf of the leg.

GLIAL CELL: Supporting and nutritive cell of the central nervous system; intervenes between nerve cells and fibers.

GLIOBLASTOMA: A malignant cerebral tumor.

GLIOSIS: Scar transformation of an area of brain through accumulation of reactive glia.

GLOMERULUS: Any tuft or cluster, nervous or otherwise, that can be seen microscopically within a body tissue.

GOLGI TYPE II NEURON: A neuron having an axon that arborizes in the immediate region of the soma.

GRAND MAL: A generalized tonic-clonic epileptic attack (*see* Chapter II for more detail).

GRANULE CELL: A small neuron scarcely larger than a red blood cell.

GRAY MATTER: That part of the brain which has a grayish appearance due to a chief composition of neuronal and glial cells, axon origins and terminals, and relative absence of myelin sheaths.

HEMIPLEGIA: Paralysis of arm and leg resulting from an opposite-side cerebral lesion.

HIPPOCAMPUS: A curved structure lying in the wall of the inferior horn of the lateral ventricle in each hemisphere. Also called *Ammon's horn* or *cornu Ammonis.*

HIRSUTISM: Excessive hairiness of skin.

HISTAMINE: An amine found in all animal and vegetable tissues, as brain. May have role as a neurotransmitter.

HOMUNCULUS: A little man created by the imagination; in this case he demonstrates the size of the body parts as represented in the motor and sensory areas of the human brain.

HORSERADISH PEROXIDASE: An enzyme extracted from horseradish.

HUMORAL: Pertaining to any fluid or semifluid of the body.

HYPERCARBIA: Excessive carbon dioxide in the blood.

HYPERPLASIA: Overgrowth, as of the gums, which may occur in diphenylhydantoin treatment of epilepsy.

HYPERPOLARIZATION: Acts antagonistically to depolarization by increasing the potential difference across the axon membrane. Inhibits the discharge of nerve impulses.

HYPOCARBIA: Insufficient carbon dioxide in the blood. A minimum of carbon dioxide is a necessary respiratory stimulant.

HYPSARRHYTHMIA: From *hypsi* (Greek for "high" or "lofty"), combined with *arrhythmia* (lack of normal rhythm). The type of EEG associated with *salaams, infantile spasms,* or *massive myoclonic attacks.*

IATROCHEMISTRY: A seventeenth-century school of medicine that believed the phenomena of life and death were based on chemical action. The then existing evidence was scanty, but the presumption has since been proved true.

IDIOPATHIC EPILEPSY: Of unknown causation. Sometimes called essential epilepsy.

INFLUENCE MACHINE: A machine that produces electricity by friction. Historically, it was used in electrical treatments.

INHIBITION: Functions to stop or slow action in progress at the command of neural mechanism.

INION: The back of the head.

INK-WRITER: An on-line electromagnetic device for tracing electrical brain activity. Usually multiple channel to cover several (to 20) combinations of leads applied to the head simultaneously.

INTERICTAL: Between seizures.

INTRINSIC: Situated entirely within or pertaining exclusively to a part of the nervous system.

IONIC: Pertains to an ion or ions, as sodium or potassium ions.

IONTOPHORESIS: Introduction of soluble salts into a nerve cell by use of an electric current. *See also* ELECTROPHORESIS.

LAMINAR NECROSIS: Dissolution of one of the six cerebral cortical layers, usually the third, due to severe oxygen deficit.

LARYNGEAL ELECTROMYOGRAPHY: Recording electrical potentials from laryngeal muscles during speech.

LESION: The site of damage to any tissue of the body. It usually results from infection, hemorrhage, or tumor.

LEYDEN JAR: A glass jar coated both inside and outside with metal foil and having the inner coating connected to a conducting rod passed upward through an insulated stopper. For storage of static electricity.

LIMBIC LOBE: Marginal portion of cerebral cortex on medial surface of the hemisphere.

LOBES: Subdivisions of the cerebral hemisphere into parts. There are five: frontal, parietal, temporal, occipital, and limbic.

LOW VOLTAGE FAST: EEG pattern with eyes open or during any active state. Called the activation trace in man and animals.

LUMBAR PUNCTURE (SPINAL TAP): Insertion of a needle through the spaces between the lower lumbar vertebra for diagnostic purposes to withdraw the fluid that bathes the central nervous system. Principally used diagnostically.

MARCH, MOTOR: Slow spread of seizure contraction from a beginning site, usually face, thumb-index, or great toe to become generalized. Corresponds to seizure spread across motor area of cerebral cortex. *See* CONVULSION.

MARCH, SENSORY: Slow spread of sensation from a local beginning, as in motor march. Corresponds to spread of epileptic discharge across sensory cortex. *See* CONVULSION.

MEASLES TITER: Serum with an unknown antibody content is diluted progressively, the successive dilutions being reacted with a known antigen. The titer is the greatest dilution at which a reaction is obtained.

MEDICOLEGAL: Pertaining to both medicine and law; forensic medicine.

MEMBRANE (PLASMA): Consists of a bimolecular layer of lipid flanked on either side by a monomolecular layer of what is principally protein. Invests the outside of the cell and also the nucleus and cell organelles.

METABOLITE: A substance produced by the bodily metabolism.

MICRON: One-thousandth of a millimeter. Unit of measurement used in light microscopy.

MICROSOME: One of the finely granular elements of neuroplasm.

MICROTOME: An apparatus for cutting thin sections of a tissue after freezing or embedding in paraffin, celloidin, or a plastic.

MICROVOLT: One-millionth of a volt.

MILLIVOLT: One-thousandth of a volt.

MODALITY: A sensory entity such as taste. Sensory axons are specific for the modalities they serve.

MOIETY: One of the portions into which something is divided.

MONOPLEGIA: Paralysis of arm or leg; results from opposite-side cerebral lesion.

MOTOR CORTEX: An electrically excitable area of cortex upon the convexity of the cerebral hemisphere. *See* Chapter VII for maps of localization of motor points relating to the opposite side of the body.

MOTOR ENDPLATE: Terminus of a motor fiber of peripheral nerve within a voluntary muscle fiber. Terminus contains synaptic vesicles and is comparable to a central synapse.

MYELIN SHEATH: The fatty investment of most axons of the central and many axons of the peripheral nervous system. In the aggregate these give to white matter its glistening white appearance.

MYOCLONUS: A brief and involuntary contraction of one or several muscles.

NEGATIVE VARIATION: Du Bois-Reymond's term for the action potential. Electrical signal that propagates along an axon.

NERVE CELL (NEURON): Includes the cell body and its axonal and dendritic extensions; the structural unit of nerve activity.

NERVE FIBER: An axon with its surrounding sheath, chiefly myelin. Thus, an axon surrounded by myelin is a nerve fiber.

NERVE REGENERATION: A peripheral nerve severed in its course shows axonal degeneration. Reinnervation may occur through sprouting of the central ends of cut axons and outgrowth to reach the former terminals.

NERVE ROOT: Collection of nerve filaments connecting peripheral nerves with brain or spinal cord.

NERVE SPIKE: The sum of individual nerve impulses recorded in a stimulating-recording system that provides nearly simultaneous conduction at finite rates between stimulating and recording electrodes. *See* NEGATIVE VARIATION.

NERVOUS SYSTEM: The central nervous system plus the plexuses and nerves of the peripheral system.

NEURAXIS: Abbreviation for the brain and spinal cord.

NEUROFIBRILS: Delicate filaments that run through the neuroplasm of neurons, extending from tips of dendrites to that of axon.

NEUROLOGICAL SURGEON: A specialist in the diagnosis and surgical treatment of diseases and disorders of the nervous system.

NEUROLOGIST: A specialist in the diagnosis and nonsurgical treatment of diseases and disorders of the nervous system.

NEUROMUSCULAR: Pertaining to both nerve and muscle. Axons of nerves form synapse-like endings protruding into muscle fibers.

NEUROPATHOLOGY: Study of the disease processes of the nervous system.

NEUROPHYSIOLOGY: All aspects of physiological studies, of the whole animal or its parts, using neurological, including electrical, methodologies.

NEXUS: Connecting link.

NONFOCAL: Describes abnormal patterns in the human electroencephalogram that are diffusely evident, not lateralized or localized.

NONMYELINATED NERVE FIBERS: Fibers whose axons are not invested by a myelin sheath. Fibers of Remak.

NONPOLARIZABLE: Term applied to electrodes. Sheer metal in contact with tissue may be electrolyzed and produce artificial voltages. Nonpolarizable electrodes may be coated with a salt, as of the metal (e.g., silver chloride for silver electrodes), which makes them resistant to polarization.

NUCLEUS (OF A CELL): A spherical body within a cell containing characteristic organelles. In neurons the nucleus has lost its power to initiate cell division, differentiating the nerve from germinal and most other body cells.

NUCLEUS (OF A NERVE): Any aggregate of neurons that have functional properties in common.

NYSTAGMUS: Involuntary rapid movement of the eyes, vertical, horizontal, rotatory, or mixed.

OCCLUSION: Where several postsynaptic neurons share their innervation by presynaptic ones, the postsynaptic response is reduced when presynaptic axons are stimulated together rather than consecutively.

OPHTHALMOSCOPE: Instrument for inspecting the inner retinal layer of the eyeball, its vasculature, and the origin of the optic nerve.

OPISTHOTONUS: Tetanic spasm in which the head and heels are bowed backwards and the body forwards.

ORGANELLE: Any particle of organized living substance present in nearly all cells, e.g., mitochondria, ergastoplasm, lysosomes, ribosomes.

ORGANIC SYNTHESIS: The production of an organic compound by the union of elements or simpler compounds or by the degradation of a more complex compound.

PARKINSON'S DISEASE: Shaking palsy. A chronic neurological condition involving the basal ganglia.

PATELLAR REFLEX: The knee jerk.

PETIT MAL: A generalized attack of minor character. *See* Chapter II.

PHASIC: Regularly recurring cycle of change.

PHOTIC STIMULATION: Stimulation of the retina of the eye by light flashes.

PHRENOLOGY: A field of study that attempts to relate the conformation of the skull to mental traits and character.

PICROTOXIN: A powerful convulsant agent.

PIEZOELECTRIC: Electric polarity due to pressure applied to a crystalline substance.

PILE: An aggregate of similar elements for producing electricity.

PLACEBO: An inert medicament given for its psychologic effect.

PLASMA CONCENTRATION: Plasma is the fluid portion of the blood in which cells are suspended. Concentration of a drug is estimated after cells have been removed.

PLASMALEMMA: Membrane which surrounds a neuron. *See* MEMBRANE.

PLEXUSES: An anastomosing arrangement of nerve cords which intervene between the spinal roots and the peripheral nerves, and in particular those which innervate upper and lower extremities.

PNEUMOENCEPHALOGRAPHY: X-radiation of the skull to show shape and size and detect contour abnormalities in the ventricles after their fluid content is replaced with air.

PONGID: An anthropoid ape.

POTENTIALS (BIOPOTENTIALS OR VOLTAGES): Differences in potential between two points on nervous tissue, or between one point and a distant nonnervous reference. Potential change, which the experimentalist universally measures, may arise intrinsically or be engendered by a stimulus.

PREMONITORY: Serving as a warning, as of an epileptic attack.

PURKINJE CELL: A unique large neuron of cerebellar cortex having a flask-shaped body and antler-like dendrites. In the aggregate, Purkinje cells generate the outflow of cerebellar cortex.

PYRAMIDAL TRACT: Bundles of axons that extend from motor cortex of the cerebral hemisphere to spinal cord. The tract crosses at the junction of hindbrain and cord. It functions in the organization of volitional movements.

QUANTAL: Step-like versus continuous variation.

RECEPTOR SITE: Minute punctate structures facing the neuromuscular cleft from the muscular side. Serve as attachment points for transmitter quanta which have diffused across the cleft, and for some toxins which, if attached, inactivate conduction.

RECRUITING RESPONSE: Potential evoked from midline thalamus that grows in amplitude upon repetitive stimulation.

REFLEXOLOGY: The study of reflexes.

RESPIRATORY CENTER: A localized region in the medulla at the lower end of the fourth ventricle that coordinates respiratory movements.

RETICULARISTS: Those who believed that all neurons, including their axons and dendrites, form a continuous net extending through the nervous system.

RHEOSCOPE: An instrument for determining the presence and nature of static electricity (Greek *skopos,* watcher; *rheos,* current).

SECONDARY DEGENERATION: Axons separated from neurons of origin undergo degeneration and disappear. *See* NERVE REGENERATION.

SEIZURE ONSET, LOCAL OR FOCAL: Commencing on one side of face, thumb-index, or great toe. *See* CONVULSION.

SENSORIUM COMMUNE: Middle level of the nervous system.

SIGNAL FORCE: Strength of electrical signal.

SIGNAL SYMPTOM: Local convulsion that points to a special site of cortical origin on the opposite side of the brain. Usually starts at a side of the mouth, thumb-index, or great toe. Remains local or can spread, as in a *Jacksonian seizure.*

SIMUNCULUS: Small image of an ape. *See* HOMUNCULUS.

SLEEP, REM: So-called "activated sleep" of man and animals. Seen in states of transition from slow-wave sleep and occurs at intervals during nocturnal sleep in man. The usual activation pattern is accompanied by saccadic (jerky) "rapid eye movements," loss in tone of neck muscles, and low-amplitude fast components in the electroencephalogram.

SLEEP SPINDLES: Spindle-like sequences of 14 to 16 cycles per sec cerebral activity having sine-like EEG rhythmicity and occurring in light sleep.

SLOW-WAVE SLEEP: Deep sleep showing 1 to 4 cycles per sec, slow-rhythmic activity in the EEG trace.

SODIUM HYPOTHESIS: The outward movement of sodium ions in nerve excitation forced against a concentration gradient, requiring a pumping action, the energy of which comes from metabolic processes in nerve components.

SPIKE FOCUS: Epileptic EEG spiking that has a local origin from one part of one side of the cerebrum.

SPIKE-WAVE: A sharp deflection in EEG followed by a slower dome-shaped wave. This finding has strong convulsive implications.

SPINAL CORD: Lengthy cylindrical extension of the brain in which white matter encases gray. Provides connecting links and reflex mechanisms necessary for body control and collects sensory information from body surface and depth.

SPINAL ROOTS: Segmentally arranged cord has 31 pairs of spinal nerves for each side. Each half-segment has a dorsal sensory and a ventral motor root.

SPONTANEOUS: Occurring without external influence, as from activation over nervous pathways. *See* INTRINSIC.

STATIC ELECTRICITY: Stationary charge as produced by friction.

STATIC MACHINE: *See* INFLUENCE MACHINE.

STEADY POTENTIAL: By use of an amplifier that remains stable without condenser coupling and with nonpolarizable electrodes, a difference of potential can be recorded in the resting state between any two points in the nervous system, or between one point in the nervous system and one outside. A variety of changes in nervous activity serve to unbalance it, including seizure-discharge.

STEREOTAXIC: Tri-dimensional placement of an electrode within the brain using Clarke-Horsley equipment.

SUBCORTICAL: White and gray matter lying within the interior of the cerebrum.

SUMMATION: Stimulative action or effect.

SYMPATHETIC GANGLION: Collection of nerve cells lying outside the brain and spinal cord belonging to the sympathetic nerve trunk. The neurons innervate smooth, involuntary muscle and glands.

SYNAPSE: Points of contiguity between the axon terminals of one neuron and the body or dendrites of another. Conduction proceeds irreversibly from axon to body or dendrite.

SYSTOLE: Refers to the period of contraction of the heart, as diastole does to its relaxation. May be applied to other situations as well in which contraction and relaxation alternate.

TEGMENTUM: The middle of three transverse divisions of the brainstem. Contains the reticular core.

TELEMETRY: In diagnostic investigations of epilepsy, either surface or implanted depth electrodes are connected to a radio transmitter worn on a helmet. The equipment broadcasts the cerebral activity to a radio receiver which in turn can provide a write-out to an EEG machine.

TELODENDRIA: Terminal arbor of an axon arising from a neuron situated elsewhere in the nervous system.

TEMPORAL LOBE: Lower, lateral lobe of the cerebral hemisphere; contains the hippocampus.

TEMPORAL LOBE SEIZURE: Epileptic seizure in which the neuronal discharge or the lesion provoking it has been objectively confirmed to be situated in the temporal lobe.

TETANUS (TETANY): A spasm of voluntary muscle or a rapidly repeating electrical stimulus of sufficient strength to produce such a spasm.

THERMOELECTRIC EFFECT: The production of a potential difference between two different metals when they are heated.

TIGHT JUNCTION: A fusion point between tri-laminated cell membranes of adjoining cells that produces a quintuple-layer spot *without* a slender intervening cleft. Occurs commonly in the CNS and elsewhere. Seen by electron microscopy.

TISSUE: An aggregate of similarly specialized cells that perform a common function.

TONIC: Continuous tension or contraction.

TORPEDO: A fish belonging to the ray family. It has an electric organ, the discharge of which benumbs its prey.

TRACT: A collection of nerve fibers (axons) that have a like origin and destination within the central system.

TRANSPORT: In the axon, refers to transport of cellular products synthesized in the soma (body) which move at definite rates toward the terminals of dendrites and axon; the neurotubular mechanism plays a role. The term more commonly refers to ion transport and its mechanism.

TREPHINE: A crown saw for removal of a circular disc of bone from the cranium. The process is variously called trephination or trepanation.

VAGAL: Pertains to the vagus nerve which has a wide visceral distribution, inhibiting the heart among other actions.

VOLTAIC ELECTRICITY: Electricity that flows in circuits.

WHITE MATTER OF BRAIN AND SPINAL CORD: Those parts that are composed largely of sheathed axons. The fatty sheaths give the white matter its appearance.

Index of Names

Subject Index